ABCs *of* FOOD

*Boost Your Energy, Confidence
and Success with the Power of Nutrition*

~

*Learn the Language of Health, Happiness
and Prosperity for You and the Planet*

PATRICIA CONLIN, RHN

Book: ISBN 978-0-9940136-1-3
E-Book: ISBN 978-0-9940136-0-6

Edited by: Catherine Leek of **Green Onion Publishing**
Cover Design: Cindy Cake of **WeMakeBooks.ca**
Interior designed and formatted by: Heidy Lawrance of **WeMakeBooks.ca**

Printed in Canada

This book is dedicated to my parents, family, and children. Also to all children as they are the seeds for the future health of the planet. Eat well, move well, think well ... be well.

"The doctor of the future will give no medicines but will interest his patients in the care of the human frame, in diet, and in the causes of disease."
Thomas Edison
(1847-1931, American inventor and businessman)

.

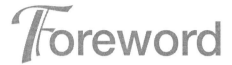

Foreword

I met Tish (Patricia) Conlin through a professional nutritionists' conference and could see immediately that she was an energetic and incredibly knowledgeable individual with a big heart and intentions to make a difference in the world. She may be petite but she is a passionate dynamo.

Today we are facing not only a global obesity crisis but a human energy crisis of epidemic proportions. It's all being driven by the fact that we are eating what I call a "Lethal Recipe" of processed foods that is toxic, addictive and leaving most people (even the affluent) malnourished. The antidote is to return to eating real food as close to nature as we can source it and in a genuine context – how it is found in nature.

Given the effects of the Western diet and the ensuing escalating health care costs, Tish's book, *ABCs of Food*, delivers practical tips for cooking, eating, and health, while sharing inspiration to make positive changes in your life.

When you return to eating real food it will nourish, energize and protect your body so that it can perform at a higher level, achieve more, live longer – and you will have greater quality of life along the way.

ABCs of Food is ideal for busy working professionals and anyone who wants an easy-to-read book that offers more than simple nutrition but includes ways to cope with your busy life and the plethora of information that comes at us about nutrition and health.

Enjoy the stories, gain insight from the articles, inspect the real foods, peruse the nutritional information and try out the recipes and make them your own. Dip into the book as you need inspiration or become inspired to try out a new food that may just contain the nutrients your body is craving.

I know that if you take the information in this book and use it to replace even one processed meal a day, you will notice a difference in your energy levels and your waistline; two meals a day and you will start to think more clearly and perform at a higher level. If you replace all three meals a day with real food, it will dramatically change your life for the better. *ABCs of Food* is a great tool to start you on that process.

May you enjoy every bite of your return to eating real food!

Sherry Strong
Author of *Return to Food — the life-changing anti-diet*
www.returntofood.com

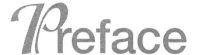reface

Yes, it is true! You are what you eat!

I am sure you have heard that before but really think about it for a minute. *ABCs of Food* will set out to answer some basic questions about common foods and show you the benefits of eating a diet rich in real food. In addition, I will introduce you to some new foods that might be healthy, fun, and delicious to try out with your family and give you some delicious recipes at the end. Eating well is one the best things you can do not only for yourself but for the health of your community, country and planet. There is a link between you and the food you eat that is powerful and we will explore some ideas to help keep healthy living a key goal for you and your family.

Before I go too far, I want to make a big confession. I have always loved food and eating. In my life it has been an on-going joy and fascination. But, a number of years ago, I started taking shortcuts, even though I *thought* I was eating healthy food. As a mother and small business owner, I was more concerned about how *fast* I could get something ready for dinner than cooking myself, using fresh ingredients. I assumed processed food would be just as nourishing and children who are picky eaters made cooking dinner more frustrating. Sure I have always loved vegetables and did cook occasionally but cooking wasn't part of my daily routine. I simply felt I didn't have time and I am sure you might feel the same way.

For me, being a sports lover, working out used to be a priority and I started putting exercise ahead of cooking for health benefits. This was a big mistake. I realize now that you need to both spend time cooking and eating homemade meals *and* exercising but it doesn't have to be a gourmet dinner or a marathon. Simply learning a few good solid recipes each year for breakfast, lunch, and dinner along with simple exercise like walking, gardening, yoga, swimming, cross-country skiing or whatever you enjoy a few times a week should be plenty. Focus on what you can do that makes you feel good and eat better!

The last few years, I have returned to my love affair with food and my interest in learning more about the food industry. I went back to school and became a Registered Holistic Nutritionist (RHN) and have spent years voraciously reading about and studying food, health, diets, agriculture, and many aspects of the current food model, as well as investigating leading experts' advice of the best ways to eat and live today for longevity and happiness. I hope to pass along some of my insights to you so you can consider implementing small regular changes to your family's diet and making cooking with fresh whole ingredients a cornerstone of every day – or at least every week! For me I noticed a huge difference in my health and stress levels almost immediately when I upgraded my diet and I hope you will too!!

Even if you can't change your eating habits and health habits all at once, you can make a commitment to change in small realistic ways and challenge yourself to do more each year. Every effort is a success and nothing should feel impossible or overwhelming. Making changes to your diet doesn't have to be expensive either. Buying better quality food or growing and storing your own can actually *reduce* your grocery bill!

We all need food to survive and food is also a great source of community and joyful celebration in cultures around the world. Daily preparations and conversations when eating food are truly one of our greatest pleasures in life! Let's all strive to eat better, cook more, and eat healthy food on a more regular basis. When we go out, let's frequent local restaurants that serve nutritious, delicious, local ingredients and support small-scale food production everywhere!

Improving your health with better food choices *will* make you healthier and happier so let's get to it!

Contents

S

T

U

V

W

X

Y

Z

What *Your* Body Needs *and* Why

Recipes from $\mathcal{A}$ to $\mathcal{Z}$

Introduction

*"While we have extended the human life-span,
we have not extended the human health span."*

John Robbins

(1947-, American writer)

Let's take a moment to step back. What is food exactly?

Foods are comprised of substances called carbohydrates, fats, proteins, vitamins and minerals and, of course, water. A healthy diet has components of all these substances in the right measure. It sounds easy to get the right amount of all these substances but is it? Why do we hear about diseases related to our so-called Western diet more and more and what can we do about it?

First of all let's examine an important difference between two cultures – North American and Asian. Food is often considered just fuel in North America. We tend to think quick energy when we grab a burger at a drive-through restaurant to supply energy and calories for survival. On average the North American diet consists of a limited supply of vegetables and fruit and focuses on eating large amounts of highly processed grains. The popular choices are wheat, soy and corn, which are in many of the packaged goods. North Americans also eat huge volumes of processed foods containing many synthetic additives and preservatives and large amounts of factory-raised meat produced with antibiotics and hormones.

In Asia, food is eaten for health and longevity. A daily diet of over 20-30 different fresh herbs and spices, vegetables, lean protein sources and fish with limited amounts of white flour, processed foods or vegetable oils is typical. More time spent cooking and eating meals, which are smaller in portions. The studies show a significant improvement in health and fewer diseases like cancer, diabetes, obesity and other diet-related illnesses appear in Asian households. For example, a typical Okinawan may live for about 110 years of healthy productive life. Research on the Okinawan population suggests that the most important factor influencing their longevity is the food they eat.

Bradley Willcox, MD, D. Craig Willcox, PhD and Makoto Suzuki, MD, are advocates of the Okinawan diet and detail their findings in *The Okinawa Program*. The key differences are a calorie restricted diet, antioxidant-rich foods, low amounts of processed fat and sugar, and more vegetarian and seafood meals along with fermented foods like miso to support immune and optimal "gut" health and build healthy gut flora.

In *ABCs of Food*, I will go over a lot of information, but you do not need to remember it all at once. In the following pages, I will cover a variety of real, nutrient-dense foods along with health information.

I'll start by listing each food – from A to Z – providing a classification (is it a fruit, vegetable, meat, etc.). I'll go on to describe the main nutrients, listing them in descending order according to the amount contained in that particular food. I may also provide information on how the food might benefit your body and health and/or how the food may be used medicinally according to studies or historical information about the food. I will conclude each alpha-section with a Food for Thought and go on to provide some thoughts on how food impacts you or your environment and offer health tips at the end of each section.

In the second part of *ABCs of Food* I provide specific information on carbohydrates, protein, fats, vitamins and minerals, and phytonutrients (which contain the powerful antioxidants we hear about that are important for our health). I will provide detailed information on the primary role of each vitamin or mineral and give you facts on how deficiencies in the diet can affect the body and overall health. Don't worry about remembering it all at once as it is for reference purposes only. You can easily refer back to this section at any time.

At the end of the book, you'll find an A-Z recipe section with a range of choices for meat eaters, vegetarians, those who favor a gluten-free diet, as well as those with a sweet tooth so that everyone can find something new to try with their family or friends.

The main goal of *ABCs of Food* is to help you find easy, simple, and affordable ways to eat healthier and support a healthier food system. You will notice that your energy will naturally increase with a healthier diet as will your natural joy as well! However, if you are having any trouble and desire nutritional advice or any other health-care guidance, please seek out a professional. Now let's get started on the exciting A-Z journey through the amazing world of food.

Please email me at *tish@abcsoffood.com* if you find any foods that I have missed and I will include them in revised additions!

Bon appetite and good reading!

A–Z
of
Foods

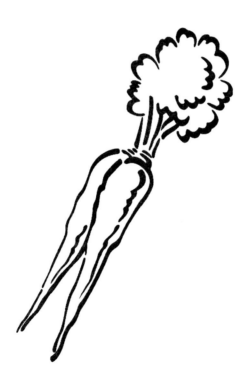

"Let Food Be thy medicine and medicine be thy Food."
Hippocrates
(460-377 BC, Greek physician and Father of Medicine)

Almonds – Soaking Delight

I used to soak raw almonds overnight and eat them in the morning. While at a soccer tournament with my team, I endured endless teasing for this unusual practice. But then I bumped into a woman from India who said eating soaked almonds for memory and health has been practiced for centuries and is known to be effective! Some members of my team even tried it after I shared that story! I still eat a lot of almonds but now I don't have time to soak them. I do eat a lot of other memory supporting foods though and play Sudoku regularly!

It is interesting to note that the production of almonds and more than 100 of our food crops depends on bees as the fruit will only set if their flowers are cross-pollinated between two different varieties. Honeybees are our tiny farmworkers who carry the pollen from one tree to another as they search for food. Almond production is especially dependent on bees and is vulnerable due to the mysterious syndrome called Colony Collapse Disorder, or CCD, which is drastically affecting bee colonies.[1]

REAL "A" FOODS

Arborio Rice [*Grain*] Arborio rice contains fiber and very small amounts of protein and iron. It is a carbohydrate-rich short-grain rice that is starchier than most rice. Traditionally, it is used to make the popular and creamy Italian dish, risotto, a rice and broth dish with parmesan cheese. See also "Rice" and "Grains" for nutrients and information.

Acai Berries [*Fruit*] Acai berries come from palm trees and contain fiber, carbohydrates, good amounts of Vitamins C, K, B3 (niacin), B2 (riboflavin) and some minerals, potassium, manganese, copper, iron and magnesium. Acai is also a source of omega fatty acids (6 and 9) and many antioxidants, including resveratrol and anthocyanins. Acai contains tannins, which are known to have anti-inflammatory properties. These berries are unique to the Amazon rain forest in Brazil and are considered a power food by many health food enthusiasts. Acai juice can be found in the grocery store. See also What Foods Fight or Help Prevent Cancer? under Food and You or Your Environment, under "C" and also Understanding Ancient Foods Today under Food for Thought, under "U."

Acerola [*Fruit*] Acerola, also known as West Indian Cherry, contains fiber, carbohydrates, a huge amount of Vitamin C and small amounts of Vitamin A and minerals magnesium, copper and potassium. Acerola cherries provide more Vitamin C than any other food source. Evergreen acerola trees thrive in the warm climates of South America, Central America, California, Texas and Florida. The fruits deteriorate rapidly once removed from the tree so they are usually found in jam, syrup, and juice but not in their natural state.

Acorn Squash. See "Squash" for nutrients and information.

Adzuki Beans. See "Legumes" for nutrients and information. See also What Foods Fight or Help Prevent Cancer? under Food and You or Your Environment, under "C."

Agave [*Sweetener*] Agave extract comes from cactus sap makes a good substitute for sugar or maple syrup. It has good amounts of fiber, magnesium, iron and calcium and is sweeter than sugar so not as much is needed. Agave works well in porridge or any recipes as a sugar substitute. Be sure to buy a quality brand as some are highly processed and contain excessive amounts of fructose. Visit *wholesomesweeteners.com*. See "Sugar" for general information. See also Sugar – A Diet No No under Food for Thought under "S."

Albacore [*Fish*] Albacore is a good source of protein and omega-3 fatty acids. It contains good amounts of Vitamins B3 (niacin), B6 (pyridoxine), B12 (cobalamin) and the minerals selenium and phosphorus. (For information on sustainable fish see "Fish" or visit *www.msc.org/cook-eat-enjoy/fish-to-eat*.)

Alfalfa [*Vegetable*] Alfalfa can be eaten as seeds, raw or sprouted. It contains fiber, carbohydrates, some protein, small amounts of many vitamins, including A, C, K, and B-complex Vitamins (B3 (niacin), B1 (thiamine), B2 (riboflavin), B5 (pantothenic acid), and B9 (folic acid)), and small amounts of the minerals calcium, iron, manganese, magnesium, phosphorus, zinc and copper. Sprouts all of kinds are full of enzymes that help with digestion and are incredibly nutrient dense. They are great to add to salads and sandwiches. See also The Stress'll Kill Ya under Food and You or Your Environment, under "S."

Allium [*Vegetable Classification*] This category includes vegetables like chives, garlic, leek, onion, and shallot. Most of the vegetables in the allium family are considered helpful in lowering "bad" cholesterol, preventing atherosclerosis, lowering blood pressure, and reducing the risk of heart attack or stroke. They are also known to be excellent for liver support and aid in detoxification.

Allspice [*Spice*] Allspice contains fiber and protein. It has good amounts of Vitamins C, A, and B-complex Vitamins (B3 (niacin), B5 (pantothenic acid), B9 (folic acid), B6 (pyridoxine), B2 (riboflavin)), and high amounts of minerals iron, manganese, copper, calcium, magnesium, potassium, phosphorus, and zinc. The essential oil, eugenol derived from the allspice berry, is used in dentistry as a local anesthetic and antiseptic for teeth and gums. Its oil is a popular home remedy for arthritis and sore muscles. Allspice, also known popularly as Jamaican pepper or pimento, is widely used in Mexican and other Central American cuisines. Ground allspice has a strong, spicy taste that resembles a mixture of black pepper, nutmeg, cloves, and cinnamon. See "Spices" for general information and cooking suggestions.

Almonds [*Nut*] Almonds are the seeds of a fruit tree and are loaded with nutrients, containing the most nutrients in comparison to all other nuts. They are high in protein, fiber, carbohydrates, and saturated fat and are an excellent source of Vitamin E and (B2 (riboflavin), B3 (niacin), B5 (pantothenic acid), B6 (pyridoxine), B9 (folic acid) and B1 (thiamine)). Almonds are also rich in minerals, including copper, calcium, magnesium, manganese, iron, phosphorus, potassium, zinc and selenium, and they contain the antioxidant quercetin. Quercetin is a flavonoid with strong antioxidant powers and eating quercetin-rich foods can help reduce the effects of free radical damage on cells from UV exposure. Studies also link almonds to improved memory! Try them raw (unroasted and unsalted) for maximum health benefits. See "Nuts" for general information. See also How Can We Hold onto Yesterday's Memories? under Food and You or Your Environment, under "Y."

Aloe Vera [*Herb*] Aloe Vera contains fiber, carbohydrates, Vitamins A, C, E, B12 (cobalamin), essential fatty acids and is naturally rich in protein, calcium, magnesium, zinc and amino acids. Aloe Vera has a minimum of three anti–inflammatory fatty acids that help in the smooth functioning of the stomach, small intestines and colon. It has a natural property to alkalize digestive juices and prevents over-acidity, which is one of the common causes of digestive ailments. Aloe Vera juice concentrates are high in essential enzymes that stimulate digestion and liver functions and it is known as a good liver-cleansing agent. Aloe Vera supplements also contain a rare natural ingredient that works to flush out waste products and toxins. It's great for those with acid reflux and stomach ulcers. See "Herbs" for general information. See also Herbaceous Cooking under Healthy You, under "H."

Amaranth [*Grain*] Amaranth has fiber and carbohydrates, is a good source of Vitamin B6 and B9 (folic acid) and a great source of the minerals manganese, magnesium, iron, phosphorus, calcium, copper, zinc, selenium and potassium. The leaves of the amaranth plant contain high amounts of Vitamins C and A, as well as calcium and iron. Amaranth is a gluten-free grain packed with nutrients and contains more protein than rice, corn or wheat (and a high amount of the amino acid lysine – making it a more complete protein). Amaranth is native to Central America, where it was domesticated over 8,500 years ago. To the Aztecs, amaranth was just as valuable as corn.[2] Today, amaranth is once again being grown on farms throughout the world and this drought-resistant crop is gaining popularity as one of the most nutritious grains under cultivation, which makes an excellent flour and bread. See also "Grains" for general information. See also Dandelions and Other "Weeds" under Food and You or Your Environment, under "D."

Anchovy [*Fish*] Anchovies are high in protein and omega-3 fatty acids. They contain large amounts of Vitamin B3 (niacin), good amounts of other B-complex Vitamins (B12 (cobalamin), B6, B2 (riboflavin)) and the minerals selenium, phosphorus, iron, calcium, zinc, copper, magnesium and potassium. (For information on sustainable fish see "Fish" or visit *www.msc.org/cook-eat-enjoy/fish-to-eat*.)

Anise [*Spice*] Anise seeds contain good amounts of fiber, protein, and Vitamins C, A, and B-complex Vitamins (B6 (pyridoxine), B1 (thiamine), B2 (riboflavin), B5 (pantothenic acid), and B3 (niacin)). Anise has huge amounts of minerals iron, manganese, copper, calcium, phosphorus, zinc, potassium, magnesium, and some selenium. Anise preparations are an excellent remedy for asthma, bronchitis, and coughs as well as digestive disorders, such as flatulence, bloating, colicky stomach pain, nausea, and indigestion. The seeds are chewed after a meal in India to refresh the breath. See "Spices" for general information and cooking suggestions.

Antioxidants. See What Your Body Needs and Why.

Apple [*Fruit*] Apples contain fiber, carbohydrates and large amounts of Vitamin C and beta-carotene along with small amounts of B-complex Vitamins (B2 (riboflavin), B1 (thiamine), B6 (pyridoxine) and the minerals potassium, phosphorus and calcium. The high amounts of quercetin and Vitamin C found in apples are powerful antioxidants and boost your body's immunity. Antioxidants help your body repair damage to cells caused by free radicals. Quercetin is also considered very helpful for allergies. Raw apple cider vinegar is known for its many health benefits (see "Vinegar"). See Amazing Apples under Food for Thought, below. See also Menopause – Can Food Help the Transition? under Food and You or Your Environment, under "M" and also How Can We Hold onto Yesterday's Memories? under Food and You or Your Environment, under "Y."

Apricot [*Fruit*] Apricots contain fiber, carbohydrates, are rich in Vitamins A and C and a good source of minerals (potassium, iron, zinc, calcium and manganese). Apricots contain the antioxidants lutein, beta-carotene, zeaxanthin, as well as lycopene and tryptophan, important amino acid that also boost mood! Dried apricots are often treated with sulfites to extend their shelf life by preventing oxidation and bleaching of colors, as in the case of other dried fruits like figs. Sulfite-treated, bright orange-colored fruits can cause bronchospasm in sensitized people who suffer from asthma. Therefore, sulfite-sensitive people should purchase unsulfured dried fruits that are brown in color but taste even more delicious. Note: sulfites have become a very common allergy. See Allergies under Food and You or Your Environment, below.

Arctic Char [*Fish*] Arctic Char is a good source of protein and omega-3 fatty acids. It also contains good amounts of B3 (niacin), B12 (cobalamin), B6 and the minerals selenium and phosphorus. (For information on sustainable fish see "Fish" or visit *www.msc.org/cook-eat-enjoy/fish-to-eat*.)

Arrowroot [*Spice*] Arrowroot comes from a tuber and contains fiber and some protein. It has B-complex Vitamins (B6 (pyridoxine), B9 (folic acid), B1 (thiamine), B3 (niacin), B2 (riboflavin)) and minerals iron, phosphorus, copper, and magnesium. It has relatively more protein than that of other tropical food sources like yam, potato, cassava, plantains, etc. Its easy digestibility and ability to mix well with a wide range of food ingredients makes it the most sought-after starch in the food industry for infant formulas, confectionaries, and as a thickener and stabilizing agent. See "Spices" for general information and cooking suggestions. See also Root Vegetables under Food for Thought, under "R."

Artichoke [*Vegetable*] Artichokes are high in fiber, Vitamin C and B-complex Vitamins (B9 (folic acid), B6 (pyridoxine), B5 (pantothenic acid), B1 (thiamine), B3 (niacin)) and minerals (copper, iron, magnesium, manganese, phosphorus with some calcium). Artichokes are known to help lower blood sugar and are a member of the thistle family.

Arugula [*Vegetable*] Arugula, also known as salad rocket or garden rocket, contains fiber and high amounts of Vitamins K, A, C and B9 (folic acid) along with small amounts of B5 (pantothenic acid) and B2 (riboflavin). It also contains good amounts of minerals calcium, iron, magnesium, and manganese, and antioxidants beta-carotene, lutein, and zeaxanthin.

Asparagus [*Vegetable*] Asparagus is rich in fiber, carbohydrates, Vitamins K, A, C, some E and B-complex Vitamins (B9 (folic acid), B2 (riboflavin), B1 (thiamine), B6 (pyridoxine) and B3 (niacin)). It contains the minerals copper, iron, manganese and phosphorus and small amounts of potassium, zinc and selenium. Asparagus has good amounts of the antioxidants lutein, beta-carotene and zeaxanthin and is considered a mild diuretic (it can increase urine production). It is a perennial plant, which means it will come up again each year once established. See also How Can We Hold onto Yesterday's Memories? under Food and You or Your Environment, under "Y."

Astragalus [*Herb*] Astragalus contains trace amounts of potassium, zinc, copper, iron and choline, a mineral vital to your body's central nervous system. It is used in Eastern medicine to boost energy, support the immune system and strengthen and repair tissues. Cancer care centers also use it to treat certain cancers, according to *asbestos.com,* and it is used for stress management and adrenal support as well. See "Herbs" for general information. See also Herbaceous Cooking under Healthy You, under "H."

Autumn Squash. See "Squash" for nutrients and information.

Avocado [*Fruit*] Avocados contain fiber, carbohydrates and have the highest protein content of any fruit. Avocados are great source for Vitamins C, K and E and have good amounts of B-complex Vitamins (B9 (folic acid), B6, B3 (niacin), B2 (riboflavin), B1 (thiamine), B5 (pantothenic acid)). Avocados contain potassium, magnesium, copper, manganese, phosphorus and small amounts of zinc and iron. They provide an excellent plant-based source of good fats, especially oleic acid (omega 6) which helps reduce bad fats in the body! Avocados are known to improve liver health through detoxification and help to lower blood pressure. See also What Foods Fight or Help Prevent Cancer? under Food and You or Your Environment, under "C," What's to be Done about the Rise in Heart Disease? under Food and You or Your Environment, under "H," and also Are Rheumatoid Arthritis and Autoimmune Diseases on the Rise? under Food and You or Your Environment, under "R."

FOOD FOR THOUGHT

Amazing Apples

Everyone knows the saying, "An apple a day keeps the doctor away!" But do you know where they come from? Trees? Seeds? Johnny Appleseed?[3]

> Apples are one of nature's most delicious and nutritious fruits.

Actually, all of the apples we eat, whether we buy them at the store or pick them off a tree, are clones! Grafting – an ancient way of cloning plants – allows plant scientists to create new consistently high quality varieties of apples and is over 2,000 years old! The selected genetic traits allow trees to make better-tasting fruits. The process involves placing/grafting the shoots and branches of an existing apple tree, called a scion, onto a new trunk and root system and planting the hybrid in the ground. Making an identical copy of the preferred fruit is a way to get a consistent apple taste and quality but also makes it more susceptible to viruses and blight.

Scientists are now trying to determine the links between specific genes and the most desirable apple traits, especially disease resistance. Apple trees absorb and store carbon from the atmosphere and they offer a perennial bounty of fruit using the energy from the sun. They have deep roots that help to stabilize the soil, which makes them a sustainable crop.[4]

Here are some quick facts about apples, one of nature's most delicious and nutritious fruits.

- The most popular are Red and Golden Delicious, Granny Smith, Gala and McIntosh.
- The science of growing apples is called pomology.
- The largest apple ever picked weighed three pounds.
- There are over 7,000 varieties of apples grown around the world.
- The ancient Greeks, Etruscans, and Romans all practiced grafting their favorite apple varieties to other apple rootstocks.
- Many commercially grown apples receive a post-harvest wax treatment using carnauba (from palm trees), shellac (from beetles), beeswax, or petroleum wax. Waxing protects fruits and makes them shiny but adds no nutritional value.
- Apples are one of the worst fruits for containing pesticide residues so it is well worth buying organic bagged apples. They may be duller in appearance and of a more varied size but they'll be much tastier and contain higher levels of nutrients! They are at the top of the dirty dozen list (see Is Organic Really Better for You under Food and You or Your Environment, under "O.")

FOOD AND YOU OR YOUR ENVIRONMENT

Why Are Food Allergies on the Rise?

Food allergies are on the rise globally. Allergic reactions are severe adverse effects that occur when the body's immune system overreacts to a particular food or ingredient.

In North America, the nine main food allergens are peanuts, tree nuts, sesame seeds, milk, eggs, seafood (fish and shellfish), soy, wheat, and sulfites (a food additive). Most allergies affect the digestive system, respiratory system, or skin. Some allergens, like peanuts, can cause an overreaction of the immune system that, in a small percentage of people, may lead to severe physical symptoms. The most severe allergic reactions can result in anaphylaxis, an emergency situation requiring immediate medical attention and treatment with epinephrine shots. Sufferers must completely exclude the food from their diets. Many schools have strict policies in place to protect children with these severe allergies and are peanut-free environments.

According to the Centers for Disease Control, between 1997 and 2007 food allergies in the U.S. increased nearly 20%, with peanut allergies nearly tripling during that same period. It is believed by some that the increased use of GMO (Genetically Modified Organisms) seeds in the U.S have contributed to the increase in allergies. Proteins are the most common part of a food that can cause an allergic reaction and are also most commonly altered through genetic modification, increasing the potential for triggering an allergic reaction. While a GMO protein may not always result in a food allergy, individuals with pre-existing food sensitivities are at a particularly high risk for more reactions. A study conducted by the York Laboratory in 1999 found a link connecting an increase in GMO soy imports into the U.K. to a 50% increase in the nation's soy allergies.

> **The Nine Main Food Allergens: peanuts, tree nuts, sesame seeds, milk, eggs, seafood, soy, wheat, and sulfites.**

According to Carolee Bateson-Koch in *Allergies: Disease in Disguise*, we sometimes aren't even aware that we have developed a food intolerance. Certain foods can even become addictive, especially the ones to which we are experiencing an allergic reaction.

Food elimination can help you figure out which foods are causing allergies. Start with a simple diet and slowly add suspected problem foods one at time and monitor your reactions. Using a food journal can be very helpful at figuring out which foods cause the most difficulty. Other ways to reduce allergy symptoms include taking a digestive enzyme to aid with the digestion of protein, supporting the immune system and gut health with probiotic-rich foods, like yogurt, kefir, and fermented vegetables, as well as eating a whole-food diet low in processed foods and high in antioxidant-rich fruits and vegetables. A supplement called quercetin (found in apples, chamomile tea, onions and capers) also shows promise in acting like a natural antihistamine. Other natural ways believed to help reduce allergy symptoms include: eating more omega-3 fatty acids to reduce inflammation in airways and body tissue; Butterbur extract, nettle root tea, and a neti pot which can wash allergies out of your nose. A daily teaspoon of local honey or 1/2 teaspoon of bee pollen has been helpful to many with seasonal allergies as well![5]

HEALTHY YOU

Keep It Real!

Eliminate aspartame and artificial additives from your diet completely! Aspartame is used in diet foods and considered a health risk by some doctors and scientists. Aspartame is known to cause allergy symptoms, decreased production of the happy hormone, serotonin, and may increase cravings for carbs. Other artificial additives to eliminate or reduce in your food include food colorings, aspartame, monosodium glutamate (MSG), high fructose corn syrup (HFCS), sodium benzoate, sodium nitrite, and trans fats. Next time you go to the grocery store, shop the outside, focusing on whole foods like vegetables, fruit, milk, yogurt, and lean meat along with foods with less than three ingredients and zero additives. (See Controversial Ingredients or Additives under Food for Thought, under "I.")

"Few of us are aware that the act of eating can be a powerful statement of commitment to our own well-being, and at the same time the creation of a healthier habitat. Your health, happiness, and the future of life on earth are rarely so much in your own hands as when you sit down to eat."

John Robbins

(1947- , American writer)

Why Bananas at Finish Lines?

I love bananas because they are tasty and rich in potassium, a mineral and electrolyte that plays a large role in metabolism, muscle contractions, nerve impulses and regulation of heartbeat and blood pressure. Deficiencies of potassium have been linked to an increased risk of hypertension, kidney stones, osteoporosis, stroke and cardiovascular disease. After or during a workout they taste delicious and really keep my energy up. When I ride or run to support charities, I always reach for a banana as I cross the finish line.

Did you know that the term "banana republic" was coined because of the poor working conditions on banana plantations? Today banana republic is used to describe a politically unstable country that economically depends upon the exports of a limited resource (e.g., fruits, minerals), and usually features a society composed of an impoverished working class and a ruling dictatorship. Bananas are the world's fourth largest crop. The most common variety grown is called "Cavendish"

and it is cultivated through cloning. This variety has become susceptible to "Panama Fungus," a blight that has threatened production in
Asia and Australia.

REAL "B" FOODS

Bamboo [*Vegetable*] Bamboo shoots contain fiber, carbohydrates,
and small amounts of protein. They have small amounts of Vitamins C, E, and B-complex Vitamins (B6 (pyridoxine), B1 (thiamine), B2 (riboflavin), and B3 (niacin)) along with good
amounts of minerals copper, manganese, and some iron and zinc.
Bamboo contains the antioxidant beta-carotene and, in Asia, tender shoots are featured in soups, noodles, salads, and stir-fry.

Banana [*Fruit*] Bananas contain fiber, carbohydrates, good amounts
of Vitamin C and B-complex Vitamins (B6 (pyridoxine), B5
(pantothenic acid), B9 (folic acid), B2 (riboflavin)), and minerals
potassium, phosphorus, and manganese. Bananas contain antioxidants, including beta-carotene, lutein, and zeaxanthin. They are
a great addition to smoothies or fruit salads. See also Happiness
and Foods that Create Bliss under Food for Thought, under "H."

Banana Peppers. See "Hot Peppers" for nutrients and information.

Banana Squash. See "Squash" for nutrients and information.

Barberries [*Fruit*] The barberry fruit is a small berry that is red or
dark blue in color. Barberries are long and narrow fruits like a
bar, hence the name barberry. They are used to make jams and
infusions. They are rich in vitamin C. See "Berries" for nutrients
and information.

Barley [*Grain*] Barley is one of the oldest cultivated grains. It contains fiber (insoluble and soluble), carbohydrates, Vitamin E, B-
complex Vitamins (high in B3 (niacin) and B1 (thiamine)), and
minerals selenium, iron, magnesium, zinc, phosphorus and copper. Barley contains lignans, a phytochemical with antioxidant
abilities and cancer prevention properties. The high fiber content

has been shown to help reduce the risk of certain cancers, including colon cancer. See also "Grains" for general information. See also What's to be Done about the Rise in Heart Disease? under Food and You or Your Environment, under "H."

Barracuda [*Fish*] A good source of protein and omega-3 fatty acids, barracuda contains good amounts of Vitamins B3 (niacin), B12 (cobalamin) and B6 (pyridoxine) and minerals selenium and phosphorus. (For information on sustainable fish see "Fish" or visit *www.msc.org/cook-eat-enjoy/fish-to-eat*.)

Barramundi [*Fish*] This fish is a good source of protein and Omega-3 fatty acids. It contains good amounts of Vitamins B3 (niacin), B12 (cobalamin) and B6 (pyridoxine) and minerals selenium and phosphorus. (For information on sustainable fish see "Fish" or visit *www.msc.org/cook-eat-enjoy/fish-to-eat*.)

Basil [*Herb*] Rich in antioxidants and fiber, fresh Basil contains small amounts of Vitamins A and C, large amounts of Vitamins K and B9 (folic acid), and minerals manganese, copper, magnesium, iron, calcium, potassium, phosphorous and calcium. Most commonly used in tomato sauces, soups and salads, basil is used for a variety of ailments, including fever, colds, flu, and digestion. It is worth buying organic as traditional farming significantly reduces the antioxidant content. See "Herbs" for general information. See also Herbaceous Cooking under Healthy You, under "H."

Basmati Rice [*Grain*] This long-grain rice contains fiber, carbohydrates and B-complex Vitamins (B1 (thiamine), B3 (niacin), and B9 (folic acid)) along with some iron and protein. Basmati rice is aromatic rice grown in India and Pakistan that has a nut-like texture and a buttery flavor. Basmati is lower in starch and does not raise blood sugar as quickly as other rice varieties. See also "Rice" and "Grains" for general information.

Bass [*Fish*] Bass is a good source of protein and omega-3 fatty acids. It contains good amounts of Vitamins B3 (niacin), B12 (cobalamin),

B6 (pyridoxine), and B1 (thiamine) and minerals selenium, phosphorus, magnesium, potassium, and iron. (For information on sustainable fish see "Fish" or visit *www.msc.org/cook-eat-enjoy/fish-to-eat.*)

Bayberries [*Fruit*] These berries are native to China and are deep red in color, or in the range from white to purple. They can be eaten as is or used for different purposes like jams, pickles, wine, and juice. See "Berries" for nutrients and information.

Beans, Dried. See "Legumes" for information, varieties, and nutrients.

Beans, Green and Yellow [*Vegetable*] Beans contain fiber, Vitamins C, A, K, and B-complex Vitamins (B2 (riboflavin), B1 (thiamine), and B9 (folic acid)). They also provide minerals iron, manganese, calcium, magnesium, and potassium along with the antioxidant zeaxanthin.

Bearberries [*Fruit*] These berries are reddish or brown in color. They have many medicinal uses, like its consumption lowers the uric acid content in the body. It also helps bring relief from pain due to kidney stones. Herbal tea made from bearberries is used to cure nephritis. See "Berries" for nutrients and information.

Beef [*Meat*] Beef is high in protein and saturated fat and contains good amounts of Vitamins D, E, K, and B-complex Vitamins (B12 (cobalamin), B9 (folic acid), B1 (thiamine), B2 (riboflavin)) along with good amounts of minerals iron, potassium, calcium, phosphorus, magnesium, and selenium. Organic, grass-fed or free-range beef is much higher in nutrients, in particular omega-3 fatty acids, and better for your health. See Beef: Grass-Fed Versus Grain-Fed under Food for Thought, below. See also Happiness and Foods that Create Bliss under Food for Thought, under "H."

Beets [*Vegetable*] Beets contain fiber and carbohydrates and are an excellent source of Vitamin B9 (folic acid) and a good source of complex carbohydrates, fiber, Vitamin C, and B-complex Vitamins (B6 (pyridoxine), B2 (riboflavin), and B5 (pantothenic acid)) and minerals iron, calcium, magnesium, manganese, potassium, and copper. Beet tops are good in salads and a source of Vitamin A. Beets are an excellent anti-inflammatory, high antioxidant and detoxification support food (traditionally used to detoxify the liver). They are the main ingredient in the popular East European dish Borscht. See also Root Vegetables under Food for Thought, under "R."

Belgium Chicory. See "Endive." See also "Lettuce" for general information.

Berries [*Fruit*] Berries are high in fiber, carbohydrates, and most contain good amounts of Vitamins C, E, K, and B-complex Vitamins. They are a good source of minerals potassium, phosphorus, copper, and magnesium, along with potent antioxidants that support health. A berry is a fruit that has a fleshy, edible outer wall that usually covers one or many seeds and is small, juicy, colorful, and has a fleshy texture. The fruit has no core and is completely edible. The list of berries is long and includes: true berries, grapes, elderberries, tomatoes, barberries, honeysuckle, Oregon grape, nanny-berries, gooseberries, mayapples, seabuckthorn berries, red and black currants (contain iron as well!), wild rose, drupes, hackberries, sugarberries, persimmon, Barbados cherries, goji berries (also known as wolf berries), Indian plums, chokeberries, ligonberries, cranberries, bearberries, crowberries, blueberries, huckleberries, bilberries, juniper berries (used to season meat and cabbage), raspberries, strawberries, blackberries, dewberries, salmonberries, boysenberries, bayberries, mulberries, cloudberries, chehalem berries, loganberries, thimbleberries, wineberries, juneberries, serviceberries, marionberries, tayberries, youngberries, Saskatoon berries, and olallieberries. Some berries are, of course, poisonous. Some poisonous berries conform to the botanical definition and some are just thought to be berries. Definition apart, these are poisonous berries that should not be consumed: baneberries (or bugbane), holly berries, yew berries, pokeberries, Jerusalem cherries, and daphne berries.[6] See What Foods Fight or Help Prevent Cancer? under Food and You or Your Environment, under "C."

Bibb Lettuce. Also known as Boston and Butterhead. See also "Lettuce" for nutrients and information.

Bilberries. See "Huckleberries."

Bison. See "Buffalo."

Black Beans [*Vegetable (Legume)*] Also referred to as Black Turtle Beans, these legumes provide an excellent plant source of fiber, carbohydrates, and protein. Black Beans also contain B-complex Vitamins (B1 (thiamine) and B9 (folic acid)), minerals manganese, magnesium, phosphorus, iron, and are also packed with antioxidants. See also "Legumes" for general information.

Blackberries [*Fruit*] Blackberries contain fiber and carbohydrates and are an excellent source of Vitamins K, C, E, A, and some small amount of B-complex Vitamins (B9 (folic acid), B5 (pantothenic acid), and B3 (niacin)) along with excellent amounts of minerals copper and iron and small amounts of potassium, calcium, and magnesium. Blackberries also contain antioxidants beta-carotene, lutein, zeaxanthin, quercetin, and tannins. See also "Berries" for general information.

Black Currant [*Fruit*] Black currants are packed with Vitamins C and B5 (pantothenic acid), and minerals potassium, phosphorous, and iron. This popular flavored berry is like the red currant in appearance. It is used in jams, pies, ice creams, tarts, etc. See also "Currants."

Black Jostaberries. See "Currants."

Black Pepper [*Spice*] Black Pepper contains very high amounts of fiber, protein, and Vitamin K, and good amounts of Vitamins C,

E and B-complex Vitamins (B6 (pyridoxine), B2 (riboflavin), B1 (thiamine), and B3 (niacin)). It has huge amounts of minerals manganese, iron, copper, magnesium, calcium, phosphorus, potassium, and zinc. It is also rich in the flavonoid polyphenol and antioxidants beta-carotene, zeaxanthin, and lycopene. Peppers have been in use since ancient times for their anti-inflammatory, antiflatulent properties but pepper should be avoided in individuals with stomach ulcers, ulcerative colitis, and diverticulitis conditions as it can cause gastrointestinal irritation. See "Spices" for general information and cooking suggestions.

Blueberries [*Fruit*] Blueberries contain fiber, carbohydrates and small amounts of Vitamins C, A, K, and B-complex Vitamins (B3 (niacin), B2 (riboflavin), B6 (pyridoxine), B5 (pantothenic acid), and B9 (folic acid)). Blueberries are known as a power food and contain good amounts of manganese and some iron and zinc. They are very high in antioxidants like anthocyanin, beta-carotene, lutein, quercetin, and tannins and they are believed to be a natural pain killer. Anthocyanins have also been linked to an increase in neuronal signaling in brain centers and are an anti-Alzheimer food. See "Berries" for general information. See also Can Certain Foods Make Us More Intelligent? under Food and You or Your Environment, under "I" and also Are Rheumatoid Arthritis and Autoimmune Diseases on the Rise? under Food and You or Your Environment, under "R."

Boar [*Meat*] Boar, also referred to as wild pork, is considered "game," or free range, as it can live in the wild. Boar meat is high in protein and Vitamins E, K and B-complex Vitamins (B12 (cobalamin), B2 (riboflavin), B1 (thiamine), B3 (niacin), B6 (pyridoxine), and B9 (folic acid)), and contains high amounts of minerals zinc, potassium, magnesium, phosphorus, iron, and selenium.

Bok Choy [*Vegetable*] Bok Choy, also known as Pak Choy, is a leafy cabbage most commonly associated with Chinese cuisine. It contains high amounts of fiber, carbohydrates, Vitamins A, C, K, B9 (folic acid), and some B2 (riboflavin) and B6 (pyridoxine). It has moderate amounts of calcium, iron, magnesium, phosphorus, potassium and is high in antioxidants. It is a cruciferous vegetable and tastes great in a stir fry. See What Foods Fight or Help Prevent Cancer? under Food and You or Your Environment, under "C."

Bone Marrow[7] [*Meat*] Bone marrow is the fatty and gelatinous matter inside large bones that becomes soft when roasted and can be spread on toast. It is high in protein and contains good amounts of the mineral calcium. It also has high amounts of CLA (Conjugate Linolenic Acid), which has powerful antioxidant properties, and good amounts of omega-3 fatty acids known to be excellent for health. It is a traditional ingredient in many cuisines, including Vietnamese and French. Bone broth is excellent to heal a damaged intestine from allergies or pathogens.

Boston Lettuce. Also known as "Bibb Lettuce." See "Lettuce" for nutrients and information.

Boysenberries [*Fruit*] Boysenberries contain fiber, carbohydrates, Vitamins K, C, E, and some B-complex Vitamins (B9 (folic acid), B1 (thiamine), and B3 (niacin)), along with good amounts of manganese and small amounts of iron, copper and magnesium. See also "Berries" for general information.

Brassica/Cruciferous [*Vegetable Classification*] This category includes vegetables like bok choy, broccoli, Brussels sprouts, cabbage, cauliflower, collard greens, kohlrabi, mustard greens, rapini, rutabaga, and turnip. Brassica/cruciferous vegetables contain high amounts of antioxidants such as zeaxanthin and lutein that are believed to possess anti-cancer properties. They also contain a sulfur-rich substance called glucosinolate that helps stimulate the activation of liver detoxifying enzymes that help flush out toxins. In addition they are rich in Vitamin K, a direct regulator of the inflammatory system response that have been studied in connection with lowering the risk of stroke. See specific foods for particular nutritional information. See What Foods Fight or Help Prevent Cancer? under Food and You or Your Environment, under "C."

Brazil Nut [*Nut*] Brazil nuts are high in protein, fiber, saturated fats, and contain Vitamin E and B-complex Vitamins (especially B1 (thiamine), B6 (pyridoxine) and B9 (folic acid)). They also have huge amounts of selenium and good amounts of other minerals such as copper, phosphorus, potassium, magnesium, manganese, potassium, calcium, iron, and zinc. Selenium is very important in liver detoxification and two Brazil nuts a day is enough selenium for your body. Selenium also helps those with an underactive thyroid as it increases the uptake of iodine which helps improve thyroid function. See "Nuts" for general information.

Broccoli [*Vegetable*] Broccoli is a powerhouse of nutrients. It contains fiber, carbohydrates, high amounts of Vitamins C, K, A, and B-complex Vitamins (B9 (folic acid), B3 (niacin), B5 (pantothenic acid), B6 (pyridoxine), B2 (riboflavin), and B1 (thiamine)) and minerals potassium, manganese, phosphorus, copper, magnesium, selenium, and zinc. Broccoli contains antioxidants, including quercetin, lutein, beta-carotene, and zeaxanthin. It also the boasts the mineral chromium, which helps regulate blood sugar. Broccoli sprouts contain up to 100 times the amount of nutrients than the mature plant. Considered an anticancer food, it contains a sulfur-rich compound that helps in detoxification. Broccoli is a cruciferous vegetable along with cauliflower, Brussels sprouts, and cabbage, all of which have anticancer properties. See What Foods Fight or Help Prevent Cancer? under Food and You or Your Environment, under "C."

Broccoli Rabe. See "Rapini." See What Foods Fight or Help Prevent Cancer? under Food and You or Your Environment, under "C."

Brown Rice [*Grain*] Brown rice contains fiber, carbohydrates, and B-complex Vitamins (B1 (thiamine), B3 (niacin), and B9 (folic acid)), along with some iron and protein. Brown rice contains the whole grain: the bran, germ, and endosperm, which supply higher levels of nutrients than white rice. See also "Rice" and "Grains" for general information.

Brown Sugar. See "Sugar." See also Sugar – A Diet No No under Food for Thought under "S."

Brussels Sprouts [*Vegetable*] These mini-cabbages are high in fiber, carbohydrates, Vitamins C, K, A, and contain good amounts of all B-complex Vitamins. Brussels sprouts are a good source of minerals iron, manganese, phosphorus, copper, potassium, and magnesium. They contain several antioxidants, including beta-carotene and lutein and, like all cruciferous vegetables, they are known as an anticancer and liver supporting food. See What Foods Fight or Help Prevent Cancer? under Food and You or Your Environment, under "C."

Buckwheat [*Fruit*] Despite its name buckwheat is a fruit, but it is generally regarded as a grain. It is gluten free and high in fiber, carbohydrates, omega-6 fatty acids, and protein. It is high in B-complex Vitamins (B3 (niacin), B2 (riboflavin), B6 (pyridoxine), B5 (pantothenic acid), B9 (folic acid) and B1 (thiamine)), as well as minerals magnesium, phosphorus, copper, zinc, potassium, and iron. It is part of the plant family that also includes rhubarb and sorrel. Buckwheat is hardy, tolerates poor soil, thrives without chemicals, and is resistant to damage, making it inexpensive and easy to grow. Buckwheat is popular in Japan for soba noodles. See also "Grains" for general information. See also Happiness and Foods that Create Bliss under Food for Thought, under "H."

Buffalo [*Meat*] Buffalo (or Bison) are known as ruminants and are grazing animals that create meat that is high in protein and omega-3 fatty acids. It tends to be raised in a more sustainable way with less antibiotics. Buffalo/bison has similar vitamins and minerals to beef (above) except it is much lower in fats.

Bulgur [*Grain*] When wheat kernels are boiled, dried, cracked, and then sorted by size, the result is bulgur. Bulgur contains fiber, carbohydrates, protein, and some B-complex Vitamins (B3 (niacin), B6 (pyridoxine), B9 (folic acid), B1 (thiamine)). It has some minerals, including magnesium, iron, phosphorus, zinc, and copper. Bulgur is wheat in its whole form and contains substances called lignans that protect against cancer. Bulgur is believed to block the process that coverts nitrites in processed foods into harmful substances in the body. Toss uncooked bulgur into soups, stews, or chili and simmer until it's soft. Use it for cereal or a side dish, the same way you'd use oats and brown rice. See also "Grains" for general information.

Bulrush [*Grain*] The shoots of this marshy plant contain Vitamins B3 (niacin), B1 (thiamine), and C, minerals potassium and phosphorus, and the antioxidant beta-carotene. The rootstock can boiled or it, along with the rhizomes and stem, can be eaten raw. Boil the leaves like you would spinach. The flower spike, which looks a little like a corn-dog, can be broken off and eaten like corn on the cob in the early summer. See also Dandelions and Other "Weeds" under Food and You or Your Environment, under "D."

Burdock Root [*Vegetable*] This root contains fiber, carbohydrates, Vitamins C, K, E, B6 (pyridoxine), B9 (folic acid) in small amounts along with minerals potassium, magnesium, phosphorus, manganese and small amounts of calcium, iron and copper. Burdock root contains inulin, a type of beneficial fiber linked to the promotion of the growth of bifidobacteria in the large intestine. It can be eaten raw or cooked. See also Dandelions and Other "Weeds" under Food and You or Your Environment, under "D" and also Root Vegetables under Food for Thought, under "R."

Butter [*Fat*] Butter is a saturated fat that contains Vitamins A, E, K2, and D along with minerals selenium, manganese, chromium, zinc, and copper. It also contains cholesterol and omega-3 and omega-6 fatty acids. Cultured and unsalted butter is healthier for you than regular salted butter as it contains probiotics and less sodium. All saturated fats are best consumed in small amounts as they are calorie dense. See War of the Spreadable Oils under Food for Thought, under "O."

Butter Beans. See "Lima Beans."

Buttercup Squash. See "Squash" for nutrients and information.

Butterhead Lettuce. Also known as "Bibb Lettuce." See "Lettuce" for nutrients and information.

Buttermilk [*Dairy*] Buttermilk contains protein and Vitamins A, C, E, and B-complex Vitamins (B2 (riboflavin), B12 (cobalamin), and B1 (thiamine)). It contains minerals calcium and phosphorus, as well as saturated fats (omega-3 and 6 fatty acids in almost equal amounts). Homemade buttermilk is the slightly sour, residual liquid that remains after butter is churned – that is, milk from the butter or buttermilk. The flavor of buttermilk is similar to yogurt and the texture is thicker than regular milk but not as heavy as cream.

Butternut Squash. See "Squash" for nutrients and information.

Button Mushrooms. See "White Button Mushrooms." See also Marvelous Mushrooms – The Magic Food under Food for Thought, under "M."

FOOD FOR THOUGHT

Beef: Grass-Fed Versus Grain-Fed

Are we splitting the wheat from the chaff? No, there is a difference in the nutrient content.

Grass-fed/pasture-raised beef is higher in B-complex Vitamins, beta-carotene, Vitamins E, K, and trace minerals like magnesium, calcium, and selenium than grain-fed beef. Studies show grass feeding results in higher levels of omega-3 fatty acids and lower total levels of saturated, monounsaturated, and polyunsaturated fats. Grass-fed meat also contains Conjugated Linoleic Acid (CLA), an omega-6 essential fatty acid, which is said to burn fat, build muscle, and fight cancer. CLA has been called "the fat that makes you thin." Some researchers attribute the rise of obesity in America to the consumption of less and less CLA.

In Mark's Daily Apple[8] he writes:

> Grass-fed cows eat hundreds of different species of grasses. Cows will also chew on shrubs, clover, and random leaves or anything green, and leafy. All these "greens" are very high in nutrients which means a healthier cow and better quality beef. Also, pasture-raised animals live their natural lives and their excrement is converted into healthy fertilizer which enriches the soil instead of being a toxic waste.

Grain-fed cows on the other hand spend little time grazing in the field and then move to feed lots (also called Concentrated Animal Feed Operations or CAFOs). Animals housed in CAFO lots live in constant stress, resulting in poor health and they often require antibiotic shots due to the cramped and unsanitary conditions. Concentrated feed can mean any number of things, but the base food is always a grain slurry including corn and corn by-products (husks, cobs), soy and soy hulls, and other cereals that are very hard for cows to digest and can cause extreme discomfort and bloating.

> Grass-fed cows graze on a variety of
> nutrient-rich greens, producing healthier
> beef and a healthier you.

According to Vandana Shiva in her book *Staying Alive*,[9] CAFO-industrial animal farms are a negative, unsustainable food system because they consume more food than they produce. Buying grass-fed beef is a good choice for the family and the environment. Cows have an incredible 3-stomach digestive system built for grass. Humans cannot digest grass so they don't compete for the same food!

Buying grass-fed beef can be pricey at grocery stores and butchers, but as more people request it prices will drop. Find a farmer who will sell to you directly a half or quarter side of grass-fed beef that you can store in your freezer for an affordable price. In the meantime, eat smaller portions that will allow you to afford this nutrient-dense meat. I love wild game for the same reason! If you are a vegetarian, that is fine. If you love meat, try grass-fed for your health and enjoy the rich taste.

FOOD AND YOU OR YOUR ENVIRONMENT

Where Have the Bees Gone?

Bees are amazing insects. Honeybees do not exist for themselves but work together for a common good. The queen bee devotes her entire life to laying as many as two million eggs. Scout bees are sent out to search for food – nectar and pollen – and return to perform a complex "waggle dance" for other forager bees to indicate where to find the food.

Honeybees are required for the pollination of many vegetable and fruit crops. Without adequate populations of bees, the production of these and other crops would be very difficult. In addition, bee colonies are maintained for their honey and wax production. Bees swallow, digest, and regurgitate nectar to make honey; this nectar contains almost 600 compounds. To make one pound of honey, bees must collect nectar from over 2 million individual flowers.

Bees have amazing healing properties. Propolis,[10] the "caulk" honeybees use to patch holes in their hives, may also slow the growth of prostate cancer. When low oral doses of a propolis extract were given to mice with prostate tumors, growth slowed by 50% and daily ingestion of the substance after that caused tumors to stop growing! Propolis also has powerful immune-modulating effects, along with its potent antioxidant and antimicrobial action and its healing, analgesic, anesthetic, and anti-inflammatory properties!

> Propolis, the "caulk" honeybees use to patch holes in their hives, may also slow the growth of prostate cancer.

Bee pollen, the food for young bees, is almost 40% protein. About half of the protein is in the form of free amino acids and enzymes that make it easier to digest and absorb. Pollen is made up of more than 96 known nutrients, including minerals zinc, calcium, magnesium, and iron. It is often consumed by high performance athletes to boost their performance.

Honey is also useful in improving eyesight, weight loss, urinary tract disorders, bronchial asthma, diarrhea and nausea! Some varieties of honey possess large amounts of friendly bacteria. Honey has antibacterial qualities that are particularly useful for the skin, and, when used with the other ingredients, can also be moisturizing. Honey contains hydrogen peroxide that disinfects cuts and scrapes.

According to Will Allen in his book, *The Good Food Revolution*, there are only half as many honey-producing hives in the U.S. as there were in 1980. Colony Collapse Disorder (CCD) is occurring all over the world and no one knows exactly why. Some scientists are concerned that the widespread use of certain insecticides and pesticides is impacting the central nervous system of bees, impairing their ability to perform tasks necessary to survive as a colony. In creating an agriculture system that depends so much on so few crops, which are heavily sprayed with pesticides, we have also displaced the crop diversity and natural habitats necessary for bees to survive.

A simple solution would be to apply fewer chemicals to more specific parts of the plant at times of the day when honeybees are not following their daily search for food. Another remedy would be to start relying on the many beneficial insects, plants, and other biological means to deter major pests. These ideas and others are not rocket science and are starting to be implemented as "best practices" in sustainability for small- and large-scale farming operations. An exciting new bio-pesticide created using spider venom and a plant protein has been found to be safe for honeybees, despite being highly toxic to a number of key insect pests. This could pave the way for better ways to control unwanted pests in our crops![11]

Presently, many growers are successfully applying more sustainable approaches to combat pests but much more effort is required to ensure a healthy bee population for years to come. Each person can start by planting flowers and edibles around their homes to attract bees. The following herbs and plants have been found useful: basil, lemon balm, lavender, anise hyssop, borage, germander, sage, savory, chamomile, rosemary, dill, thyme, and dandelion.[12] Beneficial flowers include: clover, crocuses, foxglove, geraniums, hyacinth, marigolds, and sunflowers. Bees love the colors yellow, white, blue, and purple best so keep this in mind when planting your next garden!

HEALTHY YOU

Develop a Wild Diet!

Try cooking and eating gamier meats, including buffalo (bison), elk, venison, emu, or wild boar. Ground buffalo has less fat than regular hamburger and tastes similar. Most game is pasture raised without hormones or antibiotics. Cook game meats the same way you cook beef but because of their lower fat content, it will cook faster. Any game meat can be easily used instead of or in addition to chicken, beef, and pork to add variety to the recipes like chili, stews, etc. Game has more nutrients and omega-3 fatty acids so give it a try.

"There is no love sincerer than the love of food."
George Bernard Shaw
(1856-1950, Irish playwright)

Are Picky Eaters Just Chicken?

Chicken nuggets, chicken strips, chicken tenders, chicken … is this the only thing your kids will eat? My youngest son is a very picky eater. I can honestly relate to all the mothers out there who say it just isn't going to happen when I make some suggestions for healthier eating!

Still, I keep trying and I've managed to get him to eat a wide variety of vegetables and fruit over the years. But at 7 years old certain main courses are difficult (although my 8-year-old will eat almost any main course). He will only eat a certain kind of breaded chicken or fish. When anything else is presented he makes such a fuss that I save new food presentations for days when I have the stamina to endure the onslaught of complaints! My picky eater won't eat hamburgers or hotdogs either yet but maybe that isn't such a bad thing since he loves vegetables, fruit, and many nuts.

Patience and persistence (and a good sense of humor) are key to getting picky eaters to try new foods. Chicken is a low-fat source of protein and did you know that the world's average stock of chickens is almost 19 billion, or three per person, according to statistics from the UN's Food and Agriculture Organization.[13]

REAL "C" FOODS

Cabbage [*Vegetable*] Cabbage is a good source of fiber, carbohydrates and Vitamins C, K, and small amounts of B-complex Vitamins. It contains minerals, including iron, manganese, magnesium, and copper along with phytochemicals with antioxidant properties. It is a member of the cruciferous family which also includes cauliflower, broccoli, Brussels sprouts, and kale. The most common types of cabbage are bok choy and savoy. Cabbage has more antioxidants than green tea! Cabbage is the main ingredient in sauerkraut, a fermented cabbage dish. See What Foods Fight or Help Prevent Cancer? under Food and You or Your Environment, under "C."

Cacao (Chocolate) [*Bean*] Dry ground cacao is loaded with nutrients. The bean is harvested to make chocolate. Dark chocolate is a good source of protein, saturated fat, fiber, B-complex Vitamins (B2 (riboflavin), B3 (niacin), B9 (folic acid) and B1 (thiamine)), and large amounts of minerals, including copper, magnesium, manganese potassium, selenium, calcium, iron, phosphorus, and zinc. Cacao contains the antioxidant resveratrol that protects cells from damage. Cocoa butter, the naturally present fat in cacao beans, is considered a "good fat" by health experts as it does not increase levels of LDL-cholesterol. The amount of caffeine present in chocolate and cocoa-based products differs depending on the type and amount of chocolate ingredients. Eating dark chocolate in small amounts will improve blood flow to the brain and heart. With a low Glycemic Index (see What Does Glycemic Index (GI) Mean? under Food and You or Your Environment, under "G"), dark chocolate will not cause spikes in blood sugar and it is known as a natural cough suppressant. Cocoa also contains the amino acid tryptophan, which helps create positive feelings by making serotonin. Try eating more dark chocolate instead of sweets with refined sugar as it is an amazing and tasty power food. If you find dark chocolate too bitter, gradually increase the dark chocolate content. Buying organic and Fair Trade chocolate (and coffee) supports the workers who grow and harvest these products. See also Happiness and Foods that Create Bliss under Food for Thought, under "H" and also Understanding Ancient Foods Today under Food for Thought, under "U."

Cactus Fruit. See "Prickly Pear."

Calamari. See "Squid."

Camu Camu Berries [*Fruit*] Camu Camu berries contain fiber, carbohydrates, and a small amount of protein along with one of the highest concentrations of Vitamin C known. They contain B-complex Vitamins (B1 (thiamine), B3 (niacin), B2 (riboflavin)) and minerals calcium and potassium. Camu berry is one of the world's most abundant sources of Vitamin C with 60 times more Vitamin C than an orange! The Amazonian rainforest berry also contains beta-carotene, amino acids, and powerful phytochemicals. See also "Berries" for general information. See also The Stress'll Kill Ya under Food and You or Your Environment, under "S" and Understanding Ancient Foods Today under Food for Thought, under "U."

Canola [*Vegetable*] Canola contains Vitamins E and K, and some iron. It is commonly used for a cooking oil and, like olive oil, is very low in saturated fats. It contains both omega-6 and omega-3 fatty acids at 2:1, making it one of the healthiest cooking oils. With a smoke point of 450°F, it is ideal for frying foods. Cold-pressed oil is a stable cooking oil and gives it a very long shelf life. Canola is a member of the brassica and cruciferous families, which also include mustard, cabbage, and turnips. It was developed in Canada in 1970 by breeding out rapeseed's undesirable qualities, which made it difficult for humans and animals to consume. It is considered a food different from rapeseed. See also

"Oils." See What Foods Fight or Help Prevent Cancer? under Food and You or Your Environment, under "C."

Cantaloupe [*Fruit*] Cantaloupe contains fiber, carbohydrates and high amounts of Vitamins C, A, some K and B-complex Vitamins (B9 (folic acid), B6 (pyridoxine), B3 (niacin), and B1 (thiamine)) along with some minerals, including potassium and small amounts of magnesium, manganese, and copper. In fact, cantaloupes have more Vitamin A than that of carrots, making it great for your eyes and preventing macular degeneration. As with other melons, cutting cantaloupe causes it to lose its Vitamin C and antioxidant benefits. After 6 days, cut cubes lose 25% of their Vitamin C and 10-15% of carotenoids, so buy them whole and cut only a piece at a time!

Caraway Seed [*Spice*] These seeds are a storehouse for many vital vitamins. Vitamins A, E, C, as well as many B-complex Vitamins (B1 (thiamine), B6 (pyridoxine), B2 (riboflavin), and B3 (niacin)) are particularly concentrated in the caraway seeds. It is also an excellent source of minerals like iron and copper. Caraway seeds are known to possess antifungal properties and are used in curing gastrointestinal and digestive disorders. Because of its soothing properties, it is also used to cure stomach ulcers. Caraway seeds are commonly used in the preparation of breads, cheese, and soups. See "Spices" for general information and cooking suggestions.

Carbohydrates. See What Your Body Needs and Why.

Cardamom [*Spice*] Cardamom has good amounts of fiber, protein, and Vitamin C and B-complex Vitamins (B6 (pyridoxine), B1 (thiamine), B2 (riboflavin), and B3 (niacin)). Cardamom has incredibly high amounts of manganese (one teaspoon added to coffee has 36% of your daily needs) and high amounts of iron, magnesium, zinc, copper, calcium, phosphorus, and potassium. The therapeutic properties of cardamom oil have found application in many traditional medicines as antiseptic, local anesthetic, and an antioxidant, as well as antispasmodic, carminative, digestive, diuretic, expectorant, stimulant, stomachic and tonic. See "Spices" for general information and cooking suggestions.

Cardoon/Cardone [*Vegetable*] Cardoon contains fiber and carbohydrates and is high in Vitamin B9 (folic acid) and has some B6 (pyridoxine) and B5 (pantothenic acid). It also contains high amounts of minerals copper, magnesium, and manganese, along with some iron, potassium, and calcium. Cardoon is a leaf-stalk vegetable, well-known in the Mediterranean area, that looks like celery, but is related to artichoke. It is a popular winter season vegetable that can be sautéed, boiled in soups and stews, or baked with butter and seasonings.

Carnival Squash. See "Squash" for nutrients and information.

Carp [*Fish*] Carp is a good source of protein and omega-3 fatty acids. It contains good amounts of B-complex Vitamins (B3 (niacin), B12 (cobalamin), B6 (pyridoxine), B1 (thiamine), B5 (pantothenic acid), B2 (riboflavin), and B9 (folic acid)), some Vitamins C and K, along with good amounts of minerals selenium and phosphorus. (For information on sustainable fish see "Fish" or visit *www.msc.org/cook-eat-enjoy/fish-to-eat*.)

Carrots [*Vegetable*] Carrots contain fiber and carbohydrates and are an amazing source of Vitamin A and beta-carotene. They contain Vitamins C, K, and some B-complex Vitamins and are a good source of minerals manganese, potassium, magnesium, iron, copper, and phosphorus. Vitamin A is transformed in the retina to rhodopsin, a purple pigment necessary for night vision. Beta-carotene has also been shown to protect against macular degeneration and senile cataracts. A study found that people who ate the most beta-carotene had a 40% lower risk of macular degeneration than those who consumed little.[14] Vitamin A and antioxidants protect the skin from sun damage and prevent premature wrinkling, acne, dry skin, pigmentation, blemishes, and uneven skin tone. Carrots are great for juicing and for snacking on raw so have them prepped and ready in your fridge to access. See also Root Vegetables under Food for Thought, under "R."

Casabas [*Fruit*] Casabas are melons and contain fiber, carbohydrates, good amounts of Vitamin C, and small amounts of Vitamins K and B6 (pyridoxine) along with minerals potassium and small amounts of magnesium and copper.

Cashew [*Nut*] Cashews are high in protein, fiber, saturated fats, contain Vitamins E, K and B-complex Vitamins (B1 (thiamine), B6 (pyridoxidine), B5 (pantothenic acid), B3 (niacin) and B9 (folic acid)), and are a rich source of minerals especially manganese, magnesium, potassium, copper, iron, zinc, and selenium with some other antioxidants including zeaxanthin. Cashews grow on a tree that produces flowers that in turn produce oval structures resembling apples. However, cashew apples are not actually fruits. The real fruit of the cashew tree is the kidney-shaped formation growing at the end. These are harvested and become what we know as a cashew nut. In their raw form, the outer layer contains multiple toxins similar to those found in poison ivy that must be removed prior to eating. Roasting the cashews destroys the toxins and creates the delicious treat sold in stores. See "Nuts" for general information.

Cassava [*Vegetable*] High in carbohydrates and Vitamin C, cassava contains good amounts of Vitamin K, B-complex Vitamins (B9 (folic acid), B1 (thiamine), B3 (niacin), B6 (pyridoxine)), and minerals manganese, potassium, copper, phosphorus, and zinc. For most people, cassava is most commonly associated with tapioca, but around the world, it is a vital staple for about 500 million people. Cassava is a shrubby, tropical, perennial plant that is not well known in the temperate zone. It thrives better in poor soils than any other major food plant and, as a result, fertilization is rarely necessary. Cassava's starchy roots produce more food energy per unit of land than any other staple crop. Its leaves, commonly eaten as a vegetable in parts of Asia and Africa, provide vitamins and protein. Nutritionally, the cassava is comparable to potatoes, except that it has twice the fiber content, but has less protein than some other popular staple crops. See also Root Vegetables under Food for Thought, under "R."

Catfish [*Fish*] Catfish is a good source of protein and omega–3 fatty acids. It contains good amounts of Vitamins B3 (niacin), B12 (cobalamin), B6 (pyridoxine), and minerals phosphorus, selenium, zinc, potassium, magnesium, iron, calcium and copper. (For information on sustainable fish see "Fish" or visit *www.msc.org/cook-eat-enjoy/fish-to-eat.*)

Cattail. See "Bulrush." See also Dandelions and Other "Weeds" under Food and You or Your Environment, under "D."

Cauliflower [*Vegetable*] Cauliflower contains large amounts of fiber, carbohydrates, Vitamin C and good amounts of B-complex Vitamins (B5 (pantothenic acid), B9 (folic acid), and B6 (pyridoxine)). It has small amounts of manganese, potassium, iron, and copper. As a member of the cruciferous family, it has many antioxidant anticancer properties. Try roasting it or mixing a small amount of mashed cauliflower in with mashed potatoes to increase nutrients and flavor. See What Foods Fight or Help Prevent Cancer? under Food and You or Your Environment, under "C."

Cavena Nuda [*Grain*] Cavena Nuda is a new whole grain developed by Agriculture Canada! It looks and tastes like brown rice but is a hull-less oat that is high in fiber, iron, potassium, and protein and it is gluten free. See also "Grains" for general information.

Cayenne Pepper [*Spice*] Cayenne pepper is high in fiber and protein. It is perhaps the richest source of Vitamin A among spices and also has huge amounts of Vitamin K. Cayenne has very good amounts of Vitamins C, E, and B-complex Vitamins (B3 (niacin),

B2 (riboflavin), B6 (pyridoxine), B1 (thiamine), and B9 (folic acid)), and very high amounts of minerals iron, manganese, potassium, copper, magnesium, phosphorus, zinc, selenium, and some calcium. It also contains high amounts of antioxidants, including beta-carotene, lutein, and zeaxanthin. Cayenne contains the alkaloid compound capsaicin, which studies on experimental mammals suggest has antibacterial, anticarcinogenic, analgesic, and antidiabetic properties. When used regularly it is also found to reduce triglycerides and LDL cholesterol levels in obese individuals. Capsaicin and its co-compounds are used in the preparation of ointments, rubs, and tinctures for their astringent, counter-irritant, and analgesic properties. See also "Hot Peppers." See "Spices" for general information and cooking suggestions. See also What's to be Done about the Rise in Heart Disease? under Food and You or Your Environment, under "H" and also Are Rheumatoid Arthritis and Autoimmune Diseases on the Rise? under Food and You or Your Environment, under "R."

Celeriac [*Vegetable*] Celeriac is a good source fiber, carbohydrates, Vitamins K, C, and B-complex Vitamins (B6 (pyridoxine), B5 (pantothenic acid), and B2 (riboflavin)), and has minerals iron, potassium, manganese, phosphorus, copper, and magnesium in decent amounts. It is a root crop with leaves that look like those of celery. See also Root Vegetables under Food for Thought, under "R."

Celery [*Vegetable*] Celery contains fiber, carbohydrates, a decent source of Vitamins A, K, some C and B-complex Vitamins, along with minerals potassium, manganese, calcium, magnesium, phosphorus, and iron in small amounts. It is best stored whole to avoid losing nutrients through cutting. The leaves contain most of the potassium, Vitamin C, and calcium, so be sure to use them in soups and salads too. Celery is known to help lower blood pressure.

Celery Seed [*Spice*] Celery seed contains small amounts of Vitamin B6 (pyridoxine) and good amounts of iron, manganese, calcium, and some magnesium. See "Spices" for general information and cooking suggestions.

Chaga. See "Mushrooms" for nutrients and information. See also What Foods Fight or Help Prevent Cancer? under Food and You or Your Environment, under "C" and also Marvelous Mushrooms – The Magic Food under Food for Thought, under "M."

Chard. See "Swiss Chard."

Cheese [*Dairy*] Cheese is a good source of Vitamins A, B12 (cobalamin), and B2 (riboflavin), and has high amounts of minerals calcium, phosphorus, sodium, zinc, and selenium along with high amounts of saturated fat and beneficial probiotic bacteria. There are hundreds of types of cheeses produced around the world. Texture and flavor depend on the origin of the milk, whether the milk has been pasteurized, the butterfat content, bacteria and mold, and the processing and aging conditions. Cheese is an ancient food made since the beginnings of recorded history and has been enjoyed in cuisines around the world in a huge number of dishes. Cheese is classified as hard, semi-hard, semi-soft, or soft. Some of the most popular types include: asiago, blue, brie, cheddar, chevre, colby, edam, feta, gouda, gruyere, havarti, monterey jack, mozzarella, parmesan, provolone, romano, and swiss. Hard cheese has a higher nutrient content on average and contain less sodium than other cheeses.

Chehalem Berries [*Fruit*] Chehalem berries – Himalayan blackberry and Santiam berry hybrids – have a shiny black outer surface. These are well-adapted to the Pacific coast conditions and are commercially grown in Oregon to some extent. See "Berries" for nutrients and information.

Cherimoya [*Fruit*] Cherimoya contain fiber, carbohydrates and Vitamins C, E and B-complex Vitamins (B6 (pyridoxine), B2 (riboflavin), B1 (thiamine), and B5 (pantothenic acid)), and minerals copper and potassium. It also contains several potent antioxidants including beta-carotene and lutein-zeaxanthin. Cherimoya is one of the most delicious tropical fruits of Andean valley origin.

Cherries [*Fruit*] Cherries contain fiber, carbohydrates, Vitamins C, K, and minerals potassium, magnesium and manganese along with a flavonoid compound known as anthocyanin, which has powerful antioxidant capabilities. Anthocyanins are red, purple, or blue pigments found in colorful fruits and vegetables, especially concentrated in their skins. Cherries also contain other antioxidants, including beta-carotene, lutein, and zeaxanthin. Cherries are known for their ability to relieve symptoms of gout, arthritis, and kidney stones by relieving inflammation. Tart cherries are known to help induce sleep as they contain melatonin. See also Happiness and Foods that Create Bliss under Food for Thought, under "H" and also Are Rheumatoid Arthritis and Autoimmune Diseases on the Rise? under Food and You or Your Environment, under "R."

Chestnut [*Nut*] Chestnuts contain protein, fiber, saturated fat, Vitamin E and B-complex Vitamins (B6 (pyridoxine), B1 (thiamine), B2 (riboflavin), B5 (pantothenic acid), B9 (folic acid), B3 (niacin)). They are a good source of minerals such as copper, iron, magnesium, manganese and phosphorus. As compared with the protein/fat make-up of most other nuts, chestnuts are mostly starch. They are closer in composition to potatoes, corn, or plantain. See "Nuts" for general information.

Chia Seeds [*Seeds*] Chia seeds are high in protein, omega-3 fatty acids, and fiber. They contain high amounts of minerals phosphorus, manganese, calcium, and good amounts of zinc. Chia is considered a power food and good to put in cereals for extra nutrients and protein in the morning. Ancient Aztec warriors ate chia for vitality and endurance. See also Understanding Ancient Foods Today under Food for Thought, under "U."

Chicken [*Meat*] Whether free range or factory raised, chicken provides a good source of lean protein, saturated fat, and B-complex Vitamins (B3 (niacin), B2 (riboflavin), B5 (pantothenic acid)), along with minerals selenium, phosphorus, magnesium, potassium, zinc, and iron.

Chickpeas. See "Garbanzo Beans."

Chicory [*Vegetable*] Chicory contains Vitamins K, A, C, and B9 (folic acid) along with minerals manganese and copper. Chicory is also used as a coffee replacement. See also "Endive" for general nutrients. See also Dandelions and Other "Weeds" under Food and You or Your Environment, under "D."

Chili Peppers [*Vegetable*] Chili peppers contain high amounts of Vitamins A, C, K, and some B-complex Vitamins (B6 (pyridoxine), B2 (riboflavin), B3 (niacin), B9 (folic acid), B1 (thiamine)) and Vitamin E. They have small amounts of minerals iron, copper, manganese, magnesium, and phosphorus, and antioxidants beta-carotene, lutein, and zeaxanthin. Hot chili peppers have long been used as a natural remedy for coughs, colds, sinusitis, and bronchitis and are a known to help combat obesity by reducing food cravings and increasing digestive energy. Chili peppers contain capsaicin which has shown promise for reducing cancer tumors and boosting the immune system due to its anticarcinogenic, antibacterial, and antidiabetic properties.

Chili Powder [*Spice*] Chili powder contains huge amounts of Vitamins C and B6 (pyridoxine). It also has Vitamins K, E, and B-complex Vitamins (B3 (niacin), B2 (riboflavin), B1 (thiamine), and B9 (folic acid)), and small amounts of minerals iron, copper, potassium, and manganese. Chili powder contains antioxidants beta-carotene, lutein, etc. Like chili peppers themselves, the ground seeds contain capsaicin, used in the treatment of arthritic pain, post-herpetic neuropathic pain, and sore muscles. See "Spices" for general information and cooking suggestions.

Chives [*Herb*] A perennial plant that is part of the onion or allium family, chives supply many vitamins and minerals, including potassium, calcium, beta-carotene, and Vitamins B9 (folic acid) and K. Chives also supply lesser amounts of magnesium, iron, and trace amounts of several B-complex Vitamins. Chives contain many antioxidants and are known for their anticancer and antibacterial properties. See "Herbs" for general information. See also Herbaceous Cooking under Healthy You, under "H."

Chlorella [*Vegetable (Sea)*] A type of algae that grows in fresh water, chlorella is a power food that contains carbohydrates, is extremely high in protein, has huge amounts Vitamin A, good amounts of Vitamins C and E, and excellent amounts of B-complex Vitamins (B1 (thiamine), B2 (riboflavin), B6 (pyridoxine), B9 (folic acid), and B5 (pantothenic acid)), along with huge amounts of mineral iron, zinc, magnesium, phosphorus, and calcium. Chlorella products can vary significantly in nutrients depending on where they are cultivated, harvested, and processed. As a medicine, chlorella is used for preventing cancer, reducing radiation treatment side effects, stimulating the immune system, increasing white blood cell counts, preventing colds, protecting the body against toxic metals such as lead and mercury, and slowing the aging process. Chlorella is also used to increase "good" bacteria in the intestine in order to improve digestion and to help treat ulcers, colitis, Crohn's disease, and diverticulosis. The cell wall of chlorella must be broken down before people can digest it.[15] See What Foods Fight or Help Prevent Cancer? under Food and You or Your Environment, under "C."

Chocolate. See "Cacao."

Chokeberry [*Fruit*] Chokeberries contain fiber, carbohydrates, Vitamins C, E, A, and K, and minerals manganese, iron, magnesium, and copper. They also contains several potent antioxidants, including carotenes, lutein, and zeaxanthins. Zeaxanthin is known to have photo-filtering effects on UV rays and thus protects eyes from age-related macular disease. See also "Berries" for general information.

Cilantro [*Herb*] Cilantro is a perennial herb rich in many vital nutrients, including Vitamins A, C, K, and B-complex Vitamins (B9 (folic acid), B2 (riboflavin), and B3 (niacin)), and beta-carotene. It is a good source of minerals potassium, calcium, manganese, iron, and magnesium. Cilantro leaves have many known health benefits, including protection against infections and salmonella bacteria, digestion aid, anti-inflammatory properties that may alleviate symptoms of arthritis, lowers blood sugar, lowers bad cholesterol (LDL), raises good cholesterol (HDL), good source of fiber, and rich in phytonutrients and flavonoids. See also "Coriander." See "Herbs" for general information. See also Herbaceous Cooking under Healthy You, under "H."

Cinnamon [*Spice*] Cinnamon is for well-known for balancing blood sugar and lowering blood pressure. Cinnamon has huge amounts of fiber and some protein. It has Vitamins E, K, A, C and B-complex Vitamins (B6 (pyridoxine), B3 (niacin), and B5 (pantothenic acid)), along with good amounts of minerals manganese, iron, calcium, copper, zinc, magnesium, phosphorus, and potassium. Cinnamon has huge antioxidant capabilities and contains carotenes, lutein, zeaxanthin, etc. It has one of the highest antioxidant strengths of all the food sources in nature. It is obtained from the outer bark of cinnamomum trees, then dried and sold as sticks or "quills." The essential oils in cinnamon have been found to have an anticlotting action that prevents platelets from clogging inside the blood vessels, thereby helping to prevent stroke, peripheral arterial and coronary artery diseases. It is a proven blood sugar regulator and can be added to cereal, smoothies, toast, and baking. See "Spices" for general information and cooking suggestions. See also Understanding Ancient Foods Today under Food for Thought, under "U."

Citrus [*Fruit*] All citrus fruits are high in Vitamin C and citrus fruit intake is associated with a reduced risk of stomach cancer and may be useful for lowering the risk of specific types of kidney stones. Lemons have the highest concentration of citrate of any citrus fruit, grapefruit seed extract has been used to inhibit the formation of harmful intestinal organisms, including giardia, without reducing levels of healthy bowel flora. See particular species under their specific name (e.g., "Grapefruit," "Lemons," "Limes," "Oranges," "Tangerines," etc.).

Clams [*Shellfish*] Clams are high in protein and omega–3 fatty acids. They contain good amounts of Vitamins A, C, K, and B-complex Vitamins (B12 (cobalamin), B2 (riboflavin), B1 (thiamine), B3 (niacin), and choline), and minerals chromium, iron, calcium, phosphorus, potassium, and zinc. Clam is the generic name for freshwater mussels and are classified as a mollusk. (For information on sustainable fish see "Fish" or visit *www.msc.org/cook-eat-enjoy/fish-to-eat*.) See also "Shellfish" for general information.

Clementine [*Fruit*] See "Tangerine" for nutrients and information.

Cloudberries [*Fruit*] Cloudberries are high in Vitamin C and contain benzoic acids that act as natural preservatives. They are small, brown-colored berries that ripen in autumn. They are used to make jams, juices, tarts, and liqueurs. See "Berries" for nutrients and information.

Clover [*Vegetable (Legume)*] Clover is a good source of Vitamins B1 (thiamine), B3 (niacin), and C, and minerals calcium, chromium, magnesium, phosphorus, and potassium. See also Dandelions and Other "Weeds" under Food and You or Your Environment, under "D."

Cloves [*Spice*] These "flower buds" from an evergreen rain-forest tree native to Indonesia, contain some fiber and protein along with Vitamins K, C, B-complex Vitamins (B9 (folic acid), B5 (pantothenic acid), B6 (pyridoxine), B3 (niacin), and B1 (thiamine)), and minerals copper, iron, magnesium, phosphorus, manganese, selenium, zinc, and potassium. Cloves have excellent antioxidant properties and can inhibit C0X-2, a protein that sparks inflammation. The active principles in the clove may increase gut motility as well as improve digestion power by increasing gastrointestinal enzyme secretions, relieving indigestion and constipation problems. Additionally, these active principles are believed to have antioxidant, antiseptic, local anesthetic, anti-inflammatory, warming and soothing, and antiflatulent properties. Cloves are used by different African cultures as a flavor ingredient in hot tea or chai and are said to help against nausea. See "Spices" for general information and cooking suggestions.

Cobia [*Fish*] Found in warm-temperate to tropical waters, this fish is a good source of protein and omega-3 fatty acids. It contains good amounts of Vitamins B3 (niacin), B12 (cobalamin), B6 (pyridoxine) and minerals selenium and phosphorus. Cobia grows faster than salmon and has been called the fish of the future. (For information on sustainable fish see "Fish" or visit *www.msc.org/cook-eat-enjoy/fish-to-eat*.)

Coconut [*Fruit* and *Nut*] Coconut is 85% saturated fat. They contain protein, fiber, and minerals selenium, fluoride, copper, iron, potassium, phosphorus, calcium, magnesium, zinc, copper, and selenium. Coconuts also contain lauric acid, a medium-chained fatty acid that absorbs directly into the bloodstream and helps increase blood HDL, or good cholesterol, levels. Coconut oil is believed to boost metabolism, aid digestion, reduce inflammation, assist with neurological diseases, such as ALS (or Lou Gehrig's disease), Parkinson's and Alzheimer's, has antiviral and antibacterial properties, and contains caprlyic acid which helps to kill candida in the gut. Coconut is known for high quality oil with ability to withstand high cooking temperatures. It is also a great moisturizer and sunscreen as it is mostly made up of saturated fat (like our skin)! See also "Oil" for general information. See also How Can We Hold onto Yesterday's Memories? under Food and You or Your Environment, under "Y."

Cod [*Fish*] Cod is a good source of protein and omega-3 fatty acids. It contains good amounts of Vitamin D and B-complex Vitamins (B3 (niacin), B12 (cobalamin), B6 (pyridoxine), B1 (thiamine), and B2 (riboflavin)), and some Vitamin E and C, along with minerals selenium, potassium, phosphorus, and some magnesium and zinc. (For information on sustainable fish see "Fish" or visit *www.msc.org/cook-eat-enjoy/fish-to-eat.*)

Coffee [*Seed*] Coffee comes from the seed of the coffee plant, although often referred to as beans, which is ground to make hot drink that is popular around the world. It contains B-complex Vitamins (B5 (pantothenic acid) and B2 (riboflavin)) along with fiber, protein, iron, antioxidants, and caffeine. Caffeine has been shown to help improve a range of health problems, including Parkinson's disease and other age-related brain problems, and has potential benefits for improving health and reducing the risk of chronic illnesses. Coffee is the second largest food traded in the world. See also Can Certain Foods Make Us More Intelligent? under Food and You or Your Environment, under "I," and also How Can We Hold onto Yesterday's Memories? under Food and You or Your Environment, under "Y."

Collards Greens [*Vegetable*] Collard greens contain fiber, carbohydrates, high amounts of Vitamins A, K, C, E, and some B-complex Vitamins (B9 (folic acid), B6 (pyridoxine), B2 (riboflavin), B3 (niacin), and B5 (pantothenic acid)), along with minerals calcium and magnesium and high amounts of antioxidants like beta-carotene, lutein, and zeaxanthin and some omega-3 fatty acids. They are considered a cruciferous vegetable and contain phytonutrients called glucosinolates that can help activate detoxification enzymes in our bodies. See What Foods Fight or Help Prevent Cancer? under Food and You or Your Environment, under "C."

Cordycep. See "Mushrooms" for nutrients and information. See also What Foods Fight or Help Prevent Cancer? under Food and You or Your Environment, under "C" and also Marvelous Mushrooms – The Magic Food under Food for Thought, under "M."

Coriander [*Spice*] It is generally accepted that "coriander" is the dried fruit (or seed) of the cilantro plant. It contains huge amounts of Vitamins A and K, good amounts of Vitamins C, E, and B-complex Vitamins (B2 (riboflavin), B6 (pyridoxine), B5 (pantothenic acid), B9 (folic acid), B3 (niacin), and B1 (thiamine)), and good amounts of minerals iron, manganese, magnesium, calcium, phosphorus, and potassium. Coriander has high amounts of antioxidants, including quercetin, lutein, beta-carotenes, etc. Coriander seed oil has found application in many traditional medicines such as analgesic, aphrodisiac, antispasmodic, deodorant, digestive, carminative, fungicidal, and weight management. See also "Cilantro." See "Spices" for general information and cooking suggestions.

Coridus. See "Mushrooms" for nutrients and information. See also What Foods Fight or Help Prevent Cancer? under Food and You or Your Environment, under "C" and also Marvelous Mushrooms – The Magic Food under Food for Thought, under "M."

Corn [*Vegetable* and *Grain*] Corn is a source of carbohydrates, fiber, B-complex Vitamins (B1 (thiamine), B3 (niacin), B6 (pyridoxine), B2 (riboflavin), and B9 (folic acid)) and some Vitamin A. Corn has minerals iron, magnesium, manganese, phosphorus, zinc, copper, potassium, and selenium along with some protein and omega-6 fatty acids. Many people consider it a grain because it is sugary and starchy but others view it as a vegetable. Corn was originally grown in South America and is a staple in Latin America. Most corn grown in the U.S. is used to feed cattle and to make sweeteners. Gluten free, officially corn is a fruit! See also "Grains" and "Sweetener" for general information. See also Mountains of Corn under Food for Thought, below. See also Sugar – A Diet No No under Food for Thought, under "S."

Courgette. See "Zucchini."

Covalo Nero. See "Kale." See What Foods Fight or Help Prevent Cancer? under Food and You or Your Environment, under "C."

Crab [*Shellfish*] High in protein and omega-3 fatty acids, this shellfish (also known as crayfish) contains Vitamin B12 (cobalamin) in good amounts and small amounts of other B-complex Vitamins and Vitamin C, along with good amounts of minerals zinc, copper, selenium, iron, potassium, and calcium. (For information on sustainable fish see "Fish" or visit *www.msc.org/cook-eat-enjoy/fish-to-eat*.) See also "Shellfish" for general information.

Cranberries [*Fruit*] Cranberries contain fiber, carbohydrates, and are a good source of Vitamins C, K, and the mineral potassium. They are used to treat urinary tract infections due to their antiviral properties. In disease-fighting antioxidants, cranberries are more potent than many fruit and vegetables, including strawberries, spinach, broccoli, red grapes, apples, raspberries, and cherries. Add dried cranberries to your favorite cereal, porridge, or baked recipes for added flavor and nutrients. See also "Berries" for general information.

Crayfish. See "Crab."

Cremini [*Fungi*] This mushroom is a power food loaded with B-complex Vitamins (B2 (riboflavin), B5 (pantothenic acid), B3 (niacin), B1 (thiamine), and B6 (pyridoxine)), and some B12 (cobalamin), depending on growing conditions. These B vitamins are necessary for carbohydrate, protein, and fat metabolism. They also contain good amounts of fiber and protein as well as minerals zinc, copper, manganese, magnesium, potassium, iron, calcium, and phosphorus, and also the amino acid tryptophan, which helps create the serotonin which regulates mood. For women who are at risk of hormone-dependent breast cancer, cremini mushrooms have promise as they are a significant source of conjugated linoleic acid (CLA) which is a unique type of fatty acid that can bind onto aromatase enzymes and lessen the production of estrogen.[16] Since some breast cancer tumors are dependent upon estrogen for their growth, this blocking of the aromatase enzyme by CLA may lower risk of this breast cancer type. Preliminary research shows that cremini mushrooms may be an important food in a diet that is geared towards protecting against all cancer. Extracts of cremini mushrooms have been found to protect DNA from oxidative damage. See "Mushrooms" for general information. See also Marvelous Mushrooms – The Magic Food under Food for Thought, under "M."

Cress. See "Watercress." See also "Lettuce" for general nutrients.

Cruciferous. See "Brassica."

Crustacean [*Shellfish*] This particular classification includes crabs, crayfish, lobster, and shrimp. See particular species under their specific name. (For information on sustainable fish see "Fish" or visit *www.msc.org/cook-eat-enjoy/fish-to-eat*.)

Cucumbers [*Vegetable*] Cucumbers contain fiber, carbohydrates, Vitamins K, A, C, and small amounts of B-complex Vitamins. They have small amounts of minerals, including potassium, magnesium, and phosphorus. Cucumbers (with peel) contain tryptophan, one of the ten essential amino acids that the body uses to synthesize the proteins it needs. Tryptophan serves as a precursor for serotonin, a neurotransmitter that helps the body regulate appetite, sleep patterns, and mood. Because of its ability to raise serotonin levels, tryptophan has been used therapeutically in the treatment of a variety of conditions, including insomnia, depression, and anxiety. Other rich vegetable sources of tryptophan include asparagus, beets, broccoli, cauliflower, cucumbers with peel, peppers, cabbage, eggplant, pumpkin, potatoes with skin, mushrooms, and winter and summer squash, although the best sources are meat and nuts. Cucumbers are also used for skin healing in many cultures and are in many facial products. Cucumbers are great to add to water to improve taste!

Cumin [*Spice*] Cumin seeds are actually the dried fruit of the cumin plant. This spice has high amounts of fiber and some protein. It is a good source of Vitamins A, E, C, and B-complex Vitamins (B6 (pyridoxine), B1 (thiamine), B3 (niacin), and B2 (riboflavin)), contains excellent amounts of minerals iron, manganese, and good amounts of magnesium, copper, calcium, phosphorus, zinc, and potassium. An excellent anti-inflammatory, it also contains antioxidants, including beta-carotenes, lutein, zeaxanthin, etc. The health benefits of cumin include its ability to aid in digestion, improve immunity, and treat piles, insomnia, respiratory disorders such as asthma, bronchitis, and colds. It is used in the cuisine of many cultures, including India, Middle Eastern countries, North Africa, and Europe. See "Spices" for general information and cooking suggestions. See also Root Vegetables under Food for Thought, under "R."

Currants [*Fruit*] Currants (or black and red jostaberries) contain fiber, carbohydrates and are high in Vitamin C and potassium along with several powerful antioxidants. They have been proven to have anti-inflammatory benefits. They are dried and used like raisins. See "Berries" for nutrients and information.

FOOD FOR THOUGHT

Mountains of Corn

Corn is one of the most widely eaten vegetables in North America – and I don't mean niblets or tacos even though both are tasty! Corn is now added to a ton of foods in the form of High Fructose Corn Syrup (HFCS) and it really isn't that good for our health. Why are we so in love with corn?

> In 1985 North Americans consumed about 45 pounds of high-fructose corn syrup. In 2006 that number jumped to 58 pounds, mostly from soft drinks!

In 1985 North Americans consumed about 45 pounds of high-fructose corn syrup. In 2006 that number jumped to 58 pounds, mostly from soft drinks! At the same time period childhood obesity rose from 5.8% of the population in 1971-1974 to 17.3 % in 2003-2006. Corn is in a huge number of processed foods, and can be found in the ingredient list under various names, including corn syrup, high-fructose corn syrup, dextrose, modified corn starch, glucose, polysorbate 60, and cornstarch.

According to Michael Pollan, in his book *The Omnivore's Dilemma*, corn goes into making things you can imagine and more things you can't: canned and frozen corn, snack food, cosmetic powders, livestock feed, and soup mixes, breakfast cereal, pet food, floor wax, hand soap, baby food, paper products, pharmaceuticals, potato chips, margarine, vitamin carriers, cheese spreads, prepared egg products, extracts, flavorings, peanut butter, soft drinks, wine products, canned fruit, condiments, bakery products, engine fuel, plastics, antibiotics, chewing gum, insecticides, sandpaper, wallpaper, glue, aspirin, disinfectants, detergents, crayons and chalk, precooked frozen meals, and, of course, candy to name a few![17] In addition, in North America our gas stations are turning into processed corn stations with ethanol gas on the outside for the car and high fructose corn syrup products inside.

Corn is a staple crop for many farmers but it is also a thirsty crop that depletes the soil. Farmers who grow corn rely on artificial fertilizer to replant crops each year. Corn accounts for about 40% of herbicide and insecticides (soybeans account for 22% of herbicides and of insecticides) used by farmers.[18] This makes corn a leading contributor to soil erosion and groundwater pollution.

Don't get me wrong, I love eating corn, especially in the summer when you get fresh corn on the cob, but do we need corn in all our processed foods and consumer products, particularly when drought is a growing concern in many parts of the world? I think it is time that we all ask why we need to have so much corn. The big agribusinesses are certainly happy with soaring profits but the rest of us may be left with poorer health and poorer soil as a result. That is certainly food for thought!

Next time you are at the grocery store, try reading the labels of the processed foods to see how many corn additives you find. To avoid corn by-products in your food, shop the outside, first, focusing on whole foods. Similarly use the middle aisles for whole foods, including whole grain bread, pasta, and rice, oils and herbs, and buy pickles and other condiments in the refrigerated section.

Go ahead and enjoy whole corn products like fresh corn from the vegetable section or treat yourself to the occasional taco dinner or tortilla chip and salsa snack … guilt free! I love Neil Brothers tortillas with flax along with salsa and guacamole. Now that is what corn was made for in my humble opinion.

FOOD AND YOU OR YOUR ENVIRONMENT

What Foods Fight or Help Prevent Cancer?

The statistics are staggering. Over 40.8% of the North American population will be diagnosed with a cancer at some point in their lifetime. North America leads the world in the rate of cancers diagnosed in adults, followed closely by Western Europe, Australia, and New Zealand, according to a recent estimate of worldwide cancer rates. The most common cancers in North America are breast, prostate, lung, and colon and some people believe these are connected to too many hormones in our food system and immune issues that effect our metabolism and our digestive and elimination systems.[19]

The World Health Organization and the Canadian Cancer Society claim that one-third of all cancers can be prevented with a healthy diet and lifestyle. Given the overwhelming evidence that certain foods help treat and prevent cancer, it's never too early to add cancer-fighting foods into your daily diet. In addition, certain foods and beverages and exercise can help flush toxins out of the body and stress management techniques will keep you healthy mentally and emotionally as well. No one knows for sure what causes cancer and even the healthiest of us can become a victim of this terrible disease, but our bodies are amazing machines that are built to be healthy, so let's start now by incorporating the following anti-cancer foods into our daily diets to help prevent or combat cancer.

- **Adzuki and Mung Beans:** Foods like meat, cheese, and many grains are acid forming in the body, which can cause inflammation and too much inflammation can cause problems in our bodies. Choosing a more alkaline diet with foods like fresh vegetables, fruits, and legumes will protect the body against inflammation and cancer. Beans (especially adzuki and mung) contain phytic acid, which is a cancer inhibitor, and are high in protein and minerals.

- **Berries:** Berries are loaded with antioxidants that fight cancer. Although all berries have some antioxidants, goji and acai berries from the Himalayas are considered the highest in antioxidants. Berries freeze well for the winter and can easily be added to smoothies or served with cereals or porridge.

- **Chlorella and Kelp:** As a medicine, chlorella is used for preventing cancer, reducing radiation side effects, and stimulating the immune system. Kelp and other sea vegetables are high in iodine which boosts our thyroid function, regulating metabolism. Kelp helps to break down tumors and binds with radioactive molecules so they can be easily excreted. Kelp shakers can be found in stores to add to food.

- **Cruciferous Vegetables:** Cruciferous vegetables like broccoli, cauliflower, Brussels sprouts, cabbage, bok choy, etc., contain sulfur chemicals that are proven to inhibit cancer in the bladder, breast, colon, liver, and stomach according to the National Cancer Institute. They do this by protecting cells from DNA damage, inactivating carcinogens, and inhibiting tumor vessel formation. To protect against cancer we need a healthy immune system and liver so food like cruciferous vegetables, which are great for the liver, will help ward off cancer and inflammation by boosting our liver function.

- **Garlic, Onions, and Leeks:** Garlic has incredible healing properties and is a potent antiviral and antibacterial agent. Garlic contains hydrogen sulfide that has been shown to help prevent prostate, breast, and colon cancer and is recognized by the National Cancer Institute as a powerful anti-cancer food.

- **Healthy fluids/Green tea:** Filtered water is a great way to flush the body of toxins and hydrate it at the same time. Green tea has incredible antioxidants that have been shown in numerous studies to prevent and reverse cancer, particularly prostate, blood, and lymph cancer and stimulate the production of T-cells that improve our immune function. Caffeine in moderation has shown to help prevent neurological issues and its antioxidants protect against cancer.

- **Mushrooms:** Shiitake, reishi, coridus, maitake, chaga, and cordyceps mushrooms are used worldwide to fight cancer and enhance and modulate the immune response. Extensive research has shown mushrooms to have anticancer, antiviral, anti-inflammatory, liver and kidney protective, and immune boosting properties. In addition, mushrooms have been used successfully to reduce the side effects of radiation and chemotherapy for cancer patients.
- **Spices and Herbs:** Turmeric, ginger, thyme, and rosemary are powerful cancer fighters and I recommend using them regularly in your cooking! Turmeric has been studied extensively for its anti-inflammatory benefits and is also being studied as a powerful cancer-fighter. It's been found to reduce tumors and even block cancer growth. Thyme and rosemary are powerful anti-carcinogens and it is a good idea to use them liberally on meat that will be BBQed to neutralize any adverse effects.[20]

> Incorporating anticancer foods and a
> positive lifestyle can help to combat
> one-third of all cancers.

In addition to a good diet with anticancer foods other proven causes of cancer include excessive amounts of meat on the BBQ or cooked at high temperatures, artificial sweeteners (aspartame, splenda, and sucralose), and excessive amounts of alcohol, tobacco, and obesity. To prevent cancer it may also be helpful to eat a minimum amount of refined and processed foods. Eating a fiber-rich diet with both soluble and insoluble fiber improves elimination of toxins and keeps us healthier.

Research shows, ensuring proper Vitamin D intake (20 minutes of sun exposure) has been shown to lower death rates for breast, colon, and prostate cancer, while boosting the immune system. Studies have shown that people with adequate levels of Vitamin D have a significantly lower risk of developing cancer, compared to those whose levels are low.[21] Vitamin D deficiency was found to be prevalent in cancer patients regardless of nutritional status in a study carried out by the Cancer Treatment Centers of America.

Finally, stress is also linked to lower immune function and increased rates of cancer so make efforts to reduce your stress load and get a proper sleep each night.

Cancer is a serious disease and some forms are linked to genetic or environmental factors outside of our control. Many scientists are working on promising drugs that will help fight this terrible disease and diet choices will help combat it as well.

HEALTHY YOU

Sugar Rehab

Look at the ingredients list of the packaged and processed foods in your local grocery store. How many corn by-products you can find? Make an effort to reduce consumption of the worst processed foods that contain high-fructose corn syrup (HFCS) like pop, candy, and ready-to-eat breakfast cereals. Switch from corn syrup and refined sugar for baking. Switch to sweeteners that contain nutrients and minerals like maple syrup, sucanat, rapadura, panela and molasses – the "whole grains" of sweeteners. They taste delicious in all recipes and can easily be substituted. Some people like non-sugar sweeteners like stevia or xylitol as well. For more rea sons to reduce sugar, check out *nancyappleton.com/141-reasons-sugar-ruins-your-health* and *www.wholesomesweeteners.com.*

"Herbs too, she knew, and well of each could speak,
That in her garden sipped the silvery dew …
The tuffed basil, pun-provoking thyme,
Fresh baum, and marygold of cheerful hue

…

And marjoram sweet, in shepherd's posie found;
And lavender, whose spikes of azure bloom
Shall be, ere-while, in arid bundles bound,
To lurk amidst the labours of her loom,
And crown her kerchief clean with mickle rare perfume."

William Shenstone
(1714-1763, English poet and landscape gardener)

Dandelion – Flower, Weed, or Vegetable?

My father remembers how Italian immigrants used to pick the dandelions from their front lawns and use them in salads. Non-Italians found this puzzling, but it turns out dandelions are a powerhouse of nutrients. Dandelions are a vegetable!?!

To your child, dandelions are a gift for Mommy; and to a homeowner they can be an irritating weed. To a smart gardener dandelions are a perennial crop and one of the most nutritious vegetables you can eat – or drink.

Grown as a crop in Belgium, Europeans love them in salads and dandelion tea is enjoyed by many. The entire plant along with its various parts, including the roots, leaves, flowers, and stems are edible and used to treat various health conditions. The root, however, is considered the most useful part of the plant.[22]

Dandelions can self-pollinate, which means they only need their own plant to reproduce, which is often why they are so hard to get out of our yards. But why are we trying to get rid of such a nutritious plant.

REAL "D" FOODS

Daikon Radish [*Vegetable*] Daikon radishes contain fiber and carbohydrates, along with Vitamin C and B-complex Vitamins, and small amounts of minerals potassium, manganese, copper, magnesium, and calcium. Daikon is the Japanese name of the white radish, also known as the Oriental radish or Chinese radish. Daikon is one of many cruciferous vegetables linked in studies with successful cancer prevention and contains great antioxidants associated with fighting free radical damage, a known cause of cancer. Research has also shown that daikon juice helps the liver process toxins. See also What Foods Fight or Help Prevent Cancer? under Food and You or Your Environment, under "C."

Dairy [*Classification*] Dairy is a classification of food that includes cheese, butter, yogurt, kefir, buttermilk, etc. This food group is high in protein, saturated fat, Vitamins A, D, and B-complex Vitamins (B12 (cobalamin), B6 (pyridoxine), B2 (riboflavin), B3 (niacin), B1 (thiamine), B5 (pantothenic acid), and B9 (folic acid)), and minerals calcium, magnesium, phosphorus, potassium, selenium, and zinc. Dairy products can also be a rich source of healthy probiotic bacteria that aids in digestion. Types of dairy include milk, yogurt, cheese, kefir, ice-cream, quark, and ricotta, mascarpone, and cottage cheeses.

Dandelion [*Vegetable*] Although many regard this plant a weed, it is a vegetable with a powerhouse of nutrients, including fiber, carbohydrates, Vitamins A, D, K and B-complex Vitamins (B1 (thiamine) and B2 (riboflavin)) along with minerals calcium, magnesium, potassium, iron, phosphorus, cooper and zinc. It is an amazing antioxidant with four times the beta-carotene of broccoli and the list of medicinal ails treated with dandelions is long, not to mention that it is considered a great liver tonic.

Dates [*Fruit*] Dates contain fiber, carbohydrates, are high in Vitamins C, E, and K, provide an excellent source of minerals calcium, iron, magnesium, phosphorus, and potassium, and a good source of trace elements zinc, cooper, and selenium. They are also high in iron and good for people with low iron or anemia. Dates are considered a source of natural aspirin.

Delicata Squash. See "Squash" for general information.

Demerara Sugar. See "Sugar." See also Sugar – A Diet No No under Food for Thought, under "S."

Dewberries [*Fruit*] These belong to the blackberry family, but are sweeter than blackberries. They are deep red in color when unripe, and dark purple when ripe. One striking feature is that the male and female plants grow separately. See "Berries" for nutrients and information.

Dill [*Herb*] Dill is a perennial plant and member of the flowering herb family that includes caraway, parsley, cumin, fennel, etc. Dill contains Vitamins A, C, and B-complex Vitamins (B3 (niacin), B6 (pyridoxine)), large amounts of minerals copper, potassium, phosphorus, and calcium, small amounts of magnesium, manganese, iron, and zinc, and antioxidants Vitamin B9 (folic acid) and beta-carotene. Dill is known for its antibacterial properties and is used to aid digestion, headaches, insomnia, hiccups, bad breathe and acid reflux! See "Herbs" for general information. See also Herbaceous Cooking under Healthy You, under "H."

Dragon Fruit [*Fruit*] Dragon fruit (also known as Sweet Pitayas) comes from the cactus family. Dragon fruit is high in polyunsaturated fats (omega-3 and omega-6 fatty acids) and contains fiber, carbohydrates, Vitamin C and some B-complex Vitamins (B1 (thiamine), B2 (riboflavin), and B3 (niacin)), along with minerals calcium, phosphorus, and iron, and the antioxidant lycopene, known to help prevent prostate cancer. The phyto-nutrient-dense fruit is grown in the tropical regions of Thailand, Vietnam, and South America.

Duck [*Meat*] Duck meat is an excellent source of protein, B-complex Vitamins (B2 (riboflavin), B3 (niacin), B1 (thiamine), B6 (pyridoxine), B5 (pantothenic acid), and B9 (folic acid)), and minerals phosphorus, iron, potassium, copper, zinc, and selenium. Duck contains more saturated fat than chicken or turkey.

Durian [*Fruit*] Widely revered as the "King of Fruits" in the southeast Asian countries, durian contains fiber, carbohydrates, Vitamin C, and B- complex Vitamins (B6 (pyridoxine), B1 (thiamine), B2 (riboflavin) and B9 (folic acid)) along with minerals copper, manganese, potassium, and magnesium. Durian seeds, which taste similar to jack fruit seeds or yam, can be eaten boiled or roasted.

FOOD FOR THOUGHT

Dandelions and Other "Weeds"

There are many wild plants that grow in your community that are a source of amazing nutritional and healing properties. Are weeds the next "power" food?

Although some wild plants are edible it is never a good idea to eat any food grown in the wild unless an educated expert assures you that it is safe. Some plants will keep you alive and are full of vitamins and minerals and some can make you ill (or in the case of some wild mushrooms might kill you).[23] If you are unsure about a plant it is better to play it safe and leave it alone. Avoid milky or discolored sap, spines, fine hairs or thorns, bulbs, seeds inside pods, and foliage that resembles dill, carrot, or parsley. There are many edible wild roots, berries, and fungi and you can learn more through

books or on a foraging outing with a trained and experienced forager (all the rage in many urban centers these days).

Below is a partial list of some of the common edibles you may
find in your own backyard or nearby forest.

- **Amaranth/Pigweed:** Native to the Americas but found on most
  continents, amaranth is an edible weed. You can eat all parts of the
  plant, but be on the lookout for spines that appear on some of
  the leaves. While not poisonous, amaranth leaves do contain oxalic
  acid (a substance that inhibits the absorption on some minerals)
  and may contain large amounts of nitrates if grown in nitrate-rich
  soil. It's recommended that you boil the leaves to remove the
  oxalic acid and nitrates and don't t drink the water after you boil
  the plant (see "Amaranth" for nutrients). Amaranth has high
  amounts of nutrients and is much easier to digest than wheat as
  it is gluten free. Many farmers consider it a huge problem weed
  and they pour volumes of herbicide on it in failed efforts to eliminate it, but some are harvesting it instead and making a profit!
- **Bulrush/Cattails:** Bulrush, also known as cattails or punks in
  North America, is usually found near the edges of freshwater.
  Cattails were a staple in the diet of many Native American tribes
  and many survival specialists view the cattail as one of the most
  important edible plants to know about. Most of a cattail is edible. The shoots provide essential nutrients such as beta-carotene,
  B3 (niacin), B1 (thiamine), potassium, phosphorus, and Vitamin
  C and tastes like a combination of cucumber and zucchini. The
  best part of the stem is near the bottom where the plant is
  mainly white. Either boil or eat the rootstock, or rhizomes, and
  stem raw. Boil the leaves like you would spinach. The corn dog-
  looking female flower spike can be broken off and eaten like
  corn on the cob in the early summer when the plant is first
  developing. See if you can recognize the corn-like taste.

- **Burdock:** Burdock is a medium to large plant with big leaves and purplish thistle-like flower heads. Burdock is a popular food in Japan. You can eat the leaves and the peeled stalks of the plant either raw or boiled. The leaves have a bitter taste, so boiling them twice before eating is recommended. The root of the plant can also be peeled, boiled, and eaten. The root contains Vitamins C, K, E, B6 (pyridoxine), and B9 (folic acid) in small amounts, along with fiber and minerals magnesium, phosphorus, manganese, and small amounts of calcium, iron, and copper. Burdock is a favorite blood purifier among Ayurvedic medicine doctors because it stimulates bile flow to help a weakened liver and purifies the blood to restore damaged cells and detoxify.
- **Chicory:** This plant is rich in Vitamins A, B, K, E, and C, and minerals calcium, copper, zinc, and phosphorus. You can eat the entire plant. It's a bushy plant with small blue, lavender, and white flowers – which you can pop in your mouth for a quick snack. The flowers and stems can be used in salads. The root can be eaten (after being boiled) or used as a coffee substitute. Pluck off the young leaves and eat them raw or boil them.
- **Clover:** Clover is a good source of calcium, chromium, magnesium, B3 (niacin), phosphorus, potassium, and Vitamins B1 (thiamine) and C. They are found just about everywhere there's an open grassy area. You can spot them by their distinctive small leaflets. You can eat them raw, but they taste better boiled.
- **Lamb's Quarters:** Lamb's quarters have amazing amounts of nutrients so next time you see one in your garden, pop it in your salad! Lamb's quarters have huge amounts of Vitamins A, C, and K and good amounts of B-complex Vitamins (B2 (riboflavin), B1 (thiamine), B6 (pyridoxine), B3 (niacin), B9 (folic acid)), and fiber. It also provides minerals calcium, magnesium, phosphorus, iron, potassium, copper, and manganese, and protein! They do have a lot of sodium though, so keep this in mind.

Even flowers are edible and a rich source of B-complex Vitamins (B9 (folic acid), B2 (riboflavin), B6 (pyridoxine), B3 (niacin)), and Vitamins E and C (and some contain Vitamin A), and minerals calcium, magnesium, and zinc. Most herb flowers are also edible, including chives, dill, marjoram, oregano, rosemary, and sage.

> **If they are pretty in your garden, imagine how pretty they could be on your plate – and good for you too!**

Here is a brief list of some other edible flowers.

- **Chive blossoms** (the purple flower of the chive herb) contain Vitamin C, iron, and sulfur, and have traditionally been used to help support healthy blood pressure levels.[24]
- **Lavender** contains Vitamin A, calcium and iron, and is said to benefit your central nervous system
- **Marigolds** have more lutein and zeaxanthin than collards, kale, or spinach.
- **Nasturtiums** contain cancer-fighting lycopene and lutein, a carotenoid that is important for vision health.
- **Rose petals** contain bioflavonoids and antioxidants, as well as Vitamins A, B3 (niacin), C, and E.
- **Violets** contain rutin, a phytochemical with antioxidant and anti-inflammatory properties that may help strengthen capillary walls.

Weeds are considered a nuisance and a threat to crops and are being sprayed heavily now. But maybe more will be cultivated in future for a high quality food source!

FOOD AND YOU OR YOUR ENVIRONMENT

Doritos, Doughnuts: Why Do We Crave Them?

I read recently that primitive man was programmed to eat as much as possible. During our development and evolution, food was in short and uncertain supply. In order to acquire energy as much as possible and conserve it as much as we could, man ate as much as possible when he found food because he did not know when he would eat again. Our ancestors had to "store up" whenever they had a chance in order to ensure survival.

In the recent century, Western countries have created a guaranteed food supply, but could our wiring still be so strong that we are tempted by the high-fat, high-sugar, and high-salt foods that are inevitably so bad for our health? Why are we pulled towards overeating? Could it be because all of our instincts tell us to eat when we see tempting (i.e., high fat or calorie) food even though we may not be "hungry?" Although our circumstances have changed, maybe our basic survival instincts have not. Some health experts say we have to actively fight against our instincts and rewire our brains to make healthy choices. So if you are struggling with your weight and junk food cravings, don't feel bad if it takes you a long time to create better habits. There are thousands of years of programming and habits pulling you in the wrong direction!

To make matters worse, food scientists know how to activate maximum pleasure in eating which makes it hard not to become addicted to those not-so healthy foods. Foods that melt in your mouth signal to your brain that you're not eating as much as you actually are, so you deceive yourself into thinking you are not consuming as many calories and you overeat. In his book *Salt, Sugar, Fat,*[25] author Michael Moss describes how hard it is to refrain from foods like chips and Cheetos with that melt-in-your-mouth, heavenly fat/salt delight and keep you reaching for more.

Overeating junk food also is triggered by stress. It is a quick and easy way to satisfy our brain's addictive call for comfort in fat and sugar when a situation seems out of control or our emotions are overwhelming us.

> Can you have just one handful of Doritos?
> There are ways to break the junk food habit.

And even our gut bacteria can influence our food choices and drive us to eat sugary or fatty foods. According to a study by the University of California, the bacteria within us outnumber our own cells about 100-fold and may be affecting our cravings and moods to get the foods they want and often drive us to obesity. When the "bad" bacteria in the gut outnumber the "good," they manipulate our decisions by releasing signaling molecules that connect to our immune system, endocrine system, and nervous system to influence us to select food that may not be good for us.[26]

But poor habits, like healthy ones, can be unlearned and the good news is that we can overcome our addiction to unhealthy junk food and feel much better for it.

The process takes commitment and it is important to celebrate the victories, like when you decide to take a walk around the block when you are stressed instead of reaching for Oreos or Doritos! As well, choose to be kind to yourself when you have a setback and binge on junk food; resolve to start over the next day instead of beating yourself up. It is always good to find a friend or coach who can help you kick the junk food habit and remember to start by buying whole fresh food so junk food isn't in your cupboard to tempt you![27]

Here are some ways to help kick the junk food habit.

- Drink more water during the day. Sometimes we confuse thirst with hunger. Our bodies are craving fluids which can cause fatigue, leading to the urge to binge on sugary foods.

- Keep healthy alternatives close by like a bowl of fruit or freshly cut vegetables like carrots, celery, peppers, etc.
- Reward yourself if you have gone a certain period without junk good by indulging in a download, new outfit, or movie out with a friend to keep yourself motivated to stay on course.
- Avoid eating in front of the TV or while driving. Practice mindfulness when eating so you eat less and pay attention to the quality and quantity of food you put in your mouth.
- Exercise more. If you're about to succumb to junk food, take a walk outside or jump on the treadmill or bike. Getting some exercise will keep your mind off unhealthy snacks and help curb your hunger.
- Take smaller portions of food and slow down when you eat.

HEALTHY YOU

Bitter but Sweet

Okay, I've talked a lot about dandelions and wild edibles being packed full of nutrients but what about other bitter greens?

There are a long list of bitter greens that you can start including in your diet on a regular basis. Some names you'll know – radicchio, watercress, beet greens, Belgian endive, mustard greens, collards, rapini, chard, kale, spinach, turnip greens – to name a few! All bitter greens are high in minerals calcium, magnesium, iron, and potassium, along with high amounts of Vitamins A, C, and K, and antioxidants. They even contain a good amount of protein that is great for vegetarian diets.

Bitter greens were included in diets of ancient civilizations because they contain phytonutrients that keep our livers working optimally, detoxify blood, balance hormones, help control blood sugar levels, and help metabolisms stay robust. Buy beet, dandelion, or other bitter greens in the grocery store and store 2-4 days wrapped in paper towel to absorb excess moisture. Add to salads and soups – or even smoothies with sweet fruit and juice, milk, or water in the morning to start your day!

"When a man's stomach is full
it makes no difference whether he is rich or poor."
Euripides
(480-406 BC, Greek playwright)

Where Did Endive Come From?

Do you remember eating endive when you were young? I certainly don't! Lettuce choices at the grocery store consisted of iceberg lettuce or iceberg lettuce!

I remember my mother serving the family the classic salad with iceberg lettuce, carrots, cucumbers, and tomatoes. Times have really changed over the decades and today salad can be purchased in plastic bags or cartons, although some prefer to buy lettuce loose. Some of the many types of greens to add to your salad include frisee, arugula (or rocket), endive (or Belgium chicory), radicchio, mizuna, escarole, beet and dandelion greens, cress, tatsoi, butterhead (or Boston) lettuce, romaine, oakleaf, looseleaf, etc.

This makes having a salad a lot more exciting than it used to be! Remember that the darker the lettuce, the more nutrient dense it is.

REAL "E" FOODS

Eel [*Fish*] Eel is very high in protein and omega-3 fatty acids, and also contains Vitamin A and B-complex Vitamins (B9 (folic acid) and B12 (cobalamin)), and minerals calcium, magnesium, phosphorus, potassium, and selenium. (For information on sustainable fish see "Fish" or visit *www.msc.org/cook-eat-enjoy/fish-to-eat*.)

Eggplant [*Vegetable*] Part of the nightshade family, this vegetable is high in fiber and carbohydrates, Vitamin K, and B-complex Vitamins (B9 (folic acid), B3 (niacin), and B6 (pyridoxine)), minerals manganese, potassium, magnesium, and cooper. It also contains antioxidants that help to lower cholesterol, but it may increase arthritic symptoms in some people as it is part of the nightshade family.

Eggs [*Classification*] Eggs contain saturated fat, omega-3 fatty acids, and are a complete and high protein source. They contain high doses of Vitamins A, D, E, and B-complex Vitamins (B2 (riboflavin), B12 (cobalamin), B9 (folic acid), B5 (pantothenic acid), B6 (pyridoxine), and B1 (thiamine)), and high amounts of minerals phosphorus, selenium, iron, calcium, zinc, copper, potassium, magnesium, manganese, and sodium. Organic, free-range, or farm-fresh options are an excellent source of choline and lutein, which helps keep skin healthy and elastic. While it's true that egg yolks have a lot of cholesterol, research shows that cholesterol in food has a much smaller effect on blood levels of total cholesterol and harmful LDL than does the mix of fats in the diet. Recent research has shown that moderate egg consumption does not increase heart disease risk in healthy individuals and can be part of a healthy diet. It is important to store eggs in the fridge and cook them until the whites and yolks are firm, to prevent food-borne illness.[28] I believe in eating the whole egg as the yolk contains most of the nutrients. See also The Egg under Food for Thought, below, and also Can Certain Foods Make Us More Intelligent? under Food and You or Your Environment, under "I" and also How Can We Hold onto Yesterday's Memories? under Food and You or Your Environment, under "Y."

Elderberry [*Fruit*] Elderberries contain fiber and carbohydrates, Vitamin A, significant amounts of Vitamin C, and some B-complex Vitamins. Elderberries are rich in flavonoids that have antioxidant qualities that protect cells against damage and infections by boosting your immune system. They also contain antiviral and anti-inflammatory properties. The elderberry shrub has been used in herbal medicine for thousands of years. It was recently discovered that the elderberry is very effective in treating the H1N1 flu and other respiratory viruses.[29] See also "Berries" for general information.

Elk [*Meat*] Elk does not contain any vitamins, but it is a good source of minerals, including potassium, phosphorus, magnesium, calcium, selenium, zinc, and trace amounts of copper and manganese. Most of the meat is pasture raised without hormones.

Emu [*Meat*] Emu is a high quality protein. Emu meat is higher in iron, protein and Vitamin C than beef and has the equivalent fat and cholesterol of poultry. Most emu is pasture raised without hormones.

Endive [*Vegetable*] Also known as Belgium chicory, contains fiber and carbohydrates, and Vitamins A, K, C, and B-complex Vitamins (B1 (thiamine), B2 (riboflavin), B9 (folic acid), B5 (pantothenic acid), and B3 (niacin)). It also has good amounts of protein, and minerals calcium, iron, magnesium, potassium, zinc, manganese, copper, and phosphorus. It is a green leafy vegetable used in salads with a hint of bitter flavor. Botanically this perennial herbaceous leafy plant belongs to the daisy family, and is closely related to chicory and radicchio.

Enoki [*Fungi*] Enoki mushrooms are high in B-complex Vitamins, especially B3 (niacin), but also have some B1 (thiamine), B5 (pantothenic acid), B2 (riboflavin), and B9 (folic acid). They contain smaller amounts of minerals potassium and phosphorus and very small amounts of iron, copper, zinc, and selenium. Enoki mushrooms have a distinctive look with ultra-small caps and a white color and are known as "snow puffs" in their native

Japan. See "Mushrooms" for general information. See also Marvelous Mushrooms – The Magic Food under Food for Thought, under "M" and also Are Rheumatoid Arthritis and Autoimmune Diseases on the Rise? under Food and You or Your Environment, under "R."

Escarole [*Vegetable*] This lettuce contains high amounts of Vitamins A, K, and C, beta-carotene, and good amounts of many essential B-complex Vitamins (B9 (folic acid), B5 (pantothenic acid), B6 (pyridoxine), B1 (thiamine), and B3 (niacin)). It also contains good amounts of minerals manganese, iron, copper, potassium, and zinc. See "Lettuce" for general nutrients.

European Blueberries. See "Huckleberries."

FOOD FOR THOUGHT

The Egg

Birds have been around longer than we know. History says that wild fowl were domesticated as early as 3200 B.C. Egyptian and Chinese records show that fowl were laying eggs for man in 1400 B.C. Europe has had domesticated hens since 600 B.C. It is believed that, on his second trip in 1493, Columbus' ships carried the first chickens to North America.

Nearly 200 breeds and varieties of chickens have been established worldwide, but only a few are economically important as egg producers. Most laying hens in the North America are Single-Comb White Leghorns[30] and can produce over 300 eggs per year.[31] The vast majority of poultry are raised using intensive farming or factory farming techniques.

> **Egg yolk is one of the few foods that
> contains Vitamin D and is the major source of
> the egg's vitamins and minerals.**

Here are some fun egg facts.

- The egg shell may have as many as 17,000 tiny pores over its surface. Through them, the egg can absorb flavors and odors. Storing them in their cartons helps keep them fresh.
- Eggs can be kept refrigerated in their carton for at least 4 to 5 weeks beyond the pack date.
- In cooking, eggs are "the cement that holds the castle of cuisine together," because of their ability to bind, leaven, thicken, emulsify, and clarify.
- A fresh egg will sink in water while an older egg will stand up. The secret: as the egg gets older the air space in the egg increases causing it to float.
- The stringy piece of material in the egg is not an embryo but rather a special protein called "chalazae" which acts as a shock absorber for the yolk so it doesn't break.
- Egg protein has the perfect mix of essential amino acids needed to build our own tissues. In addition, eggs have 13 essential vitamins and minerals. Eggs contain the highest quality food protein known, second only to mother's milk for human nutrition.
- The egg's yolk is one of the few foods that contains Vitamin D and is the major source of the egg's vitamins and minerals.
- The most expensive egg ever sold was the Faberge "Winter Egg" for $5.6 million in 1994.[32]

FOOD AND YOU OR YOUR ENVIRONMENT

Emissions, Climate Change, and Food

The Earth's average temperature has been rising since the late 1970s, with nine of the ten warmest years on record occurring recently. Some of us are happy to have warmer winters with less snow but others are worried. Climate change and agriculture are interrelated processes, both of which take place on a global scale. Global warming is projected to have major impacts on agriculture, including temperature, carbon dioxide, precipitation, and the interaction of these elements. These conditions determine the carrying capacity of the biosphere to produce enough food for the human and animal population.

There are three main types of Green House Gas (GHG) emissions produced by agriculture:

1. Carbon Dioxide (CO_2) is emitted from the burning of fossil fuels.
2. Nitrous Oxide (N_2O) is emitted when using synthetic nitrogen fertilizers, which are energy intensive and water polluting substances.
3. Methane (CH_4) is emitted from certain ruminant livestock, including cattle and sheep, as a result of the fermentation processes of their digestive systems. Methane is also emitted from decomposing manure on wet soils and flooded rice patties, etc.[33]

Rising CO_2 concentration in the atmosphere can have both positive and negative consequences. Carbon dioxide is critical to plant growth. Increased CO_2 will raise the rate of photosynthesis which could improve yields but will also speed up development. In the case of an annual crop, the duration between sowing and harvesting could shorten and this could have an adverse effect on productivity. Rachel Cernansky writes in *Grist.org* that warmer winters could ruin fruit production because fruit trees need winter temperatures to drop and remain there for a set period of time to allow the buds to go into dormancy and reset for fruit production in the spring.

> While we might enjoy the warmer temperatures of global warming, our food does not.

Weather changes and warmer weather can cause draught. Shortage in grain production crops such as sunflowers have been a result of severe drought conditions in Australia. India and the United States have suffered sharp harvest reductions because of record temperatures and drought over the past few decades. In 2003 Europe suffered very low rainfall throughout spring and summer, and a record level of heat damaged most crops from the United Kingdom, France, and Europe. Globally, 2012 was one of the hottest years on record and monocropping of thirsty crops and chemical-intensive farming can speed climate change.

Farmers are facing rising energy costs and uncertainty about future agriculture policies but are coming up with some exciting new strategies to reduce emissions in all three GHG areas.

- **Carbon Dioxide:** CO_2 emissions are being reduced. Farm vehicles using diesel are being used and run much more efficiently than those using gasoline; incentives are in place to build better insulation; natural light is being used and high efficiency heating and cooling equipment is reducing carbon footprints; farmers are reducing tillage (which means not turning the soil and exposing it to carbon loss); transportation costs are being reduced and local market distribution increased; renewable energy like wind and solar is being used; and the use of synthetic fertilizers, pesticides, herbicides is being minimized. Also there are new ways to sequester carbon (store it underground) which will help contain CO_2 emissions and are easy to implement like planting winter crops to increase annual carbon capture and having woodlots to maximize long-term carbon uptake are becoming more common.

- **Methane:** Farmers are starting to utilize new feeding strategies to reduce methane emissions with cows. That means more grass and less corn and soy which they have a hard time digesting. They are also using covered storage tanks for manure and keeping them at low temperatures, making sure manure is incorporated into soils on ideal days, and using anaerobic digesters to convert manure into energy.
- **Nitrous Oxide:** Recognizing the danger of nitrous oxide emissions, farmers are starting to use manure and composts in greater quantities instead of synthetic nitrogen fertilizers (which leach nitrogen into the atmosphere and waterways, which causes fish to die). Also they are practicing good old-fashioned crop rotation with "nitrogen fixing" legumes like peas and beans, which helps store nitrogen in the soil instead of planting the same crop on depleted soil year after year. A group of experts looked at a 3- or 4-year rotation that added oats and hay (alfalfa) to crop sequence and the result was stunning. This simple change decreased the need for synthetic fertilizer by a whopping 86% while maintaining yields, enriching the soil, breaking weed cycles, diminishing erosion, and protecting nearby waterways.[34]

A new study, published today in *Nature Climate Change*, suggests that "if current agriculture trends continue food production alone will reach, if not exceed, the global targets for total greenhouse gas (GHG) emissions in 2050." The study's authors say we should all think more carefully about the food we choose and its environmental impact. A shift to healthier diets across the world is just one of a number of actions that need to be taken to avoid serious climate change and ensure there is enough food for all. According to the co-author Professor Keith Richards, it is not a vegetarian argument; rather an argument to eat meat in more sensible amounts as part of healthy, balanced, plant-based diets." [35]

Whether climate change is something you care about or not, it is still worth looking into ways to support a reduction in emissions by eating less meat, buying more organic produce when you can, telecommuting if you can arrange it with your employer once or twice a week, reducing waste, and eating some locally grown foods when available. Small actions add up to make a big difference for everyone.

HEALTHY YOU

Desk Jobs = Smoking?!?

We all have good intentions but sometimes the long to-do list keeps us from exercising. Although we think we are being super productive working 10 hours straight at the office, humans are built to be more active. Overwhelming research today talks about sitting for prolonged periods as being the new "smoking" as extended periods of inactivity can contribute to metabolic diseases and are generally bad for our health. Regular exercise will boost our energy, endurance, and confidence so we can be more productive and successful, as well as healthy. There isn't a major health problem where exercise doesn't have a positive effect. A recent study estimates that nearly 80% of adult Americans do not get the recommended amount of exercise each week setting themselves up for years of health issues. As Bill Bowerman, founder of Nike said, "If you have a body, you are an athlete!" So get out and do exercise that you enjoy every day or week. And remember to get up from your office chair about every 20 minutes and move or do desk exercises. Try each week to spend time doing cardiovascular exercise, weight resistant exercises, and stretching for maximum benefit! Just do it!

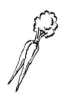

Old MacDonald

Last year I started receiving bi-weekly deliveries of vegetables from my local farmer through a CSA (Community Supported Agriculture) program and loved the taste and variety.

It felt good to get to know and help a local farmer who is making an effort to produce quality food. My farmer gave me many different new varieties. It was amazing to see purple carrots along with fabulous tasty potatoes. During the winter I stored my root vegetables in my garage as a make-shift root cellar and loved grabbing a dirty carrot and cleaning it for the most mouth-watering taste or making delicious mashed potatoes. I have received beautiful turnips, parsnips, rutabaga, onions, and garlic.

My farmer is just breaking even, so I encourage everyone to try a CSA to see if it is for them. Local, fresh, and reduced chemicals sound good to me!

REAL "F" FOODS

Fat. See What Your Body Needs and Why.

Fennel [*Herb* and *Vegetable*] Popular in Italian cuisine, this vegetable is a good source of fiber, carbohydrates, Vitamins E, K, and B-complex Vitamins (B3 (niacin), B9 (folic acid)) and minerals calcium, copper, iron, magnesium, manganese, phosphorous, potassium, selenium, and zinc. Fennel seeds are sweet, the flowers are edible in salads, the leaves are anise flavored, and the root or bulb is commonly used raw in salads and cooked as a root vegetable. The health benefits of fennel may include relief from anemia, indigestion, flatulence, constipation, colic, diarrhea, and respiratory disorders. Fennel is also used around the world in mouth fresheners, toothpastes, antacids, and in cooking, including desserts. See "Herbs" for general information. See also Herbaceous Cooking under Healthy You, under "H" and also Root Vegetables under Food for Thought, under "R."

Fiber. See What Your Body Needs and Why.

Fiddleheads [*Vegetable*] Fiddleheads are the young shoots of ferns and contain fiber, carbohydrates, very high amounts of Vitamins A, and C, small levels of some valuable B-complex Vitamins (B3 (niacin), B2 (riboflavin), and B1 (thiamine)), are a very good source of minerals potassium, iron, manganese, and copper. They are unique in their appearance and taste. They are an excellent source of many natural flavonoid compounds, such as quercetin and beta-carotenes, which convert to Vitamin A inside the body. Try pan frying them with onions and garlic.

Figs [*Fruit*] Fresh as well as dried figs contain good levels of fiber, carbohydrates, B-complex Vitamins (B3 (niacin), B6 (pyridoxine), B9 (folic acid) and B5 (pantothenic acid)), and some of Vitamins A, E, and K. Dried figs are excellent sources of minerals like calcium, copper, potassium, manganese, iron, selenium, and zinc, along with antioxidants such as carotenes, lutein, and tannins.

Fish [*Classification*] Fish is low in fat, high in protein and an excellent source of omega-3 fatty acids. Best sources of omega-3 oils come from oily fish like mackerel, sardines, and anchovies. Check for sustainable ones at local grocery stores or fish markets.

There are several main groups of fish:

- White Fish includes cod, haddock, plaice, sole, pollack, hake, monkfish, halibut, skate, sea bass, catfish, flounder, snapper, squid.
- Oily fish includes trout, mackerel, tuna, herring, sardines, swordfish, anchovies.
- Prawns and Crustaceans!–includes scampi, shrimp, crab, lobster, langoustines
- Shellfish includes shrimp, crab, crayfish, lobster, mussels, scallops, oysters, clams.

See also specific varieties for nutrients and information. See also "Shellfish."

Flax [*Seed*] Flax seeds are an incredibly nutritious food. They contain huge amounts of fiber (both soluble and insoluble), carbohydrates, omega-3 fatty acids (which reduce the risk of blood clotting), and B-complex Vitamins (B1 (thiamine), B6 (pyridoxine), B9 (folic acid), B3 (niacin), B5 (pantothenic acid), and B2 (riboflavin)). Flax seeds also have huge amounts of minerals manganese, magnesium, phosphorus, copper, iron, calcium, potassium, selenium, and zinc. These seeds are also high in lignans (up to 800 times the amount in any tested plant food). Lignans are phytoestrogen and have been called, by H. Adlercreutz (in his article "Phytoestrogens: Epidemiology and a Possible Role in Cancer Protection"),[36] natural cancer-protective and antioxidant compounds. Flax seed is also high in alpha linoleic acid (ALA) which has been found to be promising as a cancer-fighting agent too. Flax has been found to help reduce total cholesterol, LDL levels (the bad cholesterol), and triglycerides. Flax seed fiber is used to make linen and the oil extracted from the seed, linseed, is used to make paint. Flax is best ground for maximum health benefits and absorption. See also Happiness and Foods that Create Bliss under Food for Thought, under "H" and also Menopause – Can Food Help the Transition? under Food and You or Your Environment, under "M."

Flounder [*Fish*] Flounder is a good source of protein and omega-3 fatty acids. It contains good amounts of B-complex Vitamins (B3 (niacin), B12 (cobalamin), and B6 (pyridoxine)), and minerals selenium and phosphorus. (For information on sustainable fish see "Fish" or visit *www.msc.org/cook-eat-enjoy/fish-to-eat.*)

Flour [*Grain* or *Legume*] Many different grains can be used to make flour. In addition to wheat other grains like millet, spelt, kamut, quinoa, and teff are starting to be used more along with flours made from legumes and other plants. In North America, the most common form of flour is made with wheat. The wheat kernels or berries, which are ground to obtain wheat flour, consist of three distinct parts: bran, embryo, and the endosperm. Whole grain flour contains fiber, carbohydrates, vitamins, minerals, and small amounts of protein in varying amounts depending on the grain used. See also specific varieties for nutrients and information.

Flowers [*Vegetable*] Flowers, like many plant foods, often contain valuable nutrients for your health. They're also a rich source of fiber, carbohydrates and Vitamins, including B-complex Vitamins (B9 (folic acid), B2 (riboflavin), B6 (pyridoxine), and B3 (niacin)), E and C. Some flowers also some contain Vitamin A and minerals calcium, magnesium, and zinc. Certain flowers are not edible but most herbs have edible flowers and complete lists can be found online. See also Dandelions and Other "Weeds" under Food and You or Your Environment, under "D."

Frisee [*Vegetable*] Frisee is part of the chicory family. It contains high amounts of Vitamins A, B9 (folic acid), C, and K, and minerals manganese, potassium, calcium, iron, and magnesium. It is a delicate lettuce and should be torn by hand instead of cutting. Too much exposure to oxygen, as well as vinegar, can cause the leaves to wilt so add dressing just before serving. See also "Lettuce" for general nutrients.

Fruit [*Classification*] Fruits are nature's dessert and packed with vitamins, minerals, and anti-oxidants. They are full of fiber, many vitamins, particularly Vitamin C, and low in calories and fat, and a source of simple sugars. Generally fruit is easy to digest. Eating fruit helps to ward off illness as Vitamin C boosts our immunity and protects us against free radical damage in the body. Types of fruit range from berries, citrus, fleshy fruit, and melons to dried fruit, etc. Fruit doesn't take long to digest as it contains simple sugars that do not stay in the stomach for a long time. Other foods, such as foods rich in fat, protein, and starch, need to stay in the stomach for a longer period of time because they require more digestion. So it is best to eat fruit alone or limit combining it with protein-rich foods. Although tomatoes and some other foods are thought of as vegetables when it comes to cooking and eating them, they are in fact a fruit. What makes food a fruit and not a vegetable is the fact that they contain the seeds of the plant they grow on, whereas vegetables do not contain seeds. Fruits are produced after a plant flowers and the flowers have been pollinated. The pollinated flowers produce fruit that contain the seeds of the plant.

Fungi. See "Mushrooms." See also What Foods Fight or Help Prevent Cancer? under Food and You or Your Environment, under "C" and also Marvelous Mushrooms – The Magic Food under Food for Thought, under "M."

FOOD FOR THOUGHT

Food Pyramids and Food Movements

Protein Versus Carbs Versus Healthy Fats
Remember the picture of the triangle that was created to give people guidelines on healthy eating? In her book, *Food Politics,*[37] Marion Nestle writes about how the food industry influences nutrition

and health with their powerful lobbies and how developing the
Food Guide Pyramid was almost impossible as many powerful lobbies had to be satisfied along the way. No one was allowed to say
eat less, which is the obvious way to lose weight and stay healthy.

Scientists and nutritionists are now learning that the nutritional
advice given years ago may need to be updated. Food used to be
food. Now you can buy an item with the so many logos and claims
that you can get dizzy. The typical claims to fame include: low-fat,
sugar-free, organic, free-range, omega-3, heart healthy, whole grain,
sustainably harvested, fair trade, hormone and antibiotic free, etc.,
and it can get downright confusing at times.

Fat is one of the most confusing things of all. We need fat in our
diet but how much and what kind? Remember when people used
lard and tallow to cook? Fat used to be a healthy part of our diet
and then it became the evil villain as highly processed vegetable oils
started to flood the market. Which are better saturated or polyunsaturated fats? There are *experts* who loudly disagree on how much
we need.of each kind. Remember our brains our 60% fat so fat is
not the arch enemy we used to consider it to be! In addition, we
hear a lot about "healthy" fats and omega- 3s are added to eggs and
are not sure what this means or why it is healthy for us.

And what about grains? Some people promote "heart healthy"
grains and others say to reduce or eliminate grain consumption
with the growing Paleo diet and gluten-free trends! We all agree
though that consumption of refined grains is causing more people
to have digestive and health issues. Food scientists now know that
many common refined grains, like white processed wheat, are high
in sugar and can cause blood sugar fluctuations and insulin imbalances when eaten alone. There are record numbers of people in
Western countries suffering from obesity, while devastating numbers
of people in developing countries are dying from hunger. Poor
nutrition is the cause for both global epidemics. Additionally

processed grains are believed to be a contributing factor to poor nutrition in Western countries because they offer few nutrients and processing them puts stress on the body.

Protein can also be confusing. We eat so much in the Western diet (usually poor quality) but trends like the Atkins diet say it helps us to lose weight. The Paleo diet is popular but high in protein and eliminates all grains. Eating too much protein causes minerals to leach from our bones, making it difficult to maintain a proper body pH level and can contribute to systemic inflammation. Yet we are eating more meat and more high-protein bars than ever.

> So what is the food pyramid supposed to look like now? Do we eat more fat and protein and less carbs or more grain and less fat?

The Food Guide Pyramid has been replaced with a My Plate picture with half the plate showing fruit and vegetables and the other whole grains and healthy proteins that many consider an improvement over the pyramid and might be worth looking up for a reference.

However, certain nutritional recommendations do remain constant though, which is comforting. The evidence is overwhelming that it is important to enjoy a diverse diet of many colors and varieties of vegetables and fruits (preferably with a large portion of them in season). The color of vegetables reflects the different antioxidant phytochemicals they contain, like anthocyanins, polyphenols, flavonoids, carotenoids. Eating a diet that is rich in healthy fats (see War of the Spreadable Oils under Food for Thought, under "O" for more information on fats), complex carbohydrates from vegetables, and a variety of whole grains, along with smaller portions of high quality meat, legumes, or other protein, and lots of herbs and spices is certainly a recipe for good health!

Fast Versus Slow Food

We all know about fast food from years of indulging in the convenience of the drive-thru. Well now slow food is a growing international movement created by Italian Carlo Petrinin in 1986. The movement has since expanded globally to over 100,000 members in 150 countries. The Slow Food Movement strives to promote eating healthy, locally grown, and home-cooked, delicious-tasting food and enjoying the pleasure of food with family and friends. Research shows that eating a home-cooked meal with friends or family will improve your health and mood at the same time as strengthening family bonds.

Healthy and organic food is a growing segment of the market for those who can afford it or make it a priority because of their commitment to health and the environment. In his book, *The No-Nonsense Guild to World Food*,[38] Wayne Roberts describes how "Chefs are becoming celebrities and campaigners, restoring the artisanal dignity of working with honest food and the public obligation associated with the craft."

Big Business Versus Small-scale Farmers

We may or may not know about the few big agribusinesses that dominate and control food and seed supply in the world. Now a growing organization of small farmers are advocates for small, family-farm-based sustainable agriculture. Small scale farmers everywhere are seeking more ways to sell their products directly to consumers. La Via Compesina is an international movement, comprised of 148 organizations, that works to improve the rights of small-scale producers, agricultural workers, rural women, and indigenous communities all over the world. La Via Campesina advocates for small, family-farm-based sustainable agriculture with indigenous crops and was the group that first coined the term "food sovereignty." Food sovereignty refers to the right to produce food on one's own territory.

According to Barbara Kingsolver who wrote, *Animal, Vegetable, Miracle,* most people prefer farmers to be feeding those who live nearby, if international markets would allow them to do it. Food transport has become a bizarre and profitable economic equation that's no longer really about feeding anyone. In the U.S., for instance, they export 1.1 million tons of potatoes, while they import 1.4 million tons.[39] Developed nations promote domestic overproduction of commodity crops that are sold on the international market well below market price, undermining the fragile economies of developing countries. For food quality, paying more for local production but eating less could result in the same food bill and better health for you and many others

According to Vandana Shiva, Executive Director of the Research Foundation for Technology, Science and Ecology,[40] of the 80,000 edible plants used for food, only about 150 are being cultivated, and just 8 are traded globally today. In the developed world, more people are turning to planting heirloom seeds in their home gardens. There are an increasing number of sources for finding heirloom seeds, such as seed saving organizations like Seed Saver Exchange (SSE) (*www.seedsavers.org*). These organizations represent a movement of backyard gardeners who are searching the countryside for endangered vegetables, fruits, and grains. About 100 million gardeners and organic farmers keep heirloom seeds alive and consumers can be grateful as higher quality, more delicious varieties are showing up more frequently at farmers markets and grocery stores.[41]

Although food movements and trends seem to be controversial and going in different directions, it is encouraging to see how passionate people are getting about food and I applaud the dialogue that leads to improvements in quality and distribution everywhere.

FOOD AND YOU OR YOUR ENVIRONMENT

How Can I Support My Local Farmer?

Over the decades grocery stores have become the place to buy our food. But now with the greater awareness about our food systems there are many more options.

Farmers are the backbone of our healthy communities. They work long hours and sometimes face daunting challenges to bring fresh produce to our grocery stores, farmers markets, and tables. The best way to support your local farmers is to buy directly from them if possible. New programs allow you to buy fruit and vegetables from your local farmer at farmer's markets or through Community Supported Agriculture or CSA programs.

CSA farms operate like a publicly traded company. The farmer receives a set fee from you at the beginning of the growing season. In return, you receive part of the farm's produce (your dividend), but you also share in the risks that are endemic to farming, such as weather damage, pests, and other factors. Depending on the crops grown, the size of the shares, arrangements for receiving the shares, and the length of season, the share costs will vary from farm to farm. Most CSAs grow organic, or close to organic, food and provide a diversity of vegetables and herbs in season. Some farms also offer eggs and meat either as part of the share or to be purchased separately. In general, CSA farmers are dedicated to using the land in a manner that will not deplete its nutrients or value for generations to come. Healthy soil produces healthy food.

Healthy soil produces healthy food.

If we treat our farmers fairly and encourage them to grow high quality food with fewer chemical inputs, we all win. The cost of organic certification can be high so don't always insist on this if farmers are genuinely working to produce high quality, chemically reduced food for you as this is a positive step in the right direction. Governments are starting to give incentives to farmers to keep their land fertile and buyers are recognizing the challenges that come with food production and are supporting local farmers more than ever in their important work as doctors of our soil.

HEALTHY YOU

Feeling Fishy?

Eat fish at least once a week to support heart, brain, and overall health. Fish is full of omega-3 fatty acids, minerals, and high-quality protein that we need to build strong muscles and tissues. But just about all fish contains some mercury levels so aim for smaller wild-caught fish. Large fish, like tuna, swordfish, and shark, are the most contaminated so avoid or limit them in your diet. Buy wild-caught fish instead of farmed to get increased nutrients and avoid the hormones and antibiotics used frequently with farmed fish. Many companies now incorporate more sustainable practices so look for the Marine Stewardship Council (MSC) logo on the fish you buy or visit *www.msc.org/cook-eat-enjoy/fish-to-eat* or other sites to find the most sustainable types of fish to eat.

"God comes to the hungry in the form of food."

Mahatma Gandhi

(1869-1948,

preeminent leader of Indian nationalism)

Garlic – A Cure-All

I love eating garlic and use it in my cooking regularly.

Garlic is amazing! It has been used throughout recorded history for both medicinal and culinary purposes. It is known to cure a cold, get rid of acne, treat cold sores and athlete's foot, repel mosquitos, and get rid of pests in a garden without using harmful pesticides.

The only trouble with garlic is that it can leave you with the dreaded garlic breath. The benefits are too huge to ignore so I recommend the following to help neutralize the smell: parsley, fennel, lemon, or tea, especially green or peppermint. Tea contains polyphenols that reduce the sulfur compounds that garlic produces.

Garlic and onions are toxic to cats and dogs so be careful with your pets when eating it and store it away from them.[42]

REAL "G" FOODS

Ganoderma [*Fungi*] Ganoderma mushrooms are high in protein, Vitamin D, and are a good source of B-complex Vitamins, especially B3 (niacin), B2 (riboflavin), and B5 (pantothenic acid). They also have high amounts of minerals selenium and good amounts of iron, zinc, copper, and potassium. They are packed with antioxidants and are a proven immune system booster. Also known as reishi, ganoderma is a hard, bitter mushroom used to promote health and longevity in traditional Chinese medicine and generally not used for cooking. Proponents claim that ganoderma can relieve fatigue, keep cholesterol in check, curb high blood pressure, tame inflammation, build stamina, and support the immune system. See "Mushrooms" for general information. See also What Foods Fight or Help Prevent Cancer? under Food and You or Your Environment, under "C" and also Marvelous Mushrooms – The Magic Food under Food for Thought, under "M."

Garbanzo Beans [*Vegetable (Legume)*] Also referred to as chickpeas, this legume provides an excellent plant source of fiber, carbohydrates, and protein. Garbanzo beans also contain B-complex Vitamins (B9 (folic acid)), and minerals manganese, copper, phosphorus, and iron. See also "Legumes" for general information.

Garden Rocket. See "Arugula."

Garlic [*Vegetable* and *Spice*] Garlic is packed with vitamins and nutrients and contains some protein. Garlic is high in Vitamin C, B-complex Vitamins (B6 (pyridoxine), B1 (thiamine), B5 (pantothenic acid), and B2 (riboflavin)), and minerals manganese, copper, calcium, iron, phosphorus, selenium, and zinc. Garlic belongs to the onion family, which includes shallots, chives, and leek. Unlike the onion, garlic flowers are sterile and therefore do not produce seeds. New plants generally are grown from planting the individual sections of the bulb. Garlic contains compounds that help prevent nitrates in foods like bacon and cured meats to transform into dangerous compounds in the body. It is a power food for its antimicrobial, anticancer, antidiabetic, and immune-boosting and cholesterol-lowering properties. Studies show that *allicin* reduces cholesterol production. See "Spices" for general information and cooking suggestions. See also What Foods Fight or Help Prevent Cancer? under Food and You or Your Environment, under "C" and also Garlic – A

Bulb a Day under Healthy You, below. See also Root Vegetables under Food for Thought, under "R."

German Turnip. See "Kohlrabi."

Ghee [*Dairy*] Ghee is clarified butter, or butter fat. It is high is saturated fat and contains some Vitamins A and E. It is rich in antioxidants that aid in the absorption of fat-soluble vitamins and minerals. Ghee is said to stimulate the secretion of stomach acids that aid with digestion. It has been used in Indian medicine for the treatment of ulcers and constipation and the promotion of healthy skin and eyes. Chef's use clarified butter because it won't burn during frying (called a high smoking point) and has a rich flavor.

Ginger [*Spice*] Sometimes thought of as a herb, ginger is a spice because it is the rhizomes or ginger root that are used. Ginger contains Vitamin C and B-complex Vitamins (B6 (pyridoxine)), along with a small amount of minerals magnesium, manganese, potassium, and iron. Ginger has been in use since ancient times for its anti-inflammatory, anti-nausea, antiflatulent, and antimicrobial properties. Used in many countries, some say it can help cure diabetes, headaches, colds, fatigue, indigestion, bloating, nausea, and the flu when used in tea or food. See "Spices" for general information and cooking suggestions. See also What Foods Fight or Help Prevent Cancer? under Food and You or Your Environment, under "C," What's to be Done about the Rise in Heart Disease? under Food and You or Your Environment, under "H" and also Root Vegetables under Food for Thought, under "R" and also Are Rheumatoid Arthritis and Autoimmune Diseases on the Rise? under Food and You or Your Environment, under "R."

Ginseng [*Herb*] Ginseng is any one of 11 species of slow-growing perennial plants with fleshy roots. It is characterized by the presence of ginsenosides. Ginseng is one of the most popular herbal medicines in the world and is believed to increase energy, clarity of thought, vitality, and boost the immune system. This herb is classified as an adaptogen, a term that refers to substances that increase the body's resistance against fatigue, stress, trauma and anxiety. Ginseng is a powerful herb and pregnant and nursing women, kids, and people with high blood pressure and cardio-vascular diseases should avoid taking it. See also Root Vegetables under Food for Thought, under "R."

Goat [*Dairy*] Goat's milk and cheese are high in protein, omega-3 and -6 fatty acids and contains good amounts of Vitamins D, A, B2 (riboflavin), and minerals calcium, phosphorus, magnesium, and copper. A person who is lactose intolerant is deficient in levels of the enzyme that helps you digest the protein casein in milk. These people are often able to digest goat's milk and dairy products much more easily.

Goat [*Meat*] Goat meat is high in protein, B-complex Vitamins (B3 (niacin), B12 (cobalamin), B2 (riboflavin)), and minerals iron, phosphorus, copper, selenium, and zinc. Goats are browsers not grazers according to *treehugger.com* so they have a smaller impact on the land and farmers can produce more goat meat from same size pasture as they would beef. Nutritionally, goat is high in protein and very lean. It is lower in fat and cholesterol than chicken, beef, pork, or lamb.[43]

Goji Berries [*Fruit*] Goji berries are the most nutritionally dense fruit on Earth. They contain fiber, carbohydrates, and are very high in Vitamins C, A, and E, and beta-carotene. In fact, the goji berry contains approximately 500 times more Vitamin C per weight than an orange and considerably more beta-carotene than carrots. They contain minerals iron and calcium and are an excellent source of antioxidants. Goji berries are a member of the nightshade family, which contains many other common veg-etables such as potato, sweet potato, tomato, eggplant, and pep-per. Native to the Himalayan Mountains of Tibet and Mongolia, they are great to add to salads. See also "Berries" for general information. See also What Foods Fight or Help Prevent Cancer? under Food and You or Your Environment, under "C."

Goose [*Meat*] Goose meat is high in protein and fatty acids. It contains the B-complex Vitamins B3 (niacin), B2 (riboflavin), B6 (pyridoxine), B12 (cobalamin), and B5 (pantothenic acid), along with minerals iron, selenium, potassium, phosphorus, zinc, copper, and sodium. It contains more fat than some other meats but is generally healthy and tasty to many.

Gooseberries [*Fruit*] Gooseberries contain fiber, carbohydrates, Vitamins C and A, along with minerals manganese and potassium. These skin of these small round berries appears striped. These are green in color during the growing stage and ripen to become deep purple or yellow in color. See also "Berries" for general information.

Gourd [*Vegetable Classification*] This category includes vegetables like squash, pumpkin, and zucchini. See specific foods for nutrients and information.

Grains [*Classification*] Whole grains are high in fiber, carbohydrates, B-complex Vitamins (B9 (folic acid), B3 (niacin), B1 (thiamine), and B2 (riboflavin)), and contain some protein in varying amounts. They often have minerals iron, magnesium, zinc, and selenium or they are added through processing techniques. In the traditional North American diet, wheat was the main grain in use, but today many other grains are sought out for their gluten-free feature. Most grain is used to make bread, which can be high in fiber, carbohydrates and other nutrients, depending on the ingredients and the way it is made. In many cultures bread is the symbol of food. Types of bread eaten today range from white, whole wheat, multi-grain, rye, pumpernickel, sourdough, flat bread, injero, bagels, baguettes, unleavened bread, naan, etc. Artisan bakeries are slowly making a comeback and you will find these hand-crafted loaves to be of a much superior quality and taste and well worth the investment. Grains used in cooking today include amaranth, barley, buckwheat, bulgur, cavena nuda, corn, kamut, millet, oats, quinoa, rice, rye, sorghum, spelt, teff, triticale, wheat, and wild rice. See specific grains for their particular dietary qualities.

Grapefruit [*Fruit*] Grapefruit contains carbohydrates and large amounts of fiber, Vitamins C and A, and small amounts of B-complex Vitamins (B1 (thiamine), B9 (folic acid), B5 (pantothenic acid)), along with minerals potassium and small amounts of manganese. Grapefruit Seed Extract (GSE) has very high amounts of antioxidants, including the chemical component hesperidin, a natural immune-system stimulator and booster. A study by microbiologists from the University of Georgia found that GSE was a very effective non-toxic disinfectant and that GSE demonstrated a "wide spectrum of activity," including antiviral, antimitotic, and antiprotozoal capacities against many bacteria and viruses, including E.coli.[44]

Grapes [*Fruit*] Grapes contain fiber and carbohydrates and are a rich source of minerals like copper, iron, and manganese. (Iron becomes more concentrated in raisins.) Grapes also contain Vitamins C, A, K, B-complex Vitamins (B6 (pyridoxine), B2 (riboflavin), and B1 (thiamine)) and carotenes. They are a rich source of the antioxidant resveratrol (in the skin of the grape), which has been found to play a protective role against cancers, heart disease, Alzheimer's disease, and viral/fungal infections. Bioflavia™ is a new product made from organic red grapes that is a super nutrient-dense powder that has a host of antioxidant benefits. See also What's to be Done about the Rise in Heart Disease? under Food and You or Your Environment, under "H."

Grass [*Vegetable Classification*] This category includes vegetables like wheatgrass and bamboo. See specific foods for nutrients and information.

Green Melon [*Fruit*] See "Honeydew Melon."

Greens [*Vegetables*] Greens is a term given to a group of vegetables that are high in fiber, carbohydrates and many vitamins and minerals, including Vitamins B6 (pyridoxine) and B9 (folic acid), and minerals iron and magnesium. Greens include kale, Swiss chard, dandelion greens, beet greens, turnip greens, spinach, chicory, barley grass, wheat grass, lettuces like arugula, frisee, mache, radicchio, oak leaf, sorrel, escarole, endive, etc. Greens also have the antioxidant beta-carotene and are considered a power food by many health experts. See also What's to be Done about the Rise in Heart Disease? under Food and You or Your Environment, under "H."

Green Tea. See "Tea." See also What Foods Fight or Help Prevent Cancer? under Food and You or Your Environment, under "C."

Grouper [*Fish*] Grouper is a good source of protein and omega-3 fatty acids. It contains good amounts of B-complex Vitamins (B3 (niacin), B12 (cobalamin) and B6 (pyridoxine)), and minerals phosphorus, selenium, zinc, potassium, magnesium, iron, calcium, and copper. (For information on sustainable fish see "Fish" or visit *www.msc.org/cook-eat-enjoy/fish-to-eat*.)

Guava [*Fruit*] Guava contains fiber, carbohydrates, is high in Vitamins C and A, and contains some Vitamin E and B-complex Vitamins (B9 (folic acid), B6 (pyridoxine), B5 (pantothenic acid) and B3 (niacin)). It contains minerals potassium, manganese, and magnesium in small amounts and antioxidants lycopene and beta-carotene.

Guinea Fowl [*Meat*] Guinea fowl contains protein, fatty acids, and B-complex Vitamins (B3 (niacin), B6 (pyridoxine), B12 (cobalamin), B2 (riboflavin), B1 (thiamine), and B5 (pantothenic acid)). It also contains minerals phosphorus, iron, zinc, selenium, magnesium, and potassium.

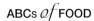

FOOD FOR THOUGHT

GMOs – Genetically Modified Organisms – Good or Bad?

Did you know that over 70% of packaged goods contain genetically modified crops? The two biggest crops today are "Bt corn" and "Roundup-Soy," which are found in countless processed foods.

Why do we have GMOs? And are they good for us?

Increasingly there is a large divide about GMOs. Some scientists view GMOs as unstable and potentially unsafe to eat, while others think they are perfectly safe. Russia has banned the import of GMO corn and countries like Peru and New Zealand are declaring their aim to be "GMO free." When given a choice between conventional corn and Bt corn, animals will not touch the GMO corn at all. Similarly wild animals will not eat soy or corn from fields planted with GMO crops.[45]

Recently, Target, Chipotle, Kroger, even General Mills and Cheerios have responded to a growing demand to eliminate and reduce GMOs in the marketplace. The potential of genetically engineered foods to cause allergic reactions is a big reason for opposition to these crops. It is also one of the concerns that led 64 countries around the world to label these foods for their citizens while 27 countries banned them entirely. The makers of GMOs claim that their crops are unique and want to patent them but they also tell us that they are the same as other crops or "substantially equivalent" so don't need a lot of testing to ensure their safety which can be confusing to consumers.

> Too much of anything can never be good for our systems. Diet variety may be a key to avoiding food sensitivities.

Joanna Blythman, a leading British investigative journalist and author of six landmark books on food issues, has provided compelling reasons why, in her opinion, GMOs just don't make any sense in our world today. Her key point is that GMO crops don't appear to have higher yields over time. Instead, the pattern is initially good harvests that decline dramatically thereafter. Even the U.S. Department of Agriculture admits that, "GMO crops do not increase yield potential." GMOs' undesirable qualities have been grouped under six categories: increased pollution, soil degradation, wildlife habitat destruction, waste of fresh water resources, loss of biodiversity, and threats posed by introducing new unstable species.[46] In 2007-08 alone, herbicide use on GMO crops in the U.S. rose by 31.4%. Sales of glyphosate, the world's biggest selling herbicide, continue to climb higher each year and the ingredient list is still highly confidential. GMO crops are linked to the emergence of devastating super-weeds. Over-use of glyphosate (Roundup), the herbicide used on GMO crops, is linked to the rapid spread of resistant weeds, such as pigweed and rye grass.

Some people fear that GMOs promote the loss of genetic seed diversity, which is a serious issue when we rely on too few crops. The Irish potato famine, which led to the death or displacement of 2.5 million people in the 1840s, is an example of what can happen when farmers rely on only a few plant species as crop cornerstones. If the Irish had planted even different varieties of potatoes, one type would have most likely resisted the blight and that would have saved countless lives.[47]

The good news is that today many scientists are using breeding techniques and less invasive genetic modification in other areas to offer improved traits that can boost food production in many harsh climates. And they are having success. Over time, other technologies to enhance nutrients or naturally lower the need for chemicals will be introduced with a positive effect on our food supply and quality of food which could greatly assist farmers.

The debate over GMOs will continue and consumers will continue to demand proper labeling. I support any technology that helps to create better quality food for populations in need without destroying the environment. The war on insects with toxic pesticides doesn't seem to be effective and changes to climate will lead to the need to plant more draught- and flood-resistant crops which already exist today without having to be rebuilt. For many people, more important than the GMO debate is making the choice to eat a varied diet and supporting biodiversity in our environment and on our plates to support a growing population.

FOOD AND YOU OR YOUR ENVIRONMENT

What Does Glycemic Index (GI) Mean?

The Glycemic Index (GI) is a ranking of carbohydrates according to the extent to which they raise blood sugar levels after eating. It uses a scale from 0 to 100, where the lower number is preferred. Foods with a high GI are those that are rapidly digested and absorbed and result in marked fluctuations in blood sugar levels. Low GI foods, because of their slow digestion and absorption, produce gradual rises in blood sugar and insulin levels, and have proven benefits for health.

Low GI diets have been shown to improve both glucose and lipid levels in people with diabetes (Type 1 and Type 2). They have benefits for weight control because they help control appetite and delay hunger. Low GI diets also reduce insulin levels and insulin resistance. Recent studies from the Harvard School of Public Health indicate that the risks of diseases, such as Type 2 diabetes and coronary heart disease, are strongly related to the GI of one's overall diet. In 1999, the World Health Organization (WHO) and Food and Agriculture Organization (FAO) recommended that people in industrialized countries base their diets on low-GI foods in order to prevent the most common diseases of affluence, such as coronary heart disease, diabetes, and obesity.

> Slow and steady wins the race and a
> low GI diet will do that for your health.

The hormones in our body that work with our digestive systems keep things operating within safe, healthy parameters like a thermostat in your house. The four main hormones that keep us healthy are insulin, glucagon, cortisol, and leptin.[48] The food we eat can affect these heating and cooling systems by stressing our hormones and causing imbalances. When we eat, our blood sugar rises and insulin is released from the pancreas to help move macronutrients (protein, fat, and carbohydrate) from the bloodstream into the cells for immediate or future use. Insulin removes sugar from the blood by creating body fat, thus earning it the nickname "the fat-storing hormone."

When we constantly eat foods that are sugary, high in carbohydrates, or have a high GI, we can develop chronically high blood sugar (hyperglycemia) that can lead to insulin resistance. Being under chronic stress releases the hormone cortisol and can also cause insulin resistance. Insulin resistance can lead to diabetes which is a disorder of metabolism – the way the body uses digested food for energy.

Diabetes develops when the body doesn't make enough insulin or is not able to use insulin effectively, or both. In diabetes, the body's cells are starved of energy despite high blood glucose levels. The two main types of diabetes are Type 1 and Type 2 diabetes. Diabetes can be caused by hereditary or genetic factors (mostly Type 1) or due to poor diet and lifestyle (Type 2). This disease currently affects more than 300 million people worldwide. One doctor's team at a Greenwich University has found plants that may help diabetics. Researchers here aim to isolate and identify certain extracts from the plants *Cassia auriculata* and *Cassia alata*, which could have "active ingredients" for treating diabetes. They discovered that one of the compounds isolated from the plant, kaempferol 3-O-rutinoside, has proved to be more than eight times more potent than the standard antidiabetic drug, acarbose, which is promising news.[49]

For those of us who can, we can work to avoid any metabolic disorders by eating foods with low GIs and by combining carbs with protein to slow down the release of insulin. Low GI foods include: fish, meat, low-sugar dairy, nuts, seeds, most vegetables (except carrots, parsnips, pumpkin, and potatoes), most fruit (except pineapples, dates, raisins, and watermelons), oats, porridge, pumpernickel, sourdough rye, sourdough wheat, buckwheat, brown, wild and basmati rice, and most whole legumes. Adding certain herbs and spices, particularly cinnamon to cereal or porridge, will also help to regulate our blood sugar.

HEALTHY YOU

Garlic – A Bulb a Day

Eat liberal amounts of garlic and onions for a potent liver detoxification. Garlic, onions, and leeks all contain sulfur-bearing amino acids that help the liver detoxify.

One of garlic's most important health benefits includes the ability to enhance the body's immune cell activity. The active component in garlic is the sulfur compound called allicin. It is a powerful antibiotic and a potent agent that helps inhibit the growth and reproduction of germs. Other benefits of garlic? It helps regulate the body's blood pressure, strengthen your body's defenses against allergies, loosen plaque from the artery walls, regulate your blood sugar levels, and is the best choice for killing and expelling some parasites from the human body. If you don't use garlic much in cooking, reconsider; if you just don't like it, consider garlic supplements, especially during the winter cold season.

"My son, eat thou honey, for it is good."
King Solomon – Proverbs: 24:13

The Hamburger Challenge

When I was young I spent many hours training as a competitive gymnast and although I stood not quite 5'2" I could eat anyone under the table.

One day someone from my class decided to put me forth to challenge a big guy in a hamburger eating contest. He was very confident he would win but, sure enough, I out ate him to everyone's shock!

While hamburgers contain high amounts of protein and carbohydrates, they also contain a lot of saturated fat. Back in the day of my burger-eating contest that was especially true and the buns were always made of white, processed flour. Today we can make better choices, including the composition of the burger itself. You can find lean beef, but also turkey, buffalo, chicken and even veggie burgers in many fast-food joints. And load up on the healthy toppings like lettuce, tomato, and onions.

I still love a hamburger now and again but often place a lean grass-fed burger patty between a delicious Portobello mushroom bun or a single slice of gluten-free bread instead.

REAL "H" FOODS

Habanero Pepper. See "Hot Peppers" for general information.

Hackberries [*Fruit*] This is a winter fruit that turns red or orange when ripe. Though it is edible, it is rarely used as food. However, it is quite a hit among wildlife and birds who love to munch on hackberries all through the winter. See "Berries" for nutrients and information.

Haddock [*Fish*] Haddock is a good source of protein and omega-3 fatty acids. It contains good amounts of B-complex Vitamins (B3 (niacin), B12 (cobalamin), and B6 (pyridoxine)), and minerals selenium and phosphorus. (For information on sustainable fish see "Fish" or visit *www.msc.org/cook-eat-enjoy/fish-to-eat.*)

Halibut [*Fish*] Halibut is a good source of protein and omega-3 fatty acids. It contains good amounts of B-complex Vitamins (B3 (niacin), B12 (cobalamin) and B6 (pyridoxine)), and minerals selenium and phosphorus. (For information on sustainable fish see "Fish" or visit *www.msc.org/cook-eat-enjoy/fish-to-eat.*)

Hazelnut [*Nut*] Hazelnuts are high in protein, fiber, and fat. They are a rich source of Vitamins E, K, C, and all B-complex Vitamins, and contain good amounts of minerals manganese, copper, iron, magnesium, phosphorus, zinc, and calcium. Hazelnuts contains phytochemicals, including flavonoids that may support brain health, improve circulation, and reduce symptoms associated with allergies. See "Nuts" for general information.

Hemp [*Vegetable*] Hemp is loaded with nutrients and provides a complete protein, and a balanced ratio of omega-3 and omega-6 essential fatty acids, which makes it an ideal choice for vegetarians or those who want to cut down on meat consumption. It also contains fiber and carbohydrates and many B-complex Vitamins, Vitamins A, D, and E, and minerals calcium, sodium, and iron. Hemp is a variety of the Cannabis sativa plant but is not the same as marijuana! You can also obtain many health benefits from it by adding the seeds to your diet or adding hemp powder to smoothies. See also Understanding Ancient Foods Today under Food for Thought, under "U."

Herbs [*Classification*] Herb refers to any green or leafy part of a plant used for seasoning and flavoring in a recipe, but is not used as the main ingredient. Herbs, like spices, are packed with nutrients and can easily be incorporated into cooking and meals. Many culinary herbs are perennials, like thyme or lavender, while others are biennials, such as parsley, or annuals like basil. Some perennial herbs are shrubs (such as rosemary) or trees (such as bay laurel). Some plants yield both herbs and spices, such as dill weed and dill seed or coriander leaves and seeds. See also specific varieties for nutrients and information. What Foods Fight or Help Prevent Cancer? under Food and You or Your Environment, under "C" and also Herbaceous Cooking under Healthy You, below.

Herring [*Fish*] Herring is a good source of protein and omega–3 fatty acids. It contains good amounts of B-complex Vitamins (B3 (niacin), B12 (cobalamin) and B6 (pyridoxine)), and minerals selenium and phosphorus. (For information on sustainable fish see "Fish" or visit *www.msc.org/cook-eat-enjoy/fish-to-eat.*)

Honey [*Sweetener*] Raw honey is high in carbohydrates and rich in vitamins and minerals. B-complex Vitamins (B6 (pyridoxine), B1 (thiamine), B3 (niacin), B2 (riboflavin), and B5 (pantothenic acid)) are the common vitamins found in raw honey, although amounts vary depending on the floral source. Minerals, including calcium, copper, iron, magnesium, manganese, phosphorus, potassium, sodium, and zinc, are abundant in raw honey. Made by bees, honey contains flavonoids and antioxidants that help reduce the risk of some cancers and heart disease. Some honeys have a low Glycemic Index, so they don't jolt your blood sugar. For recipes 1 cup of honey equals 11/4 cups sugar. Most health benefits come from raw, unpasteurized honey and in a solid form, not the liquid. See "Sugar" for general information. See also Where Have the Bees Gone? under Food and You or Your

Environment, under "B" and also Sugar – A Diet No No under Food for Thought, under "S."

Honeydew Melon [*Fruit*] Honeydew has substantial amounts of fiber, Vitamins A, C, and B9 (folic acid). It is a great source of minerals potassium, copper, and zinc, and digestive enzymes. The honeydew melon may be sweet but it ranks low on the Glycemic Index (GI), which is good news if you are watching your blood sugar levels.

Honeysuckle [*Fruit*] It is rich in Vitamin C, minerals calcium, magnesium, potassium, and quercetin, an acid that fights free radicals. It has been used as a traditional Chinese medicine for ages. There are some poisonous honeysuckle varieties as well. Hence it is a safer bet to buy from stores than plucking from the plant directly.

Horned Melon [*Fruit*] Also known as kiwanos, this fruit contains fiber, carbohydrates, good amounts of Vitamins C, A, and E, along with minerals potassium, zinc, and small amounts of iron.

Horseradish [*Vegetable* and *Spice*] Horseradish is a perennial plant of the Brassica family (which also includes mustard, wasabi, broccoli, cabbage, radish, kale, etc.). Horseradish contains some fiber, has good amounts of Vitamin C, B-complex Vitamins (B6 (pyridoxine), B2 (riboflavin), B3 (niacin), B5 (pantothenic acid), and B9 (folic acid)), and some vital minerals in moderation like sodium, calcium, potassium, manganese, iron, copper, zinc, and magnesium. The root contains many phytochemical compounds that give horseradish its pungent smell. It has been found that these compounds have antioxidant as well as detoxification functions that stimulate salivary, gastric, and intestinal glands to secrete digestive enzymes, thereby facilitating digestion and increasing appetite. See "Spices" for general information and cooking suggestions. See What Foods Fight or Help Prevent Cancer? under Food and You or Your Environment, under "C."

Hot Peppers [*Vegetable*] Hot peppers, like jalapeno, cayenne, banana, serrano, and habanero, all contain high amounts of Vitamins A, C, and K, and some B-complex Vitamins (B6 (pyridoxine), B2 (riboflavin), B3 (niacin), B9 (folic acid), and B1 (thiamine)) and Vitamin E. They have small amounts of minerals iron, copper, manganese, magnesium, and phosphorus, and antioxidants beta-carotene, lutein, and zeaxanthin. They get their heat from a substance called "capsaicin." According to the *Journal of Cancer Research*, capsaicin has been shown to suppress the growth of prostate cancer cells and its antioxidant nature can combat cell destruction caused by free radicals. Hot peppers have also been shown to relieve headaches and pain, lower blood pressure and cholesterol levels, and even are believed to help regulate blood sugar. See also What's to be Done about the Rise in Heart Disease? under Food and You or Your Environment, below.

Hubbard Squash. See "Squash" for nutrients and information.

Huckleberries [*Fruit*] Huckleberries contain fiber, carbohydrates, are high in Vitamins A, C, E, B3 (niacin), and minerals iron, potassium, and calcium. One serving of wild huckleberries has more antioxidant power (fight against free radicals that could cause cancer) than any other fruit or vegetable, except loganberries. Huckleberries are also believed to aid in protection against cardiovascular diseases, improve the immune system, help fight off infection, and protect against peptic ulcers, hemorrhoids, and prenatal issues. The berries look and taste similar to blueberries and can be sweet or sour to the taste. They are used to make excellent jams, pies, syrups, and preservatives and the leaves from the huckleberry bush can be dried and used to make tea.[50] See also "Berries" for general information.

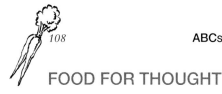

FOOD FOR THOUGHT

Happiness and Foods that Create Bliss

Did you ever notice that after you eat certain foods you may feel happy for a while, then experience a sort of low or depression? Foods you eat can powerfully influence the way you feel.

> **Can eating the right foods help you generate bliss?**

Eating sugary foods may make you happy for the moment, but after a while you feel fatigued and depressed. These foods quickly spike your blood sugar, giving you a short-lived energy rush. Then their quick digestion drastically lowers your blood sugar, resulting in lethargy. Some people call it "the sugar blues." Blood sugar levels can also impact our levels of happiness. Our brain likes a steady supply of glucose to function properly. If you ingest too many high-sugar foods (too much sugar) or skip meals (too little sugar), you will experience insulin fluctuations that can cause you to feel nervous, anxious, irritable, or tired.

For foods to make you happy, they must stimulate the neurotransmitters in your brain that control your mood. Serotonin is a neurotransmitter (brain chemical) that is involved in many vital body functions, but is very important in the regulation of mood (and sleep), resulting in a calm, happy, and relaxed feeling. Research has shown that low levels of this neurotransmitter can lead to increased symptoms of anxiety and depression. Tryptophan is an essential amino acid that is present, in different amounts, in all protein foods and is the building block for serotonin. Complex carbohydrates, such as oatmeal, whole-wheat pasta, and sweet potatoes, are digested slowly, which is better for your blood sugar, and they also stimulate serotonin in your brain. Without carbohydrates, your body cannot produce your happy hormone serotonin. New research from the University of Otago in New Zealand suggests that eating more fruits and vegetables (rich in carbohydrates) may make young people calmer, happier, and more energetic in their daily life! Now we know why!

Dopamine is another one of the brain's feel-good chemicals. In addition to simply making you feel good, dopamine helps control weight, energy levels, and supports brain and heart health. Since dopamine is synthesized from the amino acid tyrosine, you can simply consume foods rich in tyrosine to boost dopamine production or eat foods that help support dopamine production, including, fish, eggs, spirulina, red beets, bananas, strawberries and blueberries and herbs like oregano, ginkgo biloba, nettles, dandelion, and ginseng. Exercise also boosts both serotonin and dopamine levels because it causes the cells in your brain and the rest of your body to become energized or more active.[51]

In addition to foods that regulate blood sugar and the happy hormones, serotonin and dopamine, our bodies need magnesium, essential fatty acids, B-complex Vitamins, and Vitamin D to help us feel happy.

Magnesium is critical to over 300 biochemical reactions in the body from creating energy, contracting muscles, protein synthesis, regulating blood pressure to detoxification. Having enough magnesium in our diets will improve our energy levels, reduce stress, relax us, and fight fatigue, all of which will allow us to feel greater happiness. Currently, over 50% of the population is believed to be deficient in this vital mineral so by adding more greens to your diet, you will ensure you are working towards higher bliss in your life!

A major study from Harvard Medical School revealed that an omega-3 fatty acid, Eicosapentaenoic Acid (EPA), also had a very positive effect on mood. Omega-3 fatty acids help nerve cells communicate with each other and assist in serotonin production. Studies show that omega-3 supplements can reduce the risk of depression, bipolar disorder, aggression, adult ADHD (attention deficit hyper-activity disorder), and schizophrenia. A healthy brain is made of over 60% omega-3 fatty acids so we need to eat enough to keep it functioning well.

The B-complex Vitamins cannot be stored in our bodies so we need to rely on a healthy diet to supply them. They are critical for helping to convert glucose (blood sugar) into fuel, processing amino acids (the building blocks of all protein and hormones), and for manufacturing serotonin, melatonin, and dopamine (the happy hormones). Vegetables like Swiss chard, spinach, asparagus, potatoes, eggplant, and leafy greens contain high amounts of both magnesium and B-Vitamins, including Vitamin B9 (folic acid). B-complex Vitamins are depleted by alcohol, refined sugar, nicotine, and caffeine so think about your happiness when you avoid donuts and candy!

Vitamin D increases levels of serotonin and is a daily requirement. Sunlight is far more likely to provide you with your daily Vitamin D requirement than your food intake. It only takes about 10-15 minutes of sunlight for your body to take in the vitamin. You want to expose your face, hands, arms, or back at least two times a week without sunscreen to get the adequate amount of Vitamin D. After this time you can apply a sunscreen with sufficient SPF against the UVA and UVB rays, dangerous to your skin. Food sources of Vitamin D include pure cod oil, salmon, mackerel, sardines canned in oil, milk, egg yolks, beef liver, and Swiss cheese.

The way you eat can also affect your happiness levels. A recent study done at University of Toronto showed that people living in communities with a higher prevalence of fast-food restaurants were significantly less able to enjoy pleasurable activities that require us to slow down and appreciate. The study's authors propose that this occurs because fast food can incite people to feel more impatient, diminishing their ability to slow down and savor life's simpler joys.

The researchers also showed people pictures of fast food in its ready-to-go packaging which was enough to raise people's impatience and interfere with their subsequent enjoyment of photos of natural beauty or an operatic aria.[52]

Now that we know the basics of boosting joy, let's go through a list of some foods that we can eat more regularly to boost our bliss levels.

1. **Bananas:** Surprisingly bananas are high in tryptophan and also contain carbohydrates so they quickly increase serotonin levels. They are also high in sugar so be careful about eating them every day.

2. **Buckwheat:** Particularly rich in many B-complex Vitamins, buckwheat contains much more tryptophan than most other carbohydrates. Recent research has shown that certain B-complex Vitamins, particularly Vitamin B6 (B6 (pyridoxine)), are involved in proper serotonin synthesis in the brain. Carbohydrates create a small insulin spike when ingested that is necessary to clear other amino acids from the bloodstream, leaving tryptophan able to cross the blood-brain barrier where it is converted into serotonin. They assist with dopamine production as well.

3. **Dark Chocolate:** Cocoa is well known to increase serotonin levels in the brain but because it also contains sugar, you need to limit how much you eat. If you eat chocolate that contains 70% and higher cocoa content, you can have the benefits of chocolate without the downsides of insulin disruptions. Small amounts of cocoa in the diet have been shown to improve insulin sensitivity and it contains phenylethylamine, a substance that lifts your mood. When consuming cocoa, your body produces more endorphins and you experience a high, happy feeling. Women suffering from premenstrual syndrome often crave chocolate and can benefit

from consuming it, because it works as a mild antidepressant and mood lifter. Dark chocolate contains magnesium, which improves the blood flow to the brain, and caffeine, which provides an instant boost in concentration and mood and increases dopamine and serotonin transmissions within 30 minutes.[53]

4. **Flax seed/Flax seed Oil:** Flax seeds raise serotonin levels because they contain both tryptophan and high levels of omega-3 fatty acids. Sixty percent of the brain is made of structural fats, and omega-3 fatty acids make up a large proportion of brain nerve cells. Flax also contains alpha-linolenic acid (ALA) which supports happiness and reduces inflammation.

5. **Free-Range Turkey and Grass-Fed Beef:** These meats contain high levels of tryptophan, which helps make serotonin. It's important to buy good quality beef if you don't want to be ingesting a load of hormones and antibiotics.

6. **Sour Cherries:** Sour cherries contain melatonin, a hormone produced by the body when darkness hits our eyes. Melatonin helps us feel relaxed and calm and promotes sleep at night.[54]

7. **Whey Protein:** With a reputation as a super-food, whey has been shown to regulate appetite, improve insulin sensitivity and blood sugar levels, bolster the immune system, and the ideal protein source of tryptophan. Aside from these benefits, one interesting study found that whey might actually be one of the best protein foods to increase serotonin levels.[55]

Other foods that boost mood include avocado, pecans, pineapple, walnuts, oats, and coffee in moderation. Probiotic-rich foods also improve our happiness as they help maintain serotonin levels. Although serotonin is manufactured in the brain some 90% of our serotonin supply is found in the digestive tract and in blood platelets, making the expression "a gut feeling" a little clearer.[56] Of course, getting a good night's sleep and exercising are also great ways to boost mood. Some supplements like 5-HTP, SAMe, and herbs like valerian, lavender, and St. John's wort are used by many as well. (Check with a physician or health-care provider before using supplements, especially if you are taking any medications.)

Of course, we find happiness in family, friends, work and many other areas in our lives. Many articles talk about the importance of nurturing a feeling of gratitude, finding internal validation and purpose, practicing being more mindful and keeping our thoughts as positive as possible. But eating right can help to boost joy too, so give it a try!

FOOD AND YOU OR YOUR ENVIRONMENT

What's to be Done about the Rise in Heart Disease?

Did you know?[57]

- Over 600,000 people die of heart disease in the United States every year or about 1 in every 4 deaths.
- Coronary artery disease (CAD or atherosclerosis) is the most common type of heart disease, killing nearly 380,000 people annually.
- Every year about 720,000 Americans have a heart attack.
- Coronary heart disease costs the United States $108.9 billion each year.

Risk factors for heart disease include high blood pressure; high LDL cholesterol; obesity, diabetes, both due to a poor diet; excessive use of alcohol; and lack of physical activity. But how can we avoid getting heart disease in the first place? We need to remember the three important things for a healthy heart: cholesterol levels, circulation, and blood pressure.

High blood pressure, or hypertension, can be affected by your weight or other factors. If your heart has to work harder, then more pressure is placed on the walls of your arteries, which can increase your risk for blood vessel damage.

The two main kinds of cholesterol are low-density lipoprotein – LDL or the "bad" cholesterol – and high-density lipoprotein – HDL or the "good" cholesterol. When consumed in high levels, LDL cholesterol can build up in the bloodstream and calcify into hard plaque in the arteries. This plaque makes it difficult for blood to circulate through the affected arteries, increasing your risk for cardiovascular damage. Good circulation is needed to transport oxygen and nutrients to the many different cells in your body.

Although heart disease sounds scary, it is easy to avoid but cutting down on poor quality processed oils and saturated fat; eating a balanced diet with fresh fruit, vegetables, fiber; and reducing intake of salt and sugar dramatically. Exercise is also a vital key to keeping our arteries free from plaque along with diet.

> As scary as heart disease sounds,
> we can make choices to reduce the
> risk to us and our families.

Below are some great foods to include in your diet to make sure your heart is happy and healthy for many decades.

- **Avocados and Olives** are an excellent source of monounsaturated fat and can lower LDL levels while raising the amount of HDL in your body.
- **Barley** is nutritionally dense and packed with fiber. Barley's dietary fiber is rich in beta-glucan, which binds with excess cholesterol, helping to prevent its absorption. Foods rich in beta-glucan, such as barley and oatmeal, can help decrease LDL (bad) cholesterol as well as total cholesterol levels, reducing the risk of cardiovascular diseases.
- **Cayenne Pepper and other Hot Peppers,** contains capsaicin which is a compound that appears to expand blood vessels and keep them relaxed, which improves blood pressure. In addition,

cayenne pepper has been associated with increased metabolic rate and strengthening of arteries and blood vessels and has been shown to lower cholesterol and triglyceride levels. It also contains powerful phytonutrients that have anti-inflammatory effects on the blood vessels and blood cells, and anti-clotting properties.

- **Ginger** is known for increasing circulation.
- **Grapes** are packed with resveratrol, a powerful antioxidant, and flavonoids, another antioxidant that helps prevent coronary disease. Eating grapes reduces cardiovascular risk by lowering blood pressure, improving heart function, reducing inflammation throughout the body, and reducing signs of heart muscle damage. Raisins are also good for your heart as they are packed with potassium, which helps lower hypertension and increases immune-boosting antioxidants, and iron, which helps red blood cells bring oxygen to other parts of the body.
- **Oats** contain a soluble fiber called beta-glucan that helps reduce total cholesterol and LDL cholesterol. The best are steel cut oats for health and they are delicious.
- **Spinach and Leafy Greens** are packed with iron, which helps with red blood cell creation, and magnesium, which is very involved with the prevention of blood clots or platelet clumping and the regulation of heart rhythm. Magnesium also balances out excess calcium consumed to help prevent muscle spasms or tightening of the heart muscle and acts as a relaxant.
- **Sunflower Seeds** contain Vitamin E, which helps keep blood clots from forming and improves circulation. They are also a good source of protein, magnesium, and fiber.
- **Tomatoes and Watermelon** are packed with Vitamin C, a natural blood thinner that is believed to strengthen capillary walls, prevent plaque build-up (which leads to poor circulation) and reduce the risk of coronary artery disease. They also contain lycopene, an antioxidant that has been associated with reduced heart disease risk.[58]

- **Wild Salmon** is an excellent source of omega-3 fatty acids that protect your heart by reducing both inflammation and the risk of blood clots. These fats also work to keep your good cholesterol levels healthy. Salmon also has rich levels of selenium, an antioxidant that studies have shown boosts cardiovascular protection. The best fish to eat for heart health is salmon, krill, herring, and sardines. Some fish is contaminated with mercury and PCBs, particularly large fish like tuna, so keep your consumption to no more than two times a week and focus on smaller wild fish instead of farmed

Some vitamins and supplements can be very helpful for heart function. Coenzyme Q10 (CoQ10) has become one of the most popular and well-researched supplements in the U.S. and is essential to heart health and body energy production by every cell in your body. Those on a statin drug will have depleted amounts of CoQ10. In addition, drinking enough water is extremely important for circulation and cardiovascular health. Finally, avoiding trans fats at all costs is vital as they are linked to heart-related problems and increase the risk of obesity and stroke.

Research extending back as far as 1926, when Dr. Raymond Pearl published his book *Alcohol and Longevity*, has demonstrated that drinking in *moderation* is associated with a longer life-span than is either abstaining or abusing alcohol. One possible explanation is the effect of alcohol on cardiovascular disease. Moderate consumption increases your level of "good cholesterol" (HDL), clot-dissolving capacity, coronary blood flow, and insulin sensitivity while decreasing blood clotting, all and which is good for heart health. Red wine offers even greater cardiovascular protection, due to its content of polyphenols (resveratrol) contained in grape skins. Eating more grapes or other resveratrol-containing items will have the same effect on your cardiovascular system but it isn't quite as much fun.

Of course exercise is a great way to keep our arteries clear of plaque too. Even walking at a brisk pace for 3 or more hours a week lowers the risk of stroke by over 65%. So get moving and get eating well and hopefully your heart will stay healthy and happy!!

HEALTHY YOU

Herbaceous Cooking

Adding herbs to your food can be an easy way to add delicious flavor to your meals and boost your health at the same time. Below is a general guide for using herbs that might be helpful for even the best of cooks:

- **Beans** (dried): parsley, sage, savory, thyme
- **Beef:** basil, bay, cilantro, oregano, marjoram, parsley, rosemary, sage, savory, tarragon, thyme
- **Chicken:** basil, bay, dill, lemongrass, rosemary, sage, savory, tarragon, thyme
- **Eggs:** basil, chervil, chives, dill, marjoram, oregano, parsley, sage, tarragon, thyme
- **Fish:** basil, bay, chives, dill, oregano, parsley, rosemary, thyme, sage, savory, tarragon, marjoram
- **Lamb:** basil, bay, dill, marjoram, mint, oregano, parsley, rosemary, savory, tarragon, thyme
- **Pork:** caraway seeds, coriander, dill, rosemary, sage, fennel, savory and thyme
- **Potatoes:** basil, chives, dill, marjoram, oregano, parsley, rosemary, tarragon, thyme
- **Salads, Salad Dressings, and Soups:** anything including basil, chervil, chives, dill, marjoram, oregano, parsley, rosemary, sage, savory, tarragon, thyme
- **Vegetables:** you can try a wide range of herbs with various roasted vegetables, including sage, chives, oregano, thyme, rosemary, marjoram, parsley, caraway, and oregano

Other common herbs used to flavor cooking include bay leaves, marjoram (can be interchanged with oregano), tarragon, and fenugreek.

$\mathcal{I}$

*"Knowledge is knowing that a tomato is a fruit,
wisdom is not putting it in a fruit salad."*

Miles Kington

(1941-2008, British journalist, musician and broadcaster)

When in Rome … or Thailand

I remember traveling in Thailand many years ago and getting to know local tribes in Changmai in the north. One of the individuals I met took me to a local "food" market.

When we arrived, I couldn't believe my eyes. There was stall after stall of dead insects and to the people there they looked delicious!

Customers would request their favorite type of dried "meat" and the merchant would weigh them and bag them just like at a deli! I was completed grossed out at the time but have since come to respect that for many insects are a high-quality, sustainable protein source.

Insects play an important role in nutrition in many African and Asian cultures although for Westerners they sound less than delicious. But even in the West, it is impossible to eliminate pest insects from the human food chain. Insects are present in many foods, especially grains. Food laws in many countries do not prohibit insect parts in food, but, rather, they limit the quantity. Still, I am not ready to eat bug stew anytime soon.

REAL "I" FOODS

Iceberg Lettuce [*Vegetable*] Iceberg lettuce contains fiber and small amounts of Vitamins C, K, and B9 (folic acid), and small amounts of minerals potassium, magnesium, and calcium. It also has very small amounts of antioxidants beta-carotene, lutein, and zeaxanthin. See also "Lettuce" for general nutrients.

Ice Cream [*Dairy*] Ice cream is made from milk and is rich is calcium and protein but also high in sugar. See also "Milk."

Indian Plum [*Fruit*] This is an oval-shaped fruit contains fiber, carbohydrates, and B-complex Vitamins (B1 (thiamine), B3
(niacin), B2 (riboflavin)) along with minerals iron, calcium, and
phosphorus and the antioxidant beta-carotene. The fruit is
believed to remedy menstrual problems and the green fruits are
believed to act as a diuretic, laxative, and stomachic. Kernels of
the fruit have been used to treat abdominal pain and diarrhea,
and bark decoction to treat gingivitis. It turns the tongue purple
after eating and has a mixed taste of sweet-sour-astringent.

Insects [*Meat*] Insects are very high in protein and beneficial
omega-3 fatty acids. People in rice-eating regions ingest significant numbers of rice weevil larvae, suggested as an important
source of vitamins. Some of the more popular insects and arach-
nids eaten around the world include crickets, cicadas, grasshop-
pers, ants, beetle grubs, caterpillars, scorpions, and tarantulas.
Some experts suggest entomophagy – the practice of eating
insects – as a potential alternative protein source to animal livestock, citing possible benefits, including greater efficiency and
nutrition, lower resource use, increased food security, and environmental and economic sustainability.

FOOD FOR THOUGHT

Controversial Ingredients or Additives

Ingredients listed on packaged goods called "additives" perform a
variety of functions in foods such as preventing rancidity, chelating
agents to prevent discoloring, adding color, emulsifiers to keep water
and oil mixed, thickening agents, and flavor enhancers. In the U.S.,
the Food and Drug Administration (FDA) monitors the safety of
additives, while north of the border it's Health Canada. Most additives are purposely added and legal.[59] The FDA website is very

enthusiastic about all the additives, which improve safety and freshness, improve or maintain nutritional value, and improve taste, texture, and appearance.[60]

Many additives could be eliminated if we could grow our own
food, harvest and grind it, and spend many hours cooking and canning. That just isn't possible for most of us or even imaginable! Still,
why are there so many ingredients in a simple package of cookies?
Do we really need them all? Are all those hard-to-pronounce additives causing more harm than good? Why do some additives keep
being used when studies show they aren't healthy for us?

Although the FDA tries to keep a close watch over our food,
the job of strictly regulating thousands of food additives is simply
too big. Brominated vegetable oil (BVO), for instance, the subject
of a well-circulated petition in Alabama, was flagged for further
study in the '70s, but testing was never done. And butylated hydrox-
yanisole (BHA), a "probable carcinogen" according to the Department of Health and Human Services, is still allowed in some food.[61]
Similarly food colorings are thought to increase hyperactivity in
children. Red Dye was banned in the 1970s after the FDA found
large doses caused cancer in rats, but many other dyes are still being
used today. Aspartame has been linked to many health concerns
since it was introduced in 1981. It has been suspected of causing
cancer, seizures, headaches, mood disturbances, and reduced mental
performance, but is still used widely as a sugar replacement, especially in diet soft drinks.

> Remember if your food rots, then it is food and
> that is the best thing to eat for your health.

The most controversial additives today that are under scrutiny
for health issues include food colorings, aspartame, monosodium
glutamate (MSG), high fructose corn syrup (HFCS), sodium benzoate, sodium nitrite and trans fats. They are in many foods but we
can reduce our intake by sticking to a more whole food diet. Eating

food additives in moderation is not going to cause health issues so relax and don't worry if you reach for the odd donut or have to have that weekend bacon (nitrate-free bacon is now available). Other secondary additives that we are exposed to and ingest include growth hormones and antibiotics used in animal farming, pesticides and herbicides in plant-based foods, and compounds such as bisphenol A (BPA) or phthalates that enter food from packaging.

Although we have benefited enormously from the convenience of packaged goods and preservatives, it may be wise to reduce the amount we consume overall and choose whole foods to be the biggest part of our diets. Chemical preservatives in foods are designed to prevent bacteria growth and spoilage, but sometimes they can also prevent you from benefiting from the goodness of food too. Natural ingredients and additives have existed for centuries to preserve food, including salt, sugar, vinegar, and citrus juice, along with techniques like canning, pickling, drying, and lacto-fermentation (which can actually increase the available nutrients).

So remember that the goal is not to have food that can look fresh for months or years. Rather we need to buy food that actually rots because that is real, nutrient-dense food and the best kind for you because it can break down and be properly digested!

FOOD AND YOU OR YOUR ENVIRONMENT

Can Certain Foods Make Us More Intelligent?

Our brains weigh less than 2% of our total body weight, are made up of 60% fat, and play a key role as master of our bodies, health systems, and cognitive function.

From infancy to adulthood, foods that we consume can impact the level of our intelligence and our ability to think and act with clarity in our daily lives. Breast milk is nature's perfect food for babies and studies show that infants fed mostly breast milk for at least 3 months scored higher on IQ tests than did formula-fed babies. Breast feeding during infancy provides babies with other health benefits as well, including decreasing gastrointestinal tract and middle ear infections and reducing the risk of obesity and diabetes for both mothers and babies. The saturated fat in breast milk is a fundamental building block for brain cells.

As babies grow into children, a diet with reduced sugar intake will help boost intelligence as well. A study carried out by researchers from Bristol University and funded by the U.K. Medical Research Council found that eating a diet high in sugar, fats, and processed food at the age of 3 was associated with a lower IQ at 81/2 years of age. High sugar foods or high GI (Glycemic Index) foods disrupt the body's homeostasis and insulin levels, which can lead to "brain fog" and metabolic issues that effect overall energy levels and cognitive functions. Long-term over-consumption of sugar can lead to neurological problems and will reduce memory capacity. There was also an association between eating a healthy diet (including salads, vegetables, fish, and whole grains) at 81/2 years old and having a higher IQ at the same age.[62]

> **Eat powerful foods to
> increase your brain power!**

As we get older, diet plays a vital role in maintaining healthy brain and cognitive function. Poor diet along with lack of sleep, lack of exercise, over use of drugs, and lack of mental or social stimulation can have a negative impact on mental function. Foods are powerful and are brains need nutrient dense food to protect it from the toxins in our environment and nourish it so that it is sharp for a lifetime. Some of these foods will help you keep your thinking sharp and your cognitive power optimal.

1. **Blueberries** contain antioxidants that benefit the brain. Research shows that blueberries also contribute to protecting

the brain from stress induced by oxidation. Researchers think that blueberries may contribute to the reduction of the effects of age-connected conditions, such as dementia and Alzheimer's. Remember to buy organic if possible as conventional blueberries contain high amounts of pesticide residues.

2. **Coffee,** the stimulant found in coffee has been shown to improve mental acuity, when consumed in moderation and without the sugar or cream that makes it less healthy. Coffee beans contain antioxidants that support brain health and have even shown promise in warding off depression.

3. **Eggs** contain a lot of cholesterol but the body needs cholesterol to make hormones, create bile for digestion, and build a protective barrier in every cell in our bodies to keep viruses and toxins out. As we age, our brains start to shrink, but eggs contain lecithin that helps to stop this process along with Vitamin B12 (cobalamin) and choline, the building substances of brain cells that can help improve memory. (Eggs are a major animal source of choline, while wheat germ is a rich vegetarian source).

4. **Krill and sardines** are small, wild, oily fish that are full of omega-3 fatty acids, EPA and DHA, which are beneficial to our brain health and linked to improved focus and memory. These fatty acids coat the neurons in our brains with protective fats that allows for better connections and transmission of information. Omega-3 fatty acids also help more oxygen flow to the brain so we have better access to information. Small fish contain less mercury as well.

5. **Raw Vegetables** contain many phytochemicals and antioxidants that help keep our minds sharp. Like most parts of our body, our brains respond well to a variety of healthy foods and positive stimulation. Raw vegetables also have abundant sources of enzymes, which are needed to properly digest foods so we can absorb vital nutrients.

6. **Walnuts** and other high quality nuts and seeds like, Brazil nuts, cashew nuts, peanuts, sesame seeds, flax seeds, chia seeds, sunflower seeds and their oils, either raw or with minimum processing, provides your brain with Vitamin E, which has a protective effect on the brain. Walnuts contain high amounts of omega-3 fatty acids, and magnesium, which is good for memory and cognitive functions of the brain. Walnuts are full of anti-inflammatory nutrients and are the only good nut source of alpha-linolenic acid (ALA). They help promote blood flow, which in turn allows for efficient delivery of oxygen to the brain.

7. **Water** is critical to cognitive function. As little as a 2% dehydration level can result in a decrease in mental functions, according to the National Institutes of Health. *Mayoclinic.org* recommends about eight 8-oz. glasses of filtered water each day to replace lost fluids. Remember all fluids count toward that replacement, including hydrating vegetables and fruits. Caffeine, nicotine, and alcohol have a dehydrating effect on the body.[63]

Include intelligence-boosting foods in your daily/weekly diet. Encourage your kids to get more omega-3 fatty acids in their diet from wild fish, flax and pumpkin seeds, and fish oil. Sprinkle ground flax or hemp hearts on your family's cereal (when they are not looking) and try to get them to eat healthy nuts and seeds. Put ground flax on toast or add it to smoothies, pancake batter, baking, etc. Eat high quality free-range eggs every week to optimize your omega-3 fatty acids, Vitamin D and choline intake. Cut up raw vegetables for you and your family to reach for as a snack.

Besides food, intelligence can be improved through adopting a continuing learning attitude. Contrary to what was believed years ago, the brain is remarkably "plastic" and can develop and improve throughout life. Like working out our muscles, working out our brains with verbal, mental, and physical practice and challenges on a daily basis will maintain, and could even boost, intelligence throughout our entire lives.

HEALTHY YOU

International Cuisine = Variety

Who said "variety is the spice of life"? With food, the choices are endless. Eating healthy food is important, but many of us get stuck in a rut of the same meals each week. Our bodies crave variety and each food has different flavors and nutrients so mixing it up is good for your taste buds and your body.

International cuisines use a large variety of herbs and spices to create distinctive flavors and aromas. There are more types of cuisine than I could possibly list but the breadth and diversity is expressed from Ethiopian flatbread (injera) to Cajun jambalaya to German sauerbraten to Indian dahl to Portuguese fisherman's stew to Russian Borsht, to Jamaican coconut crushed Mahi Mahi to Thai green and red curries and the list goes on and on it exquisite delight.

There are many websites where you can find International recipes, including *www.epicurious.com, www.foodnetwork.ca, www.eatingwell.com, www.health.com/health/recipes, www.allrecipes.com, www.food.com,* etc. The diversity of international dishes is incredible and trying new cuisines will ensure that you are never bored of eating! If you don't want to cook, try visiting an International restaurant to sample the cuisine from other parts of the world. It will be a fun night out and your taste buds will surely thank you.

Who Doesn't Love Junk Food?

Growing up in a busy household of four girls, I must admit that I ate more than my share of junk food.

I remember going up to the cottage every weekend in the summer with six people and a dog in one average-sized station wagon and all our gear. For a treat, our parents let us go to the local store and we would each select our small paper bag and load it up with penny candy. The red licorice was always my favorite. Eating a gallon of sugar did pass the time but I didn't continue the tradition with my own children because I have learned about the dangers of excessive amounts of sugar and remember how sick I used to feel after I had overindulged in the car.

Of course, my kids love candy and other forms of junk food too. I still give my boys a treat occasionally but also insist that they eat their fruit and vegetables first!

REAL "J" FOODS

Jack Fruit [*Fruit*] Jack fruit tress produce more fruit than any other tree in the world. Jack fruit contains fiber, carbohydrates, protein, good amounts of Vitamin C and B-complex Vitamins (B6 (pyridoxine), B3 (niacin), B2 (riboflavin) and B9 (folic acid)), and minerals like potassium, magnesium, manganese, and iron. It also contains beta-carotene. The seeds are great roasted and added to curries, just as you would add lentils.

Jalapeno Peppers. See "Hot Peppers" for general information.

Jasmine Rice [*Grain*] Native to Thailand, jasmine rice contains carbohydrates, fiber and a small amount of protein. Jasmine rice contains B- complex Vitamins (B3 (niacin) and B1 (thiamine)), and some of minerals selenium, manganese and iron. Like all rice, jasmine rice is available as both white and brown types, and has more nutritional benefits as brown, wherein the rice retains its nutritious bran, has greater fiber content, and has greater amounts of nutrients. See also "Rice" and "Grains" for general information.

Jerusalem Artichoke [*Vegetable*] This root vegetable contains fiber, carbohydrates and a small amount of protein. Jerusalem artichokes contain high amounts of Vitamin K and good amounts of Vitamin C along with some B-complex Vitamins (B9 (folic acid), B3 (niacin), B2 (riboflavin) and B6 (pyridoxine)), and minerals manganese, magnesium, potassium, phosphorus, and copper. See also Root Vegetables under Food for Thought, under "R."

Jicama [*Vegetable*] Jicama contains fiber, carbohydrates, good amounts of Vitamins C and E, and some Vitamin A and B-complex Vitamins. It also has minerals iron, copper, manganese, and magnesium in small amounts along inulin. It must be well peeled when eaten. See also Root Vegetables under Food for Thought, under "R."

Juneberry [*Fruit*] These red berries turn blue-black on ripening. They are similar to the size of blueberries. They are easily distinguished by the crown on the end, away from the stock. They are great for making jams, muffins, cobblers, etc. See "Berries" for nutrients and information.

Juniper Berries [*Herb*] Usually thought of as a fruit, this herb contains fiber, carbohydrates, fat, protein, and good amounts of Vitamin C. Additionally, juniper berries have some amounts of minerals like iron, magnesium, phosphorous, cobalt, copper, chromium, potassium, and calcium. Juniper berries also contain tannins, flavonoid glycosides, and resin and are used in cooking to flavor meats and cabbage. Juniper berries have been used to treat a wide range of ailments from rheumatism to arthritis and urinary tract infections. The juice can be ingested as a digestive tonic and the berries can be crushed and applied to slow-healing wounds as an antiseptic and pain reliever. See also "Berries" for general information. See also Juniper Berries and Other Forest Foods under Food for Thought, below.

FOOD FOR THOUGHT

Juniper Berries and Other Forest Foods

The juniper is a coniferous tree and the berries have many different uses. The juniper is possibly the only conifer that is used as a seasoning and it is considered a herb even though it is a berry.

The word "gin" is derived from the Dutch word for juniper. Gin was originally developed from juniper berries as a form of medicine in the early seventeenth century. There are many health benefits of juniper berries.

Juniper berries are used in treating a variety of ailments from rheumatism, to arthritis, cystitis, and catarrh. The juice can be ingested as a digestive tonic. Juniper berries can also be used as a urinary antiseptic or can be crushed and applied topically to slow-healing wounds as they are a powerful antiseptic and pain reliever. Since juniper is also a stimulant, it helps all the various organs of the body to function more efficiently. Although there are many health benefits of juniper, it should be avoided by pregnant mothers, as well as by those with kidney problems.[64] The list of healing wonders for this tiny berry goes on and on.

As junipers are one tiny berry found in the forest, you may wonder what other amazing things can be found there. Did you know that about 1.6 billion people globally depend on forest livelihoods? Forests are the ideal place for those with limited incomes to forage with baskets for leaves and berries and drill to tap sap. It is estimated that non-wood goods from forests are valued at over $120 billion each year or more – and they're good for you.

For example, forest honey has more antioxidants than field honey, tree resin is used to make chewing gum, over 25,000 tons of Brazil nuts come from the Amazon rain forest, 1,300 tons of pine nuts come from forests in Turkey, blueberries, raspberries, and acai berries come from forests as do mushrooms and truffles (see Marvelous Mushrooms – The Magic Food under Food for Thought, under "M"), and spring greens like sorrel and fiddleheads in Canadian forests.

> It is estimated that non-wood goods from forests are valued at over $120 billion each year or more – and they're good for you.

In addition, forests provide food with medicinal properties because deep-rooted trees raise scarce minerals to the surface. Ginseng and yerba mate come from the forest as well as boars, our original wild pig! Coconut trees provide at least 45 different applications in India, from food to fuel, medicine, and fiber. Rubber tress offer similar valuable products. The wild grasslands that often neighbor forests hold a bounty of products as well, including highly valued indigenous plants (we might consider "weeds') (see Dandelions and Other Weeds under Food for Thought, under "D") that offer more nutrition than many foods found in our North American grocery stores.[65]

But forests are shrinking in South America and Africa due to deforestation for large-scale monocropping (Asia and North America are remaining steady according to recent data and the size has increased in Europe). Are we losing edible or medical treasures when we cut down our forests? The net loss of the world's forests is estimated at 7.3 million hectares (18 million acres) per year. Half the world's tropical forests have been cleared or degraded.[66]

Forests are amazing places that supply food and habitats for animals, food and medicine for humans, and carbon storage and protection from soil erosion for the planet. Many cultures revere the healing and calming powers of being in a forest. Scientists, brilliant entrepreneurs, and citizens are working to protect the forests and use our land more efficiently for growing our food so we can keep these important spaces preserved for future generations.

FOOD AND YOU OR YOUR ENVIRONMENT

Jobs and Cooking – How Can We Find the Time?

Wouldn't it be nice to have the family home at 5 o'clock to eat dinner at the same time and spend relaxing time together at night? Well at least one or two nights a week?

Many companies are now offering ways to do just that, including working from home full time or part time, job sharing, and recognizing the importance of work/life balance. Telecommuting allows people to actually get more work done by avoiding the traffic of driving to and from work to get an earlier start to the day. Telecommuting allows parents more time to cook healthy meals and save money on gas and other expenses related to traveling to and from work.

And wouldn't it be nice to get more vacation time? In European countries, many employees begin with 6 weeks' vacation! Germany has one of the world's most productive work forces and is a big advocate of taking time to recharge and relax with family and friends. One of the things people do when on vacation is take time to prepare and/or eat a nice meal with loved ones.

Right now, in North America, we are so busy that we have no time to cook. Time spent cooking at home has dropped from 2.5 hours in 1934 to 8 minutes in 2010;[67] and busy working parents have been bombarded with so-called kitchen helpers. Quick and easy tools to help reduce the time required to prepare dinner. Non-stick frying pans and microwaves have become very popular, but are all these convenience tools good for our health? Is racing ahead good for us when we are burning out?

In their book *Slow Death by Rubber Duck,*[68] Rick Smith and Bruce Lourie show the dangers of convenience tools like non-stick cookware that contains a chemical called Perfluorchemical (PFC). A known carcinogen, it accumulates in the body. Non-stick pots and pans and microwave popcorn bags (along with pizza boxes and fast food wrappers) are coated with PFC. When heated to high temperatures the coating on non-stick pans will break down and the fumes have been known to kill birds. PFC has been found to be present in every human tested. A cast iron pan will take a minute more to clean up but will last a lifetime and be better for your health and as a bonus the iron will naturally add flavor and minerals to your food and a hot-air popper makes healthier, tastier, chemical-free popcorn!

> The benefits of telecommuting for our health are twofold: time to cook healthier meals and time to spend with family.

Another modern convenience that came along years ago is plastic and it changed the way we live overnight. Plastic became the most common food container. Research on Bisphenol A (BPA) has led

Canada to take a global leadership role in banning this toxic chemical. BPA is a xenoestrogen (it mimics and disrupts the hormone estrogen) that can create an imbalance in our sex hormones and is linked to estrogen dominant cancers. Look for the number on the back of any plastic item and remember "4, 5, 1 and 2 are okay and all the rest are bad for you."[69] BPA lines most tin cans too but now many manufacturers are working hard to be BPA free so check labels when buying soup, sauces, etc. For food storage, use glass containers and never heat anything in the microwave in or on plastic!

Telecommuting means that we don't have to rush as much and we can take time to slow down and enjoy a meal together – hopefully a home-cooked meal – with our family with high quality cookware and storage containers for leftovers. The American Academy of Pediatrics examined studies about the impact of family meals on obesity, eating habits, and bonding. The results showed a 12% lower risk of being overweight, a 20% decrease in choosing unhealthy eating, and a 35% lower risk of disordered eating.[70] Eating together gives you a chance to teach your child about healthy, balanced meals. Eating meals together also has been shown to improve children's grades and strengthen family bonds. Eating without rushing as much will also help you better digest food and absorb nutrients and reduce overeating associated with eating too fast or in front of the TV.

Having enough holiday time to unwind is very important and having the time during the week to make a delicious meal and share it with your family is a great benefit for telecommuters. Those companies who offer work-from-home flexibility are more than often rewarded with grateful staff who will work extra hard to show the team that they are super productive in the home office … even if they are wearing pajamas all morning!

HEALTHY YOU

To Juice or Not to Juice?

Buy a vegetable juicer and mix up your own morning blend to drink at breakfast instead of a high-sugar pure juice. Try making a vegetable/juice blend by adding celery, spinach, or another powerhouse greens like Swiss chard, kale, or spinach, to antioxidant-rich frozen berries or your favorite fruit. Add coconut water, milk, or almond milks to create your desired consistency. Experiment until you find the winning combination for you. Add super foods like hemp hearts, chia seeds, or ground flax to get extra omega-3s in your diet. Make it creamier by adding yogurt, nut butter, or avocados. You can use pulp from your juicing machine in muffins, sauces, meat loafs, desserts and whole grain breads.

Below is a good hydration juicing recipe that is quick, easy, and will supercharge your day.

Green Juice
1/2 small-medium head organic romaine lettuce; 1 cup organic spinach; 3 cups cubed watermelon;1 cucumber (peeled if not organic); 2 small limes (peeled); 4 stalks organic celery; 4 stalks organic kale

Wash and cut to fit your juicer's shute. Start by juicing your spinach and lettuce then add the remaining ingredients. Enjoy or store up to 24 hours in an airtight container in the fridge.

K

"God made yeast, as well as dough,
and loves fermentation just as dearly as he loves vegetation."
Ralph Waldo Emerson
(1803–1882, American poet, essayist)

Kimchee from Korea

A few years ago, I discovered Kimchee, which is a traditional Korean dish made with fermented vegetables (usually cabbage like sauerkraut), garlic, ginger, chili peppers, and salt.

That might sound like an odd flavor to a traditional North American palate, but it reminded me of when I spent my third year of university in Germany. Sauerkraut, another fermented vegetable dish, seemed to be served with almost every meal! I grew to like it, and now the taste brings back fond memories.

But it isn't just the memories that draw me to fermented dishes like kimchee and sauerkraut anymore. The fermentation process of cabbage and other vegetables encourages healthy bacterial growth along the intestinal tract which is good news for our gut health. Like the healthy fats, healthy bacteria protect our bodies from damage and promote health. Experts are becoming increasingly certain that as much as 70-80% of our immune response comes from our stomachs so having healthy bacteria thriving to counter harmful intruders and help us maintain a strong intestinal barrier sounds good to me! Pass the kimchee please.

REAL "K" FOODS

Kabocha Squash. See "Squash" for general information.

Kale [*Vegetable*] Also known as Cavalo Nero and Tuscan Cabbage, kale has fiber, carbohydrates, huge amounts of Vitamins A, C, and K, and small amounts of B-complex Vitamins (B6 (pyridoxine), B1 (thiamine), B2 (riboflavin) and B9 (folic acid)). It has good amounts of minerals manganese, copper, calcium, potassium, iron, magnesium, and a balanced ratio of omega-3 and -6 fatty acids. Kale contains carotenoid and flavonoid antioxidants and is an effective anti-inflammatory food. Grown in most vegetable gardens in Tuscany, it is an essential ingredient in the signature soup of this region. While it does not lose volume like spinach when cooked, it does need to be cooked longer. See What Foods Fight or Help Prevent Cancer? under Food and You or Your Environment, under "C" and also Menopause – Can Food Help the Transition? under Food and You or Your Environment, under "M."

Kamut [*Grain*] Kamut has 20-40% more protein than wheat and is very high in fiber, carbohydrates, B-complex Vitamins (B1 (thiamine), B2 (riboflavin), B3 (niacin), B6 (pyridoxine)), and minerals magnesium, phosphorus, potassium, iron, copper, zinc, selenium, and manganese. Kamut is another example of an ancient or heirloom grain. Once pushed aside by agricultural monoculture, it is now returning to add variety to the food supply. Often called the ancient cousin of wheat, kamut is higher in protein and much lower in gluten than wheat. See also "Grains" for general information.

Kefir [*Dairy*] Kefir is fermented yogurt and high in protein, and Vitamins A, D, K, B-complex Vitamins (B2 (riboflavin), B12 (cobalamin), B1 (thiamine), B9 (folic acid) and B5 (pantothenic acid)). It also contains high amounts of minerals calcium, magnesium, and phosphorus, and is rich in tryptophan, an essential amino acid known for relaxing the nervous system. Kefir contains high amounts of probiotic healthy bacteria and enzymes that make it easy to digest. It is created by mixing milk from cows, goats or sheep with a kefir "grain" starter, a mixture of yeasts and bacteria. According to studies, kefir is known to boost immune system functions by fighting against bacteria and viruses that enter the body. Kefir has been used to treat different kinds of health problems because of its antibiotic and antifungal properties. It has been used to fight metabolic diseases, atherosclerosis, allergies, some forms of cancer, kidney stones, ulcers, osteoporosis, hypertension, tuberculosis, candidiasis, irritable bowel syndrome, diarrhea and more. Mix it in with yogurt, smoothies or have on its own with nuts, berries and granola. See also Kefir, Kimchee, Kombucha, and Vitamin K! under Food for Thought, below. See also Are Rheumatoid Arthritis and Autoimmune Diseases on the Rise? under Food and You or Your Environment, under "R."

Kelp. See "Seaweed." For nutrients and information. See also Kelp to the Rescue under Healthy You, below.

Kidney Beans (white and red) [*Vegetable (Legume)*] Whether white or red, these beans provide an excellent plant source of fiber, carbohydrates, and protein. Consuming this legume provides Vitamin K, B-complex Vitamins (B1 (thiamine) and B9 (folic acid)), and minerals manganese, iron, phosphorus, copper, potassium, and magnesium. See also "Legumes" for general information.

Kiwano. See "Horned Melon."

Kiwi [*Fruit*] Kiwis contain fiber, carbohydrates, and are rich in Vitamins C, K, E and some B-complex Vitamins (B6 (pyridoxine) and B9 (folic acid)). They also provide minerals potassium, copper, and some magnesium and manganese, along with a good amount of beta-carotene.

Kohlrabi [*Vegetable*] Fresh kohlrabi (or German turnip) is a rich source of fiber, carbohydrates, Vitamin C, good amounts of many B-complex Vitamins (B3 (niacin), Vitamin B-6 (pyridoxine), B1 (thiamine), B5 (pantothenic acid)), and has good levels of minerals copper, calcium, potassium, manganese, iron, and phosphorus. Kohlrabi leaves or tops, like turnip greens, are also very nutritious greens abundant in carotenes, Vitamins A, K, B-complex Vitamins, and minerals. It is a member of the cabbage family and is high in antioxidants. See What Foods Fight or Help Prevent Cancer? under Food and You or Your Environment, under "C."

Kombucha. See "Tea" For nutrients and information. See also Kefir, Kimchee, Kombucha, and Vitamin K! under Food for Thought, below, and also Tea, The Drink of Emperors under Food for Thought, under "T."

Krill [*Shellfish*] Krill is a good source of protein and omega-3 fatty acids. It contains good amounts of Vitamin D and B-complex Vitamins (B3 (niacin), B12 (cobalamin), B6 (pyridoxine), B1 (thiamine), and B2 (riboflavin)), and some Vitamin E and C, along with minerals selenium, potassium, phosphorus, and some magnesium and zinc. Krill is a shrimp-like animal in the crustacean family that serves as food for many sea creatures, including whales, seals, and penguins. They are small and grow to be a few inches long, and they are caught for use as bait. They are also used extensively for fish oil supplements and are preferred by some as they contain fewer calories, less odor, less mercury, and cause fewer digestive issues than some other fish oils. (For information on sustainable fish see "Fish" or visit *www.msc.org/cook-eat-enjoy/fish-to-eat.*). See also Can Certain Foods Make Us More Intelligent? under Food and You or Your Environment, under "I."

Kumquat [*Fruit*] Kumquats contain fiber, carbohydrates, and good amounts of Vitamins A, C, and E. They also contain B-complex

Vitamins (B3 (niacin), B1 (thiamine), B5 (pantothenic acid), B9 (folic acid) and B6 (pyridoxine)) and moderate amounts of minerals like copper, calcium, manganese, potassium, zinc, selenium, and iron.

FOOD FOR THOUGHT

Kefir, Kimchee, Kombucha, and Vitamin K

What do kefir, kimchee, and kombucha all have in common? Well, you can drink kefir and kombucha, but that leaves out kimchee. Puzzled? They are all fermented and help us manufacture Vitamin K!

A large number of vegetables, grains, and dairy products are fermented, including yogurt, sauerkraut, some pickles, soy sauce, cheese, wine, and sourdough bread to name a few other examples. They are a good source of Vitamin K and Vitamin B12 (cobalamin), an essential nutrient you can't get from plants (B12 is produced by animals and bacteria). They are also easy to digest and some research shows that people with wheat sensitivities are able to digest fermented sourdough bread much better than regular bread because some of the hard-to-digest proteins have been broken down during the process of fermentation. This is also true for other grains and legumes that have been fermented or even soaked overnight.

What is the difference between fermenting (yes, that sounds yucky!) and pickling? The process of pickling begins with boiling a mixture of vinegar, spices, and salt and pouring the mixture over the food. The process varies from there, but in the end the food can be stored in tightly sealed and sterilized containers for many months without need of refrigeration. In contrast, the process of fermentation generally begins with the sterilization of the containers that will hold the fermented items. The food items or beverages are then placed in the container with active cultures and allowed to ferment in a warm, dark place until obtaining the desired taste. Pickling is done to *prevent* bacteria from growing in a food; fermenting is done to *encourage* bacterial growth.[71]

> Pickling prevents bacteria from growing in food;
> fermenting encourages bacterial growth.

Fermentation not only makes the end product more digestible, it can also create improved flavor and texture, add vitamins, reduce or eliminate carbohydrates believed to cause flatulence, decrease the required cooking time, increase storage life, and replenish intestinal micro flora. Most fermentation is activated by molds, yeasts, or bacteria, working singularly or together. Fermented foods have been shown to help with irritable bowel syndrome, diarrhea, allergies, etc. Most of today's grocery store varieties of pickles, olives, yogurt, and sauerkraut are acidified and pasteurized for extended shelf life so they no longer contain beneficial bacteria. Look for fermented foods in the refrigerated section of your grocery store for a real benefit to your health.

So exactly what is it about kimchee, kefir, and kombucha that help our stomachs so much? Well, they are loaded with healthy bacteria that help us make certain B-complex Vitamins and Vitamin K and prevent the growth of unhealthy disease-causing bad bacteria and viruses. Vitamin K, which helps the liver make blood-clotting factors, can be found in green vegetables but most of it is made in our large intestines by healthy bacteria. Excessive use of antibiotics or poor diet can cause Vitamin K deficiencies.

Eating fermented foods like kefir, kombucha, and kimchee contain healthy bacteria that work to keep us healthy, strong, and help us manufacture Vitamin K. They are called probiotic foods (probiotic means "for life" in Greek) as they contain beneficial forms of gut bacteria. Other great probiotic foods include miso soup, fermented pickles (found in refrigerated section of your grocery store), sauerkraut, cheese, yogurt, and even wine! Other foods like Jerusalem artichokes and lentils (called prebiotics) contain substances that feed the healthy bacteria contained in probiotic foods and help them thrive.

Adding more probiotic and prebiotic foods to your diet will promote manufacture of Vitamin K and the growth of helpful bacteria like lactobacillus and bifidobacterium, and make a difference for your health and boost your immune system.

FOOD AND YOU OR YOUR ENVIRONMENT

Know the What, How, When, and How Much of Food?

Have you ever heard that knowledge is power? Well I firmly believe that nutritional knowledge can save lives and help create a healthier planet for future generations.

What?

We all know the importance of eating healthy foods for their vitamin and mineral content. However, in recent years, scientists have discovered that there are thousands of phytonutrients in plant food that have healing and disease prevention properties. So what are these foods? Why have we not been eating them every day?

Just as we've become a fast food society, we've also become a fast cure society. Sometimes it just seems easier to pop a pill instead of taking a long-term approach to many chronic health issues with diet and health solutions. Over-the-counter and prescription drug usage is showing alarming trends and drug misuse can cause serious side effects but what can we do about chronic pain and discomfort?

> Nutritional knowledge can save lives and help create a healthier planet for future generations.

Consulting both medical and holistic experts is a growing trend that may combine the amazing advances of medical science with the wisdom of food science to treat ailments and even support recovery with some diseases. We now know that phytochemicals in food work as antioxidants to protect our cells from damage by toxic substances and free radicals. Free radicals can damage cells in our bodies and lead to disease so what we eat can work to reduce pain and inflammation and even promote healing in the body. More and more doctors are now offering integrated medicine that combines drugs and diet, along with other therapies, to promote health for their patients and the results are impressive and noteworthy.

How?

It is also important to gain knowledge about not only to what you eat, but also how you select, cook, and combine foods.

When we choose only foods that are imported from far away, we get food with less nutrition because food loses nutrients along the journey to our grocery store. Even adding some local foods in season, will boost nutrient content when possible. Building our own gardens will also make a huge difference in fresh nutrients and the proportion of home gardens in North America is increasing steadily. According to the National Gardening Association's 2008 survey, organic gardeners are growing in numbers from 5 million house-holds in 2004 to more than 12 million just a few years later. For those who don't have time to garden, even growing herbs can add enormous nutritional value to meals and be fun.

Barbequing is delicious, but certain carcinogens in this cooking process can put harmful substances (carcinogenic compounds known as HCAs (heterocyclic amines)) in your body.[72] The good news is that there are simple ways to neutralize the carcinogenic compounds and at the same time give it extra flavor! Add rosemary. Rosemary's antioxidant blocks the HCAs before they can form during heating. Other herbs and spices rich in antioxidants include basil, mint, sage, savory, marjoram, oregano, and thyme. Marinating with any of these spices adds both protection and flavor to any grilled meat.[73]

Below is a simple marinade that is proven to eliminate carcinogens from cooking on the grill (leave it on a few hours or overnight).

> 1/2 cup packed local honey, raw sugar or sucanat
> 3 cloves crushed garlic
> 1 1/2 teaspoons salt
> 3 tablespoons mustard
> 1/4 cup apple cider vinegar
> 3 tablespoons lemon
> 6 tablespoons grape-seed oil
> 1/2 teaspoon dried rosemary or rosemary extracts

Overcooking food in general will rapidly reduce nutrients so it is best to lightly steam, bake, broil, or eat a range of raw fruits and vegetables. Many believe raw foods have many more enzymes and nutrients! Raw foods are considered to be detoxifying and cooked foods, like soups and stews, are considered to be nourishing. The ideal combination is to eat some of both – raw and lightly cooked or steamed food – every day. Fried food is delicious but keep it to a minimum. Ensure when you do fry that you use high quality cooking oils with a high smoke temperature to avoid rancidity (grapeseed, canola, peanut or coconut oils are good choices). See "Oils" for more information.

When?

Think of your digestive system as a highway. If the slower vehicles are allowed to go first, the result will be a traffic jam, but if the slower vehicles follow the faster vehicles you're highway will run smoothly and efficiently. Below is a general guide to how long certain food groups take to digest.

- Juices and water: 20-30 minutes
- Soups, fruits, or smoothies: 30-45 minutes
- Vegetables: 30-45 minutes
- Grains, starches: 2-3 hours
- Beans, poultry, meat, or fish: 3 or more hours[74]

There is conflicting evidence about food combining. Most people do just fine with just about any combination. It is always a good idea to eat fruit separately as it digests quickly and can slow down digestion of meats and legumes if eaten at the same time and cause discomfort. Also drink sparingly at meals as too much liquid can dilute the hydrochloric acid needed to digest protein in the stomach. It is important to ensure you have a good supply of enzymes needed to help with digestion and some people like to take papaya or pineapple enzymes to help digest a big meal. Raw fruit and vegetables supply many enzymes and are helpful to eat regularly to ensure good digestion.

Eating after dinner has been linked most to weight gain. In France, although they eat a lot of saturated fat, they cook from scratch more, eat less processed oils and rarely eat after dinner. Eating when you are hungry is important and not when you are tired, stressed, or bored.

How Much?

As well as how we cook food, how much and how quickly we eat can affect our digestion and overall health.

The first rule of digestion that many of us ignore is over-consumption. It may sound unbelievable, but we can survive on much less than what we currently eat and would be healthier for it! One problem is that our brains are about 10 minutes behind our stomachs. This means that once our stomachs are full, our brains don't give us that "full feeling" until 10 minutes later. To avoid over-consumption we should stop eating before we get the feeling of fullness (go for half full). In North America, overeating is a major issue.

In John Robbins book *Healthy at 100*, he studies research from societies with great longevity among their members. All of the citizens have high levels of energy in their 70s, 80s, 90s, and many into their 100s! What he noticed was that their diets were very low in sugar, processed foods, and overall calorie intake was far lower than in North America. Many different vegetables were consumed daily. Daily exercise was part of the lifestyle in these cultures along with strong social networks.

So good food (but less of it!), good exercise, and good times with good friends will not only boost your energy but help you to live longer too! That knowledge is easy to digest!

HEALTHY YOU

Kelp to the Rescue

Kelp, a brown algae, and chlorella, a green algae, are among nature's most incredible foods. They have been a part of Asian nutrition and medicine for hundreds of years. Slowly North America is learning about their health benefits, especially their ability to cleanse and detoxify the body.

Brown algae, or kelp, is one of the most common types of seaweed and is believed to rid the body of many toxins and heavy metals (like mercury, cadmium, and lead) by binding with them (chelating) and then allowing them to be expelled easily from the body as harmless salts that are easy to eliminate. Kelp is rich in minerals like iodine, calcium, and potassium and is shown to boost the body's natural immune system and improve thyroid and liver function, which also helps with detoxification. They are also rich is chlorophyll (a pigment that makes plants green) which is a natural detoxifier.

Kelp can be chopped and used in soup, added into a vegetable stew, or blended into smoothies in the morning for a period of 3–4 weeks to clean and refresh the body. Other types of common seaweed include nori, dulse, arame, wakame, and kombu. When sourcing seaweed, try to find organic sources wherever possible as seaweed will absorb components from the water in which they are grown. Consult with your health-care provider before combining any natural detoxifying seaweeds with prescription medication, particularly if you have any thyroid issues.

*"Life handed him a lemon, as Life sometimes will do.
His friends looked on in pity, assuming he was through.
They came upon him later, reclining in the shade,
in calm contentment, drinking a glass of lemonade."*

Dale Carnegie

(1888-1955, American writer and lecturer)

Local – It's Win Win Win

I decided to buy a local, quarter, grass-fed cow this year for many reasons. Grass-fed beef is very high in omega-3 fatty acids, buying in bulk came at a lower cost, and I received higher quality meat as it was raised without antibiotics or factory-style living arrangements. I was also supporting a local producer, which felt good. The farmer was very helpful and instructed me on which cuts of beef to choose.

Next, I went to the local processing facility on the day of my pick up and met the manager of the facility and the butchers. Speaking with him made me realize how important the workers are in the food processing industry and how little we actually see of them.

As I carried my boxes to my van, I imagined all the great stews and dishes I would make in the months to come.

REAL "L" FOODS

Lamb [*Meat*] Lamb is a rich source of protein and Vitamins A, B3 (niacin), B6 (pyridoxine), and B12 (cobalamin). The mineral content includes iron, zinc, phosphorous, and calcium with trace minerals being selenium, manganese, and copper.

Lamb's Quarters [*Vegetable*] Considered an edible weed in North America, lamb's quarters is cultivated in other parts of the world. It is related to quinoa and has highly nutritious seeds. It is a good source of fiber, carbohydrates, Vitamins A, C, B2 (riboflavin), and minerals phosphorus, calcium, and iron. Lamb's quarters can be found in the wild and often grows in vegetable gardens. See also Dandelions and Other "Weeds" under Food and You or Your Environment, under "D."

Leek [*Vegetable*] Leeks are a rich source of fiber, carbohydrates, and Vitamin A. They also contain Vitamins C, B9 (folic acid) and some small amounts of minerals iron, manganese, calcium, magnesium, copper, and potassium. Leeks are known to have antibacterial and diuretic properties and are a member of onion family, related to garlic and chives. See What Foods Fight or Help Prevent Cancer? under Food and You or Your Environment, under "C.

Legumes [*Vegetable*] Legumes are an excellent plant source of fiber, carbohydrates, protein, vitamins, and minerals. Although they don't offer a complete protein like meat alone, you can combine with grains to get the complete protein needed for proper health. They are one of best foods for lowering cholesterol (along with apples, barley, and oat bran). They also keep blood sugar regulated as they are low on the Glycemic Index (GI). Beans can cause digestive discomfort and therefore are best when cooked or soaked before eating. They can be purchased in cans for quick and easy use (be sure to drain and rinse first) or soaked overnight and cooked in bulk for the week ahead. The following are classified as legumes (see each listing for specific nutrients): black beans, garbanzo beans, kidney beans, lentils, lima beans, navy beans, peas, pinto beans, and soybeans. See also Eat More Legumes under Healthy You, below.

Lemongrass [*Herb*] Lemongrass is high in fiber, Vitamins C, A and B-complex Vitamins (B9 (folic acid), B5 (pantothenic acid), B6 (pyridoxine), and B1 (thiamine)), and contains many minerals (large amounts of manganese and good amounts of potassium, zinc, calcium, iron, copper, and magnesium). Lemongrass is known for having antifungal and calming properties. See "Herbs" for general information. See also Herbaceous Cooking under Healthy You, under "H."

Lemons [*Fruit*] This citrus fruit contains fiber, carbohydrates, Vitamins C, B9 (folic acid), and small amounts of minerals potassium, copper, calcium, and magnesium. They contain bioflavonoids, pectin, and limonene that promote immunity and fight infection. Known for their strong antibacterial, antiviral, and immune-boosting powers, lemons are also used for digestive and weight loss aids and as a gentle liver cleanser. The citric acid in lemon juice helps to dissolve gallstones, calcium deposits, and kidney stones.[75] See also Lemons – The Fruit that Helped Sir Edmund Hillary under Food for Thought, below.

Lentils [*Vegetable (Legume)*] Lentils are a great plant source of fiber, carbohydrates, and protein. This legume also provides a good source of Vitamin C and B-complex Vitamins (B1 (thiamine), B3 (niacin), B6 (pyridoxine), B5 (pantothenic acid), B2 (riboflavin), and B9 (folic acid)), and minerals iron, copper, manganese, magnesium, phosphorus, potassium and selenium. Lentils are the third highest source of protein from plant food. See also "Legumes" for general information. See also Eat More Legumes under Healthy You, below.

Lettuce [*Vegetable*] Lettuce now comes in many varieties and do not all rank the same in nutritional value but all contain fiber and carbohydrates. Romaine provides good nutrition but iceberg does not compared to other flavored greens like radicchio, arugula, endive, chicory, and escarole. The darker the color of the salad green, the more nutritious it is. Beta-carotene is found in the darker-colored greens. A dark-green color also indicates the presence of Vitamin B9 (folic acid) and salad greens also have notable sources of Vitamins A, C, and K. Lettuce contains small amounts of minerals copper, iron, calcium, potassium, phosphorus and manganese in varying amounts depending on type. Some of the many types of greens to add to your salad include frisee, arugula or rocket, endive or Belgium chicory, radicchio, mizuna, escarole, beet and dandelion greens, cress, tatsoi, butterhead or Boston lettuce, romaine, oakleaf and looseleaf. See also specific varieties for nutrients and information.

Lima Beans [*Vegetable (Legume)*] Also referred to as butter beans, lima beans are an excellent plant source of fiber, carbohydrates, and protein. These legumes also provide B-complex Vitamins (B1 (thiamine) and B9 (folic acid)), and minerals manganese, potassium, iron, copper, phosphorus, and magnesium. See also "Legumes" for general information.

Limes [*Fruit*] Limes contain fiber, carbohydrates, Vitamins C, B9 (folic acid), and small amounts of minerals calcium, potassium, copper, and iron. Limes are anticarcinogenic and lime juice can help prevent formation of kidney stones. The peels of citrus fruits contain an inhibitor of melanin production that can combat aging skin. Add slices of lime to water to improve taste.

Lingonberries [*Fruit*] Lingonberries are similar to cranberries in appearance. They contain fiber, carbohydrates, and good amounts of Vitamin C. They also contain minerals potassium and magnesium and good amounts of antioxidants anthocyanin and quercetin. See also "Berries" for general information.

Lobster [*Shellfish*] Lobster is an excellent source of protein, Vitamins A, E, K and B-complex Vitamins, along with minerals calcium, iron, magnesium, phosphorus, potassium, zinc, cooper, manganese, and selenium. (For information on sustainable fish see "Fish" or visit *www.msc.org/cook-eat-enjoy/fish-to-eat*.) See also "Shellfish" for general information.

Loganberries [*Fruit*] Loganberries are high in fiber, and contain carbohydrates, Vitamins C, K, and B9 (folic acid) and the mineral manganese, and some magnesium, calcium, iron, potassium, and copper. These are ruby-red, sweet, juicy berries that turn purple-red when ripe. An accidental cross between the raspberry and blackberry, this newer variety of berry is named for its creator, James Logan. See also "Berries" for general information.

Looseleaf Lettuce. See "Lettuce" for nutrients and information.

Loquat [*Fruit*] Loquat contains fiber, carbohydrates, and high amounts of Vitamin A. It also contains small amounts of Vitamins B6 (pyridoxine) and B9 (folic acid), and minerals manganese and potassium. Loquat originated in the mountainous, evergreen rain forests of southeastern China and they have a similar taste and flavor to that of apples.

Lucuma [*Fruit*] Peruvian lucuma fruit contains fiber, carbohydrates, and small amounts of protein, along with Vitamins C and B3 (niacin), and minerals iron, zinc, and calcium. It also contains high amounts of beta-carotene and is used as a low-glycemic sweetener. Lucuma has a unique maple-like taste and can be used as a sugar substitute in a variety of recipes.

Lychees [*Fruit*] Lychees contain fiber, carbohydrates, and huge amounts of Vitamin C. They also have B-complex Vitamins (B6 (pyridoxine), B3 (niacin), and B9 (folic acid)), along with small amounts of minerals copper, potassium, phosphorus, magnesium, and manganese. Lychees are a tropical fruit native to southern China.

Lycium [*Fruit*] Lycium berries contain fiber, carbohydrates, Vitamin C, and small amounts of minerals. The root is believed to have a protective effect on the liver and kidneys, nourishing them and acting as a tonic. Lycium helps relieve excessive thirst and nighttime urination.

FOOD FOR THOUGHT

Lemons – The Fruit that Helped Sir Edmund Hillary

Lemons are part of the citrus family, which includes grapefruit, kumquat, lime, mandarin, orange, pomelo, tangerine, and ugli fruit. All citrus fruits grow on trees and interestingly enough the seed from one can often grow into a tree that bears the fruit of any of the others.[76] That is why commercial growers rely of grafting or cloning (see Amazing Apples under Food for Thought, under "A.") techniques to get the same species of citrus fruit in an orchard.

Lemon juice with water makes a great organ and liver cleanser. As the primary function of the liver is to break down toxins present in the body, it is very important to overall health to keep this organ working efficiently. In the book, *Back to Eden*,[77] author Jethro Kloss touts lemon as an antiseptic and a tool to detoxify the body. Drinking lemon water daily may, over a short period of time, help maintain liver and kidney health and the antiseptic properties of lemon might stave off infections. According to "The Amazing Health Benefits of Drinking Lemon Water," by registered nurse Ann Heustad,[78] the consumption of lemons increases production of liver enzymes. If the liver does not produce enough enzymes, it is more difficult for the body to break down toxins. Lemons are acidic to the taste but one of the most alkaline-forming foods in the body, so eating or drinking them also helps to balance body pH levels and reduce inflammation.

Lemons are extremely high in Vitamin C and scurvy (caused by lack of Vitamin C) is treated with diluted lemon juice. In 1747, a naval surgeon named James Lind cured scurvy with fresh lemons. To this day, the British Navy requires ships to carry enough lemons so that every sailor could have one ounce of juice a day. In the past, lemons were replaced with limes; this is where the English got their nickname "limeys." Lemons are even believed to help with breathing at high altitude. The first man to reach the top of Mt. Everest,

Edmund Hillary, said that his success on Mother of the Universe was greatly due to lemons.[79]

> Lemons – they can keep us clean
> and our environment.

Lemons can be used in many ways besides food, but their antiseptic properties come in handy for other health benefits.

- **Cleaning Cutting Boards:** Rather than use harsh cleaners, use half a lemon to sanitize cutting boards. Rub it all over the board with the cut side of a lemon or wash it in undiluted juice straight from the bottle.
- **Keep Insects Out of the Kitchen:** Squirt some lemon juice on door thresholds and windowsills and squeeze lemon juice into any holes or cracks where ants are getting in and scatter peels around the entrance. This gets rid of ants, roaches, fleas, and other invasive insects quickly. Mix the juice of 4 lemons with rinds with 1/2 gallon of water.
- **Disinfect and Deodorize Humidifiers:** Humidifiers in winter can become breeding grounds for bacteria, so it is important to keep them clean and fresh. Pour 3 to 4 teaspoons of lemon juice into the water. Repeat every few weeks. It will disinfect the machine and give off a delightful lemon-fresh fragrance.

Lemons are truly an amazing and inspirational fruit that I now try to eat and drink and clean with more often!

FOOD AND YOU OR YOUR ENVIRONMENT

Why Do We Need More Local Food?

A common complaint about organic or local foods is that they're more expensive than "conventional" (industrially grown) foods.

Most consumers don't realize how much we're already paying for the conventional foods, before we even get to the supermarket.

According to Barbara Kingsolver, in her book *Animal, Vegetable, Miracle*,[80] our tax dollars subsidize the petroleum used in the growing, processing, and shipping of these products from locations all over the world. Additionally we're paying more each year for the environmental and health costs of that method of food production.

Many small-scale local farmers use practices that build up rather than deplete the soil, using manure and cover crops. They eliminate or reduce pesticides and herbicides by instead using biological pest controls and regular hand-weeding with a hoe. Buying some local produce is a smart investment in your health, community, and environment. Not all food can be sourced locally, so don't think you have to give up coffee or chocolate! But locally grown food is more bio diverse and usually picked at its peak of freshness so include a visit to a farmer's market when you shop whenever available where you live.

Many large-scale crops are grown using monocultures, defined as the high-yield agricultural practice of growing a single crop year after year on the same land, without rotating in other crops. Corn, soybeans, wheat, palm, cotton, and rice are the most common crops grown with monocropping techniques. In fact, corn, wheat, and rice now account for 60% of human caloric intake, according to the UN Food and Agriculture Organization. Monoculture is detrimental to the environment for a number of reasons, including depletion of soil nutrients, making crops more vulnerable to pathogens and increasing dependency of chemicals and may also threaten biodiversity and promote food sensitivities when too much is consumed.

Many small-scale local farmers are switching to a more sustainable practice of using polycultures to grow food. Polycultures try to mimic a natural ecosystem by establishing multiple species in the same area. Plants, like people, have tastes and requirements for certain nutrients, therefore a diverse group can make better use of the soil conditions than a single species. Polycultures with a diversity of plant species make a farm less vulnerable to pests and improves its ability to weather disease. Integrating appropriate grazing animals into perennial polycultures, necessary for healthy woodlands, wetlands, savannas, and prairies, will add to fertility.[81] Topsoil gets depleted by shallow rooted annual crops. Polyculture, when done well, automatically replenishes the soil with minimal effort.

In his book, internationally known farmer Joel Salatin[82] describes how his farm has sustainably developed polycultures using forest, animal grazing, and crop rotation to harness the power of the sun and create more nutritious food instead of relying on soil-depleting fossil fuels and chemicals. The result is a rich top soil that nourishes his crops year after year instead of depleted soil. His success has encouraged some governments to start rewarding local farmers who take better care of their soil and land by offering financial incentives and cash to set up nature reserves on their farms.

> Plant some edible perennial plants as borders and in gardens. They'll come up every year and delight you with their bounty and beauty.

In many local communities, there is a growing trend called "edible landscaping" that can bring both food and beauty to gardens and pathways around the home by planting edible perennial plants and trees. Given some of the ongoing concerns with food security around the world, more and more people are interested in having more local or backyard sources of fresh food. Even a herb garden or basket is a great way to get started and will add a perennial touch to your home. Each year, I try to put in more perennial plants and we now have strawberries, blueberries, raspberries, and asparagus to enjoy each year. Learning what vegetables and fruits grow best in your area will help get you started and buying extra local products to store for future use by freezing, pickling, canning, fermenting, or cellaring will lower your food bill.

Local food is a popular selling pitch in many small-scale and even some big restaurants now. Savvy owners know that most people like to support their local farmers and producers whenever they can and enjoy the added flavor and freshness that local food brings.

If you haven't visited a local farmers market yet, it may be a very fun experience and you may find that you are returning over and over for the diverse selections and personal touch that each farmer brings to your local food choices.

For some of us, eating local in the winter is pretty difficult and trying to function without some of our favorite imported foods just isn't going to happen for most of us. But supporting local farmers is really easy to do and can be a fun way to add variety to your diet while getting to know farmers whogrow all the delicious varieties for you.

HEALTHY YOU

Eat More Legumes

Beans, peas, and lentils belong to the legume family and all are great sources of protein and fiber as well as minerals iron, magnesium, and zinc. Legumes are low in fat and high in B-complex Vitamins. Legumes contain insoluble fiber that helps prevent constipation and soluble fiber that helps keep blood sugar levels balanced, and lowers cholesterol.

They are easy to add to your diet and a great replacement for meat at lunch or dinner. Combine legumes with whole grains, like brown rice, quinoa or corn, to obtain all nine essential amino acids (building blocks for protein).

If stored properly, dried beans and peas will last for a year or more. After opening, store beans in a dry, tightly closed glass jar in a cool, dark spot. When cooking with dried legumes, rinse the beans in cold water. It's best to soak your beans overnight, for 6-8 hours; they'll cook faster and you'll inactivate gas-producing compounds. After soaking, discard any beans that float to the top, then throw out the soaking water and add fresh water for cooking. Enjoy the rich flavor and variety in many dishes each week.

*"If more of us valued food and cheer above hoarded gold,
it would be a much merrier world."*

J.R.R. Tolkien

(1892-1973, English writer, poet, philologist)

More Milk Please

As a toddler, I developed hives and was diagnosed as allergic to certain dairy products, including cow's milk.

The main protein in cow's milk is called "casein" and it is hard for many people to digest. My mother gave me goat's milk instead, which is highly nutritious and much easier to digest as well as being more alkaline and higher in calcium. I grew out of my allergy but still eat a lot of dairy from goat's milk. I only eat fermented cow dairy products like kefir as it is easy to digest and is full of probiotics.

If you have a hard time with dairy, try goat dairy or fermented kefir (start with one tablespoon a day and slowly increase your intake) to help with digestive issues. Kefir has an abundance of bacteria that have pre-digested the milk protein casein and may be just what you need to get back to enjoying dairy! It has a tart flavor, a slightly sour taste somewhere between buttermilk and sour cream. I even put a tablespoon in my mashed potatoes and it makes them delicious!

REAL "M" FOODS

Maca [*Vegetable*] Maca contains fiber, carbohydrates, and good amounts of Vitamin C and B-complex Vitamins (B6 (pyridoxine), B2 (riboflavin), and B3 (niacin)), and protein. It contains huge amounts of minerals copper, iron, and good amounts of potassium, manganese, and calcium. Maca is a root vegetable that has been cultivated in the Peruvian Andes since 1600 B.C. Native Americans and indigenous Peruvians have used maca as a medicine and a source of nutritional support to stimulate the immune system, enhance memory, and alleviate menstrual disorders, menopause symptoms, infertility, sterility, and sexual disorders. Maca is widely categorized as a super food.[83]

Macadamia Nut [*Nut*] Macadamia nuts are high in protein, fiber, saturated fats, including healthy omega-7 fatty acids. They contain huge amounts of Vitamin B1 (thiamine), very good amounts of Vitamin E and other B-Complex Vitamins (B2 (riboflavin), B3 (niacin), B6 (pyridoxine), and B5 (pantothenic acid)). Macadamia nuts have high amounts of minerals copper, magnesium, phosphorus, iron, potassium, zinc, manganese, selenium, and calcium too. See "Nuts" for general information.

Mackerel [*Fish*] Mackerel is a good source of protein and omega-3 fatty acids. It contains good amounts of B-complex Vitamins (B3 (niacin), B12 (cobalamin), and B6 (pyridoxine)), and minerals selenium and phosphorus. (For information on sustainable fish see "Fish" or visit *www.msc.org/cook-eat-enjoy/fish-to-eat*.)

Mahi-mahi [*Fish*] A good source of protein and omega-3 fatty acids, mahi-mahi contains good amounts of B-complex Vitamins (B3 (niacin), B12 (cobalamin), and B6 (pyridoxine)), and minerals selenium and phosphorus. (For information on sustainable fish see "Fish" or visit *www.msc.org/cook-eat-enjoy/fish-to-eat*.)

Maitake. See "Mushrooms" for nutrients and information. See also What Foods Fight or Help Prevent Cancer? under Food and You or Your Environment, under "C" and also Marvelous Mushrooms – The Magic Food under Food for Thought, below and also Are Rheumatoid Arthritis and Autoimmune Diseases on the Rise? under Food and You or Your Environment, under "R."

Mandarin. See "Tangerine."

Mango [*Fruit*] Mangos contain fiber, carbohydrates, and high levels of Vitamins C, A, and some E, K and B-complex Vitamins (B6 (pyridoxine), B1 (thiamine), B2 (riboflavin)). They also contain copper and the antioxidant beta-carotene. They are known for clearing pores in skin. Great in smoothies.

Mangosteen [*Fruit*] Mangosteen contain fiber, carbohydrates, Vitamin C, and B-complex Vitamins (B9 (folic acid), B1 (thiamine), and B2 (riboflavin)), along with some minerals copper, manganese, and magnesium. The mangosteen plant is an evergreen commonly found in tropical rain forests in Asia.

Maple Syrup [*Sugar (Natural)*] Made from the sap of maple trees, this sweetener contains high amounts of minerals manganese, zinc, calcium, iron, potassium, magnesium, and copper. The high amount of zinc supports reproductive health and helps to keep your white blood cell count up, which assists in protection against colds and viruses. Manganese keeps bones strong and blood sugar levels normal. Maple syrup is filled with anti-inflammatory and antioxidant compounds that may help prevent several chronic and inflammatory diseases. Buy real Canadian maple syrup and use it in recipes instead of sugar and on homemade pancakes.

Maqui [*Fruit*] Maqui contains a huge amount of Vitamin C and minerals calcium, iron, and potassium, along with antioxidants and anti-inflammatory compounds. It has a fruity flavor similar to blackberries and acai. This Patagonian super berry is the fruit of an evergreen shrub. This sacred berry boasts more antioxidants than any other food on Earth. It has been used in both spiritual ceremonies and as staple food for the Mapuche Indians – one of the most ancient indigenous cultures in the world.[84]

Marionberries [*Fruit*] These berries are a cross between Chehalem and Ollallieberry. They are glossy and darker than blackberries and are used to prepare pies, ice creams, jellies, etc. See "Berries" for nutrients and information.

Marrow. See "Bone Marrow."

Marrow [*Vegetable*] Marrow squash, also known as vegetable marrow, is green in color and oval shaped. It can grow to the size of a watermelon. Marrow is a term used by the English to refer to tender vegetables, while in the U.S. the term squash is used. It is related to the zucchini. See "Zucchini" for nutrients and information.

Mashua [*Vegetable*] This tuber is rich in carbohydrates, fiber as well as other nutrients, including beta-carotene, Vitamin C, and all of the essential amino acids. Mashua contains a small amount of protein, although the foliage has a high protein content and it has been suggested that it could be grown for livestock feed. Traditionally used as a diuretic and remedy for kidney ailments, it has been shown to prevent the development of cancerous cells in the stomach, colon, skin, and prostate.[85] It thrives on marginal soils, develops rapidly, and competes successfully with weeds. See also Root Vegetables under Food for Thought, under "R."

Mate. See "Yerba Mate."

Mayapple [*Fruit*] Mayapples contain fiber, carbohydrates, Vitamins C and B5 (pantothenic acid), along with minerals potassium and phosphorous, and some iron. The mayapple plant grows in the wild, mostly covering the forest floor (of the U.S. and southern Canada). In the budding stage, the fruit is green, hard, and poisonous. However, it turns yellow and soft when ripe, and tastes like a tropical fruit. The plant produces podophyllotoxin from the flowers, a compound used in manufacturing an active ingredient in a drug used for treating lung and testicular cancer. [86]

Meat [*Classification*] All sources of food from animals, with the exception of eggs and milk (and their products) are called "meat." Meat contains many vitamins and minerals and is a complete source of protein. Organic or free-range meats have better omega-3 fatty acid profiles and have fewer hormones and antibiotic residues in them. Meat contains high levels of heme iron that is easily absorbed into our systems to help with red blood cell formation. Many North Americans consume too much meat in our current diet, which puts stress on our kidneys and other organs.

Melon [*Fruit*] Melons contain good amounts of Vitamins A, B, and C as well as containing protein, and the minerals calcium and phosphorus. This group of fruit has a high water content and is good for digestion and heartburn. See particular varieties under their specific name (e.g., "Cantaloupe," "Honeydew," and "Watermelon").

Milk [*Dairy*] Traditionally in North America, milk came from cows. Today we can find goat and sheep milk quite readily and llama, yak, and camel milk is used extensively in other cultures. Regardless of the animal, milk is a great source of Vitamins D, A, and B-complex Vitamins (B2 (riboflavin), B5 (pantothenic acid), B1 (thiamine), B12 (cobalamin)), is high in protein, and contains omega-3 fatty acids (especially if cows are allowed to graze). Milk is high in minerals phosphorus, calcium, selenium, zinc, and has some magnesium. The vitamins and minerals of most types of milk are easily absorbed into the body. Milk does contain saturated fat so many choose skim milk. Skim milk is made by separating and removing the fat content from whole milk. This process, however, also strips the milk of its fat-soluble vitamins so skim milk must be fortified with Vitamins A and D to make up for the loss of nutrition. Some health experts are starting to question the benefit of skim milk for those with no history of cholesterol issues because our bodies cannot digest the protein or absorb the calcium from milk without the fat and some research has shown that low-fat and fat-free diets do not help prevent heart disease.[87] But the debate is ongoing. Most of us buy 2%. Many people who are allergic to milk's protein, casein, are able to tolerate other kinds of milk better.

Milk Thistle [*Herb*] This edible plant is often found growing in the wild. The entire plant can be eaten – root, stem, leaves, even the spiny bracts of the flower head. It provides minerals selenium and zinc and the seeds contain iron. The power ingredient in milk thistle is silymarin, which may have protective effects on the liver due to its antioxidant and anti-inflammatory properties. Milk thistle helps boost levels of gluthione, considered one of the best antioxidants that our body produces naturally. Milk Thistle is known to improve milk metabolism in cows and lactating mothers. See "Herbs" for general information. See also Herbaceous Cooking under Healthy You, under "H."

Millet [*Grain*] Millet is a small, round, yellow-colored cereal grain. It contains fiber, carbohydrates, some protein, and small amounts of essential fatty acids. A source of B-complex Vitamins (B1 (thiamine), B2 (riboflavin), B3 (niacin), B9 (folic acid), B6 (pyridoxine)), millet contains minerals magnesium, phosphorus, manganese, copper, zinc, and small amounts of iron. It is gluten-free and high in protein compared to other grains. Millet is believed to strengthen the kidneys and immune system and be beneficial to the stomach, spleen, and pancreas. Millet is rarely served in North America except in bird feeders, but is a leading staple grain in India, and is commonly eaten in China, South America, Russia and the Himalayas. See also "Grains" for general information.

Minerals. See What Your Body Needs and Why.

Minneola [*Fruit*] Minneloas contain fiber, carbohydrates, and good amounts of Vitamins C and B9 (folic acid). They look like tangerines but have a knob-like formation near the stem and are a deep orange color.

Mint [*Herb*] A perennial herb, mint is one of the top five herbs in North America today. Varieties include spearmint, peppermint, lemon, pennyroyal, Brazilian, and Moroccan mint. This herb contains Vitamins A, C, and smaller amounts of B-complex Vitamins (B2 (riboflavin), B1 (thiamine), B12 (cobalamin), B9 (folic acid) and B2 (riboflavin)) along with minerals manganese, copper, iron, potassium, calcium zinc, phosphorus, fluoride and selenium. It is a powerful antioxidant and offers antiseptic and antiviral properties. Mint is known for its ability to relieve indigestion, bloating, congestion. A compress soaked in steeped mint tea and applied to the skin may help alleviate arthritis pain, insect sting irritation, painful burns, muscular pain, or irritation from eczema. See "Herbs" for general information. See also Herbaceous Cooking under Healthy You, under "H."

Miso [*Fermented Food*] Miso is a traditional Japanese seasoning and is produced by fermenting rice, wheat, barley, and/or soy. Loaded with nutrients but also very high in sodium, it contains high amounts of protein, fiber, omega-3 and -6 fatty acids, and huge amounts of Vitamin K. It has very good amounts of B-complex Vitamins (B12 (cobalamin), B2 (riboflavin), B1 (thiamine), B6 (pyridoxine), B3 (niacin), B9 (folic acid), B5 (pantothenic acid)) and high amounts of minerals sodium, manganese, copper, phosphorus, zinc, iron, magnesium, and potassium. Miso played an important nutritional role in feudal Japan and is still widely used in traditional and modern Japanese cooking. Miso has been gaining world-wide interest for its digestive and probiotic immune-boosting benefits. See also Kefir, Kimchee, Kombucha, and Vitamin K! under Food for Thought, under "K" and also Understanding Ancient Foods Today under Food for Thought, under "U."

Mizuna [*Vegetable*] Mizuna is an Oriental vegetable much like mustard greens with similar nutrients. It can be eaten raw or cooked. See "Lettuce" for general nutrients.

Molasses [*Sugar (Natural)*] Molasses contains B-complex Vitamins (B6 (pyridoxine), B3 (niacin), and B5 (pantothenic acid)) along with very high amounts of minerals magnesium, manganese, potassium, copper, selenium, iron, calcium, and some phosphorus. Molasses is a by-product of the sugar refining processes of sugarcane, grapes, or sugar beets and is derived from the Latin word for honey. The quality of molasses depends on the plant, the amount of sugar extracted, and the refinement method.

Mollusks [*Shellfish*] This particular classification includes squid, octopus, scallops, clams, mussels, and oysters. See particular species under their specific name. (For information on sustainable fish see "Fish" or visit *www.msc.org/cook-eat-enjoy/fish-to-eat*.)

Monkfish [*Fish*] Monkfish is a good source of protein and omega-3 fatty acids. It contains good amounts of B-complex Vitamins (B3 (niacin), B12 (cobalamin), and B6 (pyridoxine)) and minerals selenium and phosphorus. (For information on sustainable fish see "Fish" or visit *www.msc.org/cook-eat-enjoy/fish-to-eat*.)

Moose [*Meat*] Moose is extremely high in protein, B-complex Vitamins (B12 (cobalamin), B6 (pyridoxine), B3 (niacin), B2 (riboflavin), and B1 (thiamine)), and minerals zinc, iron, selenium, phosphorus, potassium, magnesium, and copper along with some healthy omega-3 fatty acids. Moose is a wild game and a healthy alternative to factory-raised meats.

Moringa [*Vegetable*] Moringa contains high amounts of fiber, protein, Vitamin A, and minerals calcium, iron, and potassium. All parts of the moringa tree are consumed as food or used medicinally, including the leaves (fresh and dried), bark, flowers, fruit, seeds, and root. Referred to as the miracle tree for third world countries because it is easy to grow and highly nutritious, it also produces animal feed, cleansers, medicine, fertilizer, and rope fiber. When used in cattle feed, moringa increases milk production up to 65% according to information from World Vision.

Mottled Beans. See "Pinto Beans."

Mulberries [*Fruit*] Mulberries contain carbohydrates, fiber, and are high in Vitamin C and iron. They contain some other B-complex Vitamins, including B2 (riboflavin), along with Vitamins E and K, and some of the minerals potassium and magnesium. Containing half the sugar found in other fruit, mulberries are high in antioxidants like resveratrol, lutein, and zeaxanthin. See also "Berries" for general information.

Mushrooms [*Fungi*] All mushrooms are high in protein, loaded with Vitamin D, and are a good source of B-complex Vitamins, especially B3 (niacin), B2 (riboflavin) and B5 (pantothenic acid) and some have very small amounts of B12 (cobalamin). Mushrooms also have high amounts of minerals selenium and good amounts of iron, zinc, copper, and potassium. They are packed with antioxidants, a proven immune system booster, and are good for your bladder.[88] Drying is the most common method of preserving mushrooms. Researchers are just starting to identify the incredible nutrition in mushrooms. There are six main types of edible mushrooms, including cremini, enoki, oyster, portobello, shiitake, and white button. Ganoderma is a bitter mushroom (also known as reishi) that has long been a popular herb in Chinese medicine and is attributed to assisting in longevity and good health but is generally too bitter to eat.[89] All varieties of edible mushrooms contain purines, which can be broken down to form uric acid, so they are not recommended for sufferers of gout or kidney stones but very safe for everyone else. See also specific varieties for nutrients and information. See also Marvelous Mushrooms – The Magic Food under Food for Thought, below. See also Are Rheumatoid Arthritis and Autoimmune Diseases on the Rise? under Food and You or Your Environment, under "R."

Mussels [*Shellfish*] Mussels are high in protein and omega-3 fatty acids. They also contain Vitamin C and B-complex Vitamins (B12 (cobalamin), B1 (thiamine), B2 (riboflavin), B3 (niacin), and B9 (folic acid)), and minerals manganese, selenium, iron, phosphorus, and zinc. (For information on sustainable fish see "Fish" or visit *www.msc.org/cook-eat-enjoy/fish-to-eat*.) See also "Shellfish" for general information.

Mustard Greens [*Vegetable*] Mustard greens are the leaves of the mustard plant and they contain fiber, carbohydrates, huge amounts of Vitamins A, K, and C, some E, and B-complex Vitamins (B1 (thiamine), B3 (niacin), B6 (pyridoxine), B2 (riboflavin), and B9 (folic acid)), along with minerals manganese, calcium, potassium, phosphorus, iron, and copper. They are rich in antioxidants, including beta-carotene, lutein, and zeaxanthin. Mustard greens are considered a power food because of their nutritional density. They are added to stews or steamed and mixed with other greens such as spinach, fenugreek, etc. Because of its high Vitamin K content, patients taking anti-coagulants such as warfarin are best to avoid this food as Vitamin K assists with building clotting factors that for most other people are highly beneficial. See What Foods Fight or Help Prevent Cancer? under Food and You or Your Environment, under "C."

Mustard Seed [*Spice*] Mustard seed contains fiber, protein, and minerals calcium, iron, phosphorus, magnesium, manganese, and good amounts of selenium. Known as a spice, they are used regularly in cooking and as oil in south Asia. See "Spices" for general information and cooking suggestions.

FOOD FOR THOUGHT

Marvelous Mushrooms – The Magic Food

Mushrooms are fungi. Fungi are as different from plants as plants are from animals. They don't get their energy from the sun but rather get nutrients they need from the ground or from the trees on which they grow. Fungi recycle plants after they die and transform them into rich soil. If it weren't for mushrooms and fungi, the Earth would be buried in several feet of debris and life on the planet would not be sustainable.

The spores of mushrooms are made of chitin, the hardest naturally-made substance on Earth. A mushroom cap is the part of the fungus that you can see; beneath the surface of the soil is the mycelium, a network of thin fibers that act as the root. This incredible mycelium can grow for years or even centuries before the mushroom pops up and can spread out over acres and acres. Mushrooms can live for an incredible length of time and certain types have been found to be thousands of years old.

Paul Stamets,[90] a mushroom expert, believes that growing more mushrooms may be the best thing we can do to save the environment as then we can capitalize on mycelium's digestive power and use it to decompose toxic wastes and pollutants (mycoremediation), catch and reduce silt from streambeds and pathogens from agricultural watersheds (mycofiltration), control insect populations (mycopesticides), and generally enhance the health of our forests and gardens (mycoforestry and mycogardening). In addition to being used to absorb and digest dangerous substances like oil, pesticides, and industrial waste, mushrooms are used extensively for their medicinal properties and, of course, for a variety of delicious and nutritious recipes and dishes.

Mushrooms – Are they really magic?

Ancient hieroglyphics from more than 4,600 years ago tell us Egyptians called mushrooms "the magic food." They believed eating them resulted in immortality, and only pharaohs were given this privilege so that they could live forever. The Romans described mushrooms as "foods of the gods" and believed that they were created by the lightning rods thrown down to earth by the god Jupiter. Other ancient civilizations in places such as Russia and Mexico thought mushrooms had ingredients that could produce superhuman strength and could even help locate lost objects.

Over the past several decades, scientific research has intensified and focused on analyzing the hundreds of unique bio-active compounds found in the medicinal shitake, reishi, coridus, maitake, chaga, and cordyceps mushrooms. There is now a wealth of impressive data that demonstrates reishi's life-extending properties but also its significant ability to stimulate brain neurons, search and destroy cancer cells, and prevent the development of new fat cells in obese individuals. In addition, these mushroom's numerous compounds show a therapeutic effect on asthma, allergies, autoimmune diseases, Alzheimer's and Parkinson's diseases, diabetes, liver disease, and more. Asians eat up to four time more mushrooms than North Americans and their health benefits from it. So eating more mushrooms may be a good idea!

Mushrooms can be highly nutritious, but some types are very deadly so foraging for wild mushrooms is best done with an expert only. Some wild mushrooms like morels are tasty and popular to "hunt" for those who are trained foragers. Mushrooms have been known in fairy tales to be magical and psilocybin mushrooms are a hallucinogenic. Some scientists suspect that mushroom spores are capable of space travel; a few even believe that some fungi found on Earth originally came from outer space![91] Mushrooms are still a great and marvelous mystery and I believe we will continue to learn more and more about their incredible nutritional, health, and environmental benefits in years to come.

FOOD AND YOU OR YOUR ENVIRONMENT

Menopause – Can Food Help the Transition?

I have talked to a lot of women lately who are complaining about menopause symptoms and are eager to find ways to reduce symptoms. One was always getting hot flashes, even at work, and had embarrassing sweat marks on her clothing. One had migraines, another had terrible mood fluctuations, and a third kept complaining of memory problems.

Menopause brings an end to the monthly menstruation cycles that women have to endure for their right to be fertile and give birth. The transition starts with perimenopause, which can last up to a year or more, during which time the body prepares gradually for the menstruation cycle to cease. The main hormone that declines during menopause is estrogen and as levels begin to decline, the brain registers the change as well, which can, in turn, effect the production of mood-regulating chemicals, including serotonin and endorphins. The most common health problems experienced during transition include hot flashes, mood swings, and memory issues.

After menopause, some women face increased risk of possible health issues, including osteoporosis, heart disease, stroke, and breast cancer. The good news is that many of the symptoms of menopause and the increased health risks can be prevented with good nutrition. Getting enough nutrition can help reduce side effects and improve mood, memory, and bone health.

> Menopause is a natural process and it can be a smooth transition with good nutrition.

Below are my top recommendations to help smoothly move your body into the next exciting life phase and make menopause an easy and natural process.

1. **Apples:** Apples contain high levels of quercetin (mostly found in the skin), an antioxidant that has been shown in recent studies to protect against memory loss. Apples also contain both soluble and insoluble fiber that helps regulate cholesterol.
2. **Ground Flax Seed:** *Ground* flax seed has omega-3 fatty acids and lignans, which act as phytoestrogens. Results from studies have been mixed, but it may help symptoms in some women. It

is also believed to help lower cholesterol. Avoid whole flax seeds because they are difficult to digest.

3. **Kale:** This leafy green contains high amounts of iron *and* magnesium, both important for our heart and circulation, supporting heart health, and regulating mood.

4. **Sage:** An herb that is high in nutrients and antioxidants, sage has been studied for its benefits on hot flashes with some promise. Other than adding it to food, it can be taken as a tea or used in cooking.

5. **Steel-cut Oats:** Also referred to as "Scottish oats," steel-cut oats are an excellent source of soluble and insoluble fiber. They are also high in B-complex Vitamins (B1 (thiamine), B2 (riboflavin), B3 (niacin), B-6 (pyridoxine) and B9 (folic acid)), which help to balance and regulate moods associated with menopause by helping with dopamine and serotonin production (the happy hormones). Besides helping balance mood, these vitamins aid in metabolism. Additionally the soluble fiber found in oats helps reduce cholesterol as it binds to cholesterol molecules in your intestinal tract, preventing it from entering your bloodstream.

6. **Tempeh:** Fermented soy has isoflavones, which are phytoestrogens (plant estrogen). Plant-based foods that have isoflavones work in the body like a weak form of estrogen and may help relieve menopausal symptoms. Some may help lower cholesterol levels and have been suggested to relieve hot flashes and night sweats.

7. **Yogurt:** A fermented dairy product, high quality plain yogurt delivers high and easily absorbable amounts of calcium and Vitamin D, both critical for bone health, which is much needed as we age. The probiotics in yogurt also boost our immune system and improve our intestinal flora. Stay away from processed brands and stick to plain varieties and add your own berries or natural sweetener for added taste.

Supplements that have been studied to help with menopausal symptoms include dong quai for balancing hormones, black cohosh for reducing hot flashes, and evening primrose oil (evening primrose oil is rich in gamma-linolenic acid (GLA), a fatty acid involved in the production of hormone-like substances called prostaglandins that are thought to help counter hormonal changes associated with menopause). Other supplements that are believed to help are eucalyptus, motherwort tea, red clover, black haw, fennel, anise, and wild yam. Always check with your doctor or health-care provider before starting any additional supplements for menopause or any health condition, especially if you are taking any medications.

Menopause can be viewed as the gateway to a new beginning. Some women will decide to use hormone replacement therapy and others will decide against it. Many women start a new career or life direction after menopause and feel a stronger sense of self and a deeper life purpose. Not having to deal with the aggravation of monthly cycles can be liberating. Taking time to meditate, connect with nature, and spend time exercising will also help the transition be easier and reduce uncomfortable side effects for most.

HEALTHY YOU

Money and Health – How to Create and Keep Both

Does having more money mean that we will be healthier? Not necessarily.

Having more money means we can buy expensive health club memberships and take time for relaxing holidays. But many wealthy people are so busy trying to maintain their wealth that they forget to look after their health or become burned out with work demands. Ed Diener, a researcher who has spent over 30 years studying well-being, postulates that a higher income may mean more work, less leisure time, and fewer strong social connections.

On the other hand, not having enough money doesn't allow us to meet our basic needs like food, shelter, and health care. Anyone with debt knows that it also contributes to stress, which can lead to health issues and that isn't good either. Buying fast food is cheaper than whole food, so rates of diabetes 2 and obesity are higher among the poor. Organic food is expensive and many of us cannot afford it on a regular basis so money helps there.

So what is the right balance?

No matter how healthy your bank account is, or isn't, take time each day to attend to your other health needs by exercising, eating better, and reducing your stress. Over time, you will develop a sustainable health-wealth equilibrium that you can maintain for a lifetime. That way when a job or other financial loss occurs, your health will not suffer since you have taken time to save for a rainy day. Likewise, if your career takes off, you will have the discipline to not let work dominate your life so you can stay focused on the most important things, including health, happiness, and taking time to be connected to the world around you in meaningful ways.

*"He who distinguishes the true savor of his food
can never be a glutton; he who does not cannot be otherwise."*
Henry David Thoreau (1817-1862,
American writer, poet, philosopher)

Nutty for Nuts

Growing up a friend of mine was hypoglycemic, meaning she had low
blood sugar. There could be serious side effects if her blood sugar
dipped too low so she would always carry around different types of
nuts in her pocket and eat them – right in class – if she felt the need!

Today, there are so many nut allergies that schools have strict policies against bringing them to school. I am careful to avoid any nut
products when I pack my sons' lunches but offer nuts to them as
snacks at night and on the weekends because they are a high quality
source of protein and loaded with nutrients.

REAL "N" FOODS

Natto [*Fermented Food*] Made from fermented soybeans, natto is
high in protein, fiber, carbohydrates, and fatty acids. It has good
amounts of Vitamins C, K, and B-complex Vitamins (B1 (thiamine), B2 (riboflavin), B6 (pyridoxine,) and some B5 (pantothenic acid) and B9 (folic acid)). It has good amounts of
minerals manganese, iron, calcium, magnesium, phosphorus,
potassium, zinc, copper, and selenium. Natto originated in Japan
around 1,000 years ago. It is made of fermented, cooked whole

soybeans and is fermented without bacteria. It has a cottage cheese-like texture and strong smell. Traditionally it is served as a topping for rice, in miso soups, or added to vegetables. In Japan, it is even eaten for breakfast with eggs. See also Kefir, Kimchee, Kombucha, and Vitamin K! under Food for Thought, under "K" and also Understanding Ancient Foods Today under Food for Thought, under "U."

Navy Beans [*Vegetable (Legume)*] Also referred to as white beans, these legumes provide an excellent plant source of fiber, carbohydrates, and protein. Navy beans are also a good source of B-complex Vitamins (B1 (thiamine) and B9 (folic acid)), and minerals manganese, phosphorus, copper, magnesium, and iron. See also "Legumes" for general information.

Nectarine [*Fruit*] Nectarines contain fiber, carbohydrates and are high in Vitamins C, K and B9 (folic acid). They also contain minerals potassium and small amounts of copper as well as naturally occurring sugars that help provide energy. Often erroneously believed to be a crossbreed between peaches and plums, nectarines belong to the same species as peaches.

Nightshade [*Vegetable Classification*] This category includes vegetables like peppers, tomatoes, and potatoes. Nightshade plants are nutrient- and antioxidant-rich and a great choice. They also have a substance that some believe may worsen degenerative joint diseases but research is inconclusive and many experts believe they have no effect on arthritis or osteoarthritis. See specific foods for particular nutritional information.

Noodles [*Grain-based*] Noodles contain fiber, carbohydrates, many B-complex Vitamins, small amounts of protein, and other nutrients depending upon the source of the flour used to produce them. The common pasta was made from Durham and semolina wheat traditionally. Today noodles can be made from many grains or legumes. The dough for East Asian noodles, for instance, can

be made from wheat, rice, buckwheat, or mung bean starch. Usually used in soups or on their own with sauces, noodles in their
many varieties are eaten in many cultures around the world.
Some of the most common Italian types of noodles made with
Durham wheat include: spaghetti (most common), spaghettini
(spaghetti's thinner cousin), vermicelli (slightly thicker than
spaghettini), capellini (thinnest of the long noodles), fusilli/rotini
(shape of coiled rods), lasagna (wide, flat noodles), fettuccine/lin-
guine (flattened ribbons), cannelloni/manicotti (large tubes
meant for stuffing), penne/rigatoni (small–medium tubes), farfalle
(butterfly or bow tie shaped), ravioli/tortellini (stuffed pasta), and
orzo (rice shaped) pasta. Other cultures also create their own
noodles made from different ingredients: spatzle (German pasta
made from Durham wheat and eggs), soba (Japanese noodles
made from buckwheat), udon (thick Japanese noodles made from
wheat), ramon (thin Japanese noodles made from wheat), bean
threads (Japanese noodles made from mung bean starch), vermicelli (thin noodles made from rice), and rice noodles (thicker
noodles made from rice). With the increase in gluten-related
issues, more noodles are being made with other gluten-free
grains, including lentils and corn.

Nori [*Vegetable (Sea)*] Nori is a red seaweed that is commonly used
in the making of sushi. It also contains good amounts of protein,
and is a good source of Vitamins A, B9 (folic acid), and B3
(niacin). Fresh nori is a good source of Vitamin C, but the shelf
life for this nutrient after processing is fairly short. A good source
of iron for people eating rice-based meals, nori consumption
could have a beneficial effect on cholesterol levels.

Nutmeg [*Spice*] Nutmeg contains good amounts of fiber, protein,
fatty acids, along with Vitamins A, C, and B-complex Vitamins
(B6 (pyridoxine), B9 (folic acid), and B1 (thiamine), and B2
(riboflavin) and B3 (niacin) in trivial amounts). Nutmeg contains

very high amounts of minerals copper, manganese, magnesium, calcium, potassium, phosphorus, and iron. This spice tree is a large evergreen plant that thrives well under tropical climates, but originated in the Indonesian rain forest. The seeds are grated to form the powdered nutmeg we use today. The active principles in nutmeg have many therapeutic applications in traditional medicines as an antifungal, antidepressant, aphrodisiac, digestive, and carminative. See "Spices" for general information and cooking suggestions.

Nuts [*Classification*] All nuts are high in protein and minerals, and rich in omega–3 fatty acids, Vitamin E, and fiber. They're a powerhouse of protein, fiber, calcium, and magnesium, and contain both healthy mono- and polyunsaturated oils. A nut is a fruit composed of a hard shell and a seed, which is edible, and the shell does not open to release the seed. Nuts are great as energy-boosting snacks and add flavor and protein to many cooked dishes. The major nuts eaten today include almonds, Brazil nuts, cashews, chestnuts, coconuts, hazelnuts, macadamia nuts, peanuts, pecans, pine nuts, pistachios, and walnuts. See particular species under their specific name.

FOOD FOR THOUGHT

Natural Remedies

Eighty percent of the world's population relies on natural remedies for their health and wellness according to *Prescription for Natural Cures*.[92] Physicians in countries from Germany to China commonly suggest herbs alongside conventional pharmaceuticals[93] and are successfully treating more aches and pains. More people in Western countries are seeking alternative therapies for a range of conditions, including chronic ones.

> Always check with your doctor before exploring alternative treatments.

Today, in an integrated health facility, a medical doctor, osteopathic doctor, naturopath, Chinese medicine or Ayurveda practitioner may recommend a herbal remedy or alternative treatment during an office visit for a specific health problem first, before prescribing drugs or offer both options to address whole health from a holistic perspective.[94] Other than biological-based healing practices, there are numerous other natural healing tools, including aromatherapy, biofeedback, detoxification, reiki massage, acupuncture, meditation, chiropractic, tai chi, etc. The most common conditions for which people seek complementary or alternative therapies are back pain, head or chest colds, neck pain, joint stiffness and arthritis, anxiety and depression, stomach or intestinal issues, migraines, pain, insomnia, high cholesterol, asthma, and menopause. It is important to always check with your doctor or health-care provider before exploring alternative treatments as even herbal remedies with scientifically proven benefits may carry hidden side effects or interfere with medication.

Below are some of the herbal or alternative remedies offered for certain ailments or diseases to help alleviate pain. It is good to buy from a high quality source to ensure maximum benefit and absorption.

- **Antibiotic Properties:** garlic, oregano oil, bee propolis, goldenseal, olive leaf, royal jelly, aloe vera, grapefruit seed extract (do not take for extended periods of time, as they will reduce healthy bacteria similarly to prescription antibiotics).
- **Anxiety:** lemon balm, linden, alfalfa, motherwort, skullcap, green tea, St. John's wort, valerian, kava root, passionflower, holy basil, California poppy tincture, lavender, gaba, natural sources of tryptophan like spirulina, mushrooms, cheese, turkey and other meat especially wild game, nuts, B-complex Vitamins, ginkgo, feverfew, l-theanine, valerian root, omega-3 fatty acids (from sources such as fish oil, flax seed oil, nuts, cold water fish), chamomile, lavender, meditation, massage, shiatsu, and tai chi.

- **Arthritis:** white willow bark, cayenne, cat's claw, yucca root tea, capsaicin, calendula, turmeric root tea or turmeric spice, bromelain (found in pineapple and papaya), glucosamine, chondroitin, acupuncture, yoga, massage, tai chi, traumeel creams, arnica cream
- **Digestion Issues:** artichoke leaf extract, peppermint tea/oil, caraway oil, ginger, astragalus, chamomile, probiotics, carob, digestive enzymes, papaya, pineapple, apple cider vinegar, grape seed extract, fennel seeds, catnip leaf, lemon balm, olive leaf extract, garlic, oregano oil, berberine, pau d'arco, aromatic bitters, reduced consumption of starchy carbohydrates
- **Fatigue:** ginseng, reishi mushrooms, herbal tea, water, coffee (only in the morning and in small quantities), yerbe mate, astragalus
- **High Cholesterol:** alfalfa, fenugreek, dandelion root, flax, pumpkin seeds, soluble fiber (psyllium, oats), carob, chocolate, apple peels, seeds, red rice yeast extract (do not take with statin drugs), Vitamin B3 (niacin), artichoke leaf, coenzyme Q10, green tea
- **Immune Boost:** aloe vera, garlic, goldenseal, licorice, echinacea, reishi, chaga and shiitake mushrooms, Vitamins A, E, C, zinc, selenium, orango-germanium, marigold, astragalus, St. John's wort, liver supporting foods such as the cruciferous vegetable family
- **Memory:** gingko biloba, panax ginseng, centella asiatica, lycopodium clavatum, peppermint, rosemary oil, basil, lemon/orange/grapefruit extract, eucalyptus, vinpocetine, soaked almonds
- **Sleep Disorders:** valerian, holy basil, chamomile, foods rich in magnesium, foods rich in tryptophan, melatonin, kava, SAM, melatonin, 5-HTP, aromatherapy, acupuncture, exercise, music, meditation and relaxation techniques, feng shui, tai chi, reduced light, elimination of caffeine after 12 noon[95]

When picking a Naturopath or Alternative Medicine practitioner, do your homework to find one with a good reputation and happy customers. Also, remember to check with your doctor to make sure natural remedies you want to try don't interfere with current medications and stop immediately if you experience any side effects. If you prefer to stick to your doctor's prescriptions, that is fine, just add healthier and nutrient-dense food to your diet and this could help you in your journey to health as well.

FOOD AND YOU OR YOUR ENVIRONMENT

Can Nature Feed the Soul?

Nature supplies us food. Humanity has eaten more than 80,000 plants through it evolution. But nature is also a major source of renewal and rejuvenation for many people.

According to Diana Beresford-Kroeger[96] humans and nature share a unique relationship. The red blood cells flowing through our bodies are made up of hemoglobin molecules, which are donut-shaped sacs. This design is similar to the green pigment in plants called a "chloroplast," which has sacs containing green chlorophyll molecules. The two molecules, hemoglobin and chlorophyll, the red and the green, have a unique and beautiful symbiotic relationship that is key to mutual survival. Without plants we simply would not survive as a species on the planet.

> **Without plants we simply would not survive as a species on the planet.**

Both red blood cells and chloroplasts have an incredibly similar design with four rings that contain nitrogen. Sitting in the center position of these rings is an atom of metal. The nitrogen in both holds the atom of iron, in the case of hemoglobin, and magnesium, in the case of chlorophyll. Both these metals work together like a great quantum pendulum. Oxygen is passed into the human hemoglobin molecule when the plant expires and carbon dioxide is passed into the plant system when humans expire. Plants breathe in CO_2, and during photosynthesis they break apart the carbon and oxygen molecules, keeping the carbon to build and fuel their bodies and releasing the oxygen for humans.[97] It is a perfect system created for life between species.

Today, many people suffer from "nature deficiency." They spend most of their time indoors, working under artificial fluorescent lights, eating and sleeping inside, commuting in the artificial environment of a car, bus or train, expending limited time in the outdoors except the odd time to mow our artificially uniform lawns.

Spending time in nature has incredible benefits, including increased exposure to Vitamin D through sunlight, which boosts immune function, and exposure to natural sounds, especially water in streams and rain, known to have a healing and relaxing effect. In addition, exposure to the different colors of nature or different wavelengths is a form of energy medicine called light therapy and spending more time outdoors allows your brain to explore a more diverse natural reality causing it to function at a higher level.[98] Being in nature also promotes physical movement and exercise comes naturally. Getting exposure to fresh air, versus sterile indoor air, is important for our lungs and breathing fresh air is energizing and healing. Getting your hands dirty is great for kids and adults alike and the current obsession with sterility and antimicrobial soaps and cleansers are not actually helpful to our health as there is concern that all these antibacterial products may actually be contributing to the resistance of bacteria to medications that we currently use to kill them.

Beyond the light, the sounds, the air, and all the other healing elements of nature, there's also something powerful, namely, the spiritual connection we feel with nature. In some way that scientists still don't understand, lush living ecosystems "recharge" the human body and mind. Spending time in nature rejuvenates your system and boost your energy. Some people say that being electrically "grounded" with the earth (through barefoot walking) makes an important difference in reducing the electric "noise" that interferes with our health. By walking barefoot over open countryside, early man was inadvertently enjoying the benefits of reflexology, a therapeutic form of foot massage.[99] A 2010 study in environmental psychology found individuals walking outdoors reported greater vitality compared with indoor walkers.

A new growing field is called "ecotherapy" and it encourages us to use nature to heal. Howard Clinebell, the first to use the term, defined ecotherapy as "healing and growth nurtured by healthy interaction with the earth."[100] For example, people report they feel more relaxed and their blood pressure levels drop after being outdoors. Adults and teens both report increased self-esteem, self-confidence, patience, cooperation, and have a more positive outlook and view of other people when they spent more time outside. Spending time in nature has positive impacts on those dealing with more serious issues, such as depression, anxiety, and ADHD. For example, in Holland, people who live within one kilometer (a little more than a half mile) of a park or wooded area experience less anxiety and depression than those living farther away. Participants in a study in England reported declines in their levels of depression when they spent time walking outside. Research also shows that being in nature can help those with concentration problems such as ADHD. Time in nature enhances our ability to focus and perform better academically, as several studies of school children have shown. In some towns, teachers are taking hyperactive children outside for a quick walk before class to help them concentrate during the school day.[101]

Humans have shared a special bond with nature for thousands of years. It can heal, restore, energize, and nourish our spirits. It might be a great idea to spend more time outside and ensure that forests are protected and diverse and majestic trees are preserved for future generations to enjoy.

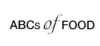

HEALTHY YOU

They're Not Just for Squirrels

Nuts are a power food and packed with health benefits. New medical research suggests that eating high-protein foods, such as nuts, can stabilize blood sugar levels, so include them as high-quality snacks daily.

Nuts do have lots of fat but it is largely polyunsaturated or monounsaturated and can actually lower your LDL, or bad, cholesterol. Nuts have huge amounts of minerals like magnesium and calcium and are packed full of protein, so they make a good vegetarian choice for meatless Mondays and help to fuel our bodies and energize us. Nuts also have large amounts of Vitamin E, a powerful antioxidant that has been identified as having anti-aging effects on the body by neutralizing damage from free radicals. They also contain gamma-tocopherol, a variety of Vitamin E, that helps protect against many cancers. They are full of anti-inflammatory omega-3 fatty acids.

Many nuts contain high amounts of salt so try to source minimally processed or salted nuts or eat them raw. The only downside is that nuts are calorie dense so don't eat a ton at once!

"I hate people who are not serious about meals.
It is so shallow of them."
Oscar Wilde, from *The Importance of Being Earnest*
(1854-11900, Irish writer and poet)

Are Organs Food?

When I was a kid we went to visit my great aunt in the city. She was an older woman and never had kids – and truth be told, I'm not sure she really liked kids – but we liked the pool located at the top of her high-rise apartment.

After our swim we went back to her apartment for lunch. She served an array of jellied salads and luncheon meats – not really great kid fare. But there, in the middle of the platter, was a meat my sisters and I had never seen before. "What is that?" my sister blurted out.

My mom took her aside and quietly told her it was tongue. "Tongue!" exclaimed my young sibling. "I'm not eating anything that came out of a cow's mouth!"

My mom quickly responded that "Organ meat was very healthy and just where did she think eggs came from anyway?"

REAL "O" FOODS

Oakleaf Lettuce [*Vegetable*] Oakleaf lettuce contains fiber, carbohydrates, and Vitamins A, C, K, and B9 (folic acid), along with very small amounts of minerals copper, iron, calcium, potassium, phosphorus, and manganese. See also "Lettuce" for general information.

Oats [*Grain*] Unique among grains, oats almost never have their bran and germ removed in processing so you are always eating the whole grain. Whole grain oats are high in fiber, carbohydrates, B-complex Vitamins (B1 (thiamine), B2 (riboflavin), B3 (niacin), B6 (pyridoxine), B9 (folic acid)), and are a good source of minerals manganese, magnesium, phosphorus, zinc, copper, selenium, and iron. Oats also contain antioxidants and in most cases are safe for gluten-sensitive individuals to consume. Steel-cut oats contain the highest level of nutrients as they are minimally processed. See also "Grains" for general information. See also What's to be Done about the Rise in Heart Disease? under Food and You or Your Environment, under "H" and also Menopause – Can Food Help the Transition? under Food and You or Your Environment, under "M."

Oca [*Vegetable*] Oca is tuber that contains high amounts of carbohydrate and small amounts of fiber. It is a good source of Vitamin A, and also contains Vitamin B6 (pyridoxine), potassium, and beta-carotene. Yellow-orange colored varieties indicate the presence of carotenoids, while red skins and red specks in flesh indicate the presence of anthocyanin. A staple of rural Andean diets for centuries, oca is important because of its role in crop rotations and its high nutritional content.

Octopus [*Shellfish*] Octopus is high in protein and omega-3 fatty acids and contains Vitamins C, A and B-complex Vitamins (B12 (cobalamin), B6 (pyridoxine), B3 (niacin), and B5 (pantothenic acid)). It also has minerals selenium, iron, calcium, zinc, potassium, phosphorus, magnesium, calcium, copper, and sodium. (For information on sustainable fish see "Fish" or visit *www.msc.org/cook-eat-enjoy/fish-to-eat.*)

Oils [*Fat*] Cooking and salad oils come about through extraction and refinement processes of fruits (oil, grape seeds, avocado), vegetables (corn), grains (canola, safflower), nuts (walnut, almond), seeds (flax seed, sesame seed), and meat (lard and rendering of products like bacon). Oils are important to our health for their essential fatty acids that cannot be made within the body. Omega-3 plays an important role in the preservation of healthy heart and brain function and the normal growth and development of the body. Oils also contain omega-6 and omega-9 fatty acids. There are two main types of oils: saturated and unsaturated (monounsaturated and polyunsaturated). While we tend to think of saturated fats (butter and lard) as coming from animal sources, there are some vegetable sources, including coconut, cottonseed, and palm kernel oils, and chocolate. Unsaturated oils come from a variety of plant sources. Monounsaturated fats include canola, olive, peanut, avocado, almond, pecan, and cashew oils. Polyunsaturated oils come from safflower, sesame and sunflower seeds, corn, soybeans, and many nuts and seeds. Some fats have a higher "smoke temperature" making them better for high temperature cooking, like frying (canola, grape seed, coconut, and peanut oils). Others are better for salads (olive, avocado, or flax seed oils) and some taste better in baking, like butter. A list of other oils used both for cooking and medicinally is long as it would also include primrose oil, borage oil, pumpkin oil, hemp oil, walnut and hazelnut oil, mustard seed oil, macadamia oil, etc. See War of the Spreadable Oils under Food for Thought, below.

Okra [*Vegetable*] Okra contains fiber, carbohydrates, and some protein and fatty acids. Also found in okra are Vitamins A, C, B6 (pyridoxine), B9 (folic acid), minerals iron, calcium, manganese, copper, and zinc, and the antioxidant beta-carotene. The leaves are eaten raw in salads. Okra grows very well in warm climates, producing high yields.

Olives [*Fruit*] Olives contain omega-6 and omega-3 fatty acids and high amounts of Vitamins E, K, and A, along with small amounts of B-complex Vitamins (B1 (thiamine), B2 (riboflavin), B3 (niacin), B5 (pantothenic acid), and B6 (pyridoxine)), antioxidants lutein and zeaxanthin, and minerals calcium, magnesium, potassium, phosphorus, and copper. While they are technically a fruit, olives are considered vegetables because of how they are used. There are many varieties of olives, including black, green, niçoise, kalamata, and manzanilla. Green olives are olives that were picked before they are ripened. Black olives were picked ripe and dipped in an iron solution to stabilize their color. Olives play a prominent role in the healthy Mediterranean diet. Greeks have been aware of the many health benefits of olive oil for thousands of years. In fact the Greek physician Hippocrates is said to have referred to olive oil as "the great therapeutic." To begin with, olive oil's high monounsaturated fat decreases LDL (bad) cholesterol while raising HDL (good) cholesterol, thereby potentially lowering the risk of heart disease.[102] In fact, the U.S. Food and Drug Administration has officially credited olive oil with decreasing the risk of coronary artery disease. This good fat also acts as an anti-inflammatory, helping to reduce and relieve symptoms caused by inflammatory diseases such rheumatoid arthritis. See also What's to be Done about the Rise in Heart Disease? under Food and You or Your Environment, under "H" and also Are Rheumatoid Arthritis and Autoimmune Diseases on the Rise? under Food and You or Your Environment, under "R."

Onion Powder [*Spice*] Onion powder contains Vitamins B6 (pyridoxine), B9 (folic acid), and a small amount of calcium. Using fresh onions is always best for nutrients and flavor. See "Spices" for general information and cooking suggestions.

Onions [*Vegetable*] Onions are a good source of fiber, carbohydrates, Vitamins A (green tops), C, K, and B-complex Vitamins (B1 (thiamine), B6 (pyridoxine), and B9 (folic acid), and minerals calcium, selenium, and chromium. Onions provide a rich source of the antioxidant quercetin, which is known to play a significant role in preventing cancer. Onions, like garlic, contain sulfur which is good for the liver and helps with detoxification. The phytochemicals in onions improve Vitamin C's function in the body, giving you improved immunity. Onions contain chromium, which assists in regulating blood sugar. For centuries, onions have been used to reduce inflammation and heal infections. They are known for antiviral, antifungal, antibacterial, and improved blood circulation properties. Raw onion encourages the production of good cholesterol (HDL), thus keeping your heart healthy. Onions scavenge free radicals, thereby reducing your risk of developing gastric ulcers.[103] Onions are a power food but sometimes people avoid them for fear of bad breathe. Sucking on a lemon, eating parsley or mint, or drinking green or mint tea can quickly neutralize any odor in the mouth. See What Foods Fight or Help Prevent Cancer? under Food and You or Your Environment, under "C" and also Root Vegetables under Food for Thought, under "R."

Orange Roughy [*Fish*] Orange roughy is a good source of protein and omega-3 fatty acids. It contains good amounts of B-complex Vitamins (B3 (niacin), B12 (cobalamin), and B6 (pyridoxine)), and minerals selenium and phosphorus. (For information on sustainable fish see "Fish" or visit *www.msc.org/cook-eat-enjoy/fish-to-eat*.)

Oranges [*Fruit*] The most popular of the citrus fruits, oranges contain fiber, carbohydrates, Vitamins C and A, and good amounts of B-complex Vitamins (B1 (thiamine), B5 (pantothenic acid), and B9 (folic acid)) along with small amounts of minerals calcium, magnesium, copper, and potassium. The peel or zest can be used to prepare delicious dishes and dried orange blossoms and leaves are used in herbal teas.

Oregano [*Herb*] A perennial herb, oregano is a particularly good source of iron, manganese and Vitamin K, as well as fiber, Vitamins

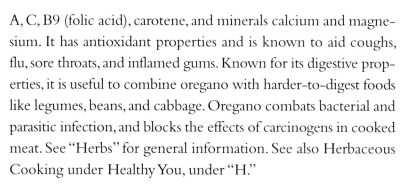

A, C, B9 (folic acid), carotene, and minerals calcium and magnesium. It has antioxidant properties and is known to aid coughs, flu, sore throats, and inflamed gums. Known for its digestive properties, it is useful to combine oregano with harder-to-digest foods like legumes, beans, and cabbage. Oregano combats bacterial and parasitic infection, and blocks the effects of carcinogens in cooked meat. See "Herbs" for general information. See also Herbaceous Cooking under Healthy You, under "H."

Oregon Grape [*Fruit*] They have a grape-like appearance and are purple or blue in color. They look as if they are covered in powder. They are known to be anti-inflammatory and antibacterial in nature. See "Berries" for nutrients and information.

Organ Meats [*Meat*] Organ meats such as liver, heart, and kidney contain the highest concentrations of many daily requirements of nutrients, including Vitamin A (431% of daily requirement), B12 (cobalamin) (800% of daily requirement), Vitamin D (30%), B-complex (B1 (thiamine), B2 (riboflavin), B3 (niacin), B6 (pyridoxine), and B5 (pantothenic acid)), iron (25%), copper (486%), selenium (35%). They are also a good source of other minerals zinc, manganese, and phosphorus, and are high in protein. Always buy organic as organs accumulate more toxins than muscle tissue.

Ortaniques [*Fruit*] Ortaniques are hybrids between oranges and tangerines. See "Orange" for nutrients.

Ostrich [*Meat*] Ostrich is a red meat that is high in protein, iron, and contains less saturated fat than other red meats. It also contains minerals phosphorus and selenium in good amounts.

Oyster Mushrooms [*Fungi*] Oyster mushrooms contain Vitamins B3 (niacin), B2 (riboflavin), B1 (thiamine), B6 (pyridoxine), B9 (folic acid), B5 (pantothenic acid), and minerals iron, magnesium, phosphorus, potassium, zinc, manganese, and selenium. See "Mushrooms" for general information. See also Marvelous

Mushrooms – The Magic Food under Food for Thought, under "M" and also Are Rheumatoid Arthritis and Autoimmune Diseases on the Rise? under Food and You or Your Environment, under "R."

Oysters [*Shellfish*] Oysters are high in protein, healthy omega-3 fatty acids, and Vitamins A, C, D, and B-complex Vitamins (B12, B3 (niacin), B9 (folic acid), and B2 (riboflavin)). They are high in minerals iron, magnesium, calcium, and are especially high in zinc. They are considered to be great for the male libido as zinc supports sperm production and helps with prostate issues. (For information on sustainable fish see "Fish" or visit *www.msc.org/cook-eat-enjoy/fish-to-eat*.) See also "Shellfish" for general information. See also The Stress'll Kill Ya under Food and You or Your Environment, under "S."

FOOD FOR THOUGHT

War of the Spreadable Oils

Fats are important in our body as they act as a secondary source of energy after carbohydrates. They also provide insulation and protection for the body, including the organs, help regulate body temperature, transport fat soluble vitamins (A, D, E, K), provide structure for all cell walls, and support brain health (the brain is 60% fat!). Certain fats are definitely not healthy and should be avoided (trans fats and hydrogenated fats), especially for those with high cholesterol or heart disease but others help heart disease (omega-3 fatty acids). But for healthy individuals, fat is not an enemy and actually supports growth and maintenance functions, so a small amount of the right kinds each day is good for us.

Butter or margarine? Which is better for me and which should I use for cooking?

With so many types of spreadable oils – olive oil, safflower oil, canola oil – it can get quite confusing for a consumer. The most popular oils are butter and margarine. Butter is saturated which is the "bad" fat and margarine is made of healthy polyunsaturated fat so is better right? Well, according to Stephen Byrnes, ND, RNCP, butter is by far the healthier choice and he has some great reasons why you should consider switching back to this tastier spread – in moderation of course because all fats are high in calories!

- **Vitamins:** Butter is a rich source of easily absorbed Vitamin A, fat soluble Vitamins E and K, and one of the very few food sources of Vitamin D, all needed for a wide range of functions in the body, from maintaining good vision, to keeping our hormones balanced.
- **Minerals:** Butter is rich in trace minerals, especially selenium, a powerful antioxidant. Butter has more selenium per gram than either whole wheat or garlic. Butter also supplies iodine, needed in the thyroid gland.
- **Fatty Acids:** Butter has good amounts of butyric acid, used by the colon as an energy source. This fatty acid is also a known anticarcinogen and antifungal substance. Butter also contains conjugated linoleic acid (CLA) that is believed to provide protection against cancer (CLA is also found in high amounts in grass-fed beef). Butter also has small, but equal, amounts of omega-3 and -6 fatty acids, the so-called essential fatty acids.

According to the Weston A. Price Foundation, when eaten in small amounts quality saturated fats from grass-fed or pasture-raised animals can be healthier than poor quality processed polyunsaturated fats (which are prone to going rancid during the extraction process) because they are more natural and the body knows how to use them. In their book *Nourishing Traditions*,[104] Sally Fallon and

Mary G. Enig offer a compelling argument in favor of small to moderate saturated fat consumption.

Before a researcher in the 1940s coined the "lipid hypothesis" condemning saturated fat, most people ate larger amounts of saturated fats than they do today. Once saturated fat was declared the enemy of health, vegetable oil manufacturers started processing low cost grains into margarine and shortening. Heart disease has since gone up not down in North America. Clogged arteries today are more common and heart disease causes at least 40% of all deaths.

A multi-year British study was conducted involving several thousand men. Half were asked to reduce saturated fat and cholesterol and increase consumption of fat like margarine and refined vegetable oil. Those on the "good" diet had 100% more deaths than those on the "bad" diet.[105] Greeks, Austrians, and French also have long life-spans and consume high saturated fat diets![106]

That doesn't mean you can eat all the fat you want without consequence but a small amount of good quality saturated fats is now being considered useful for our bodies in moderation along with high quality, minimally processed unsaturated oils. Who knows for sure what the best ratio of saturated to polyunsaturated to monounsaturated is, but the debate certainly rages on. For me, I love the taste of butter and so prefer to bake with it and use it as my topping of choice – especially for baked potatoes! I buy unsalted, cultured butter because it is a whole food with minimal ingredients and an additional probiotic punch but you can make your own choice!

Guide to Using Oils

When buying polyunsaturated vegetable oils, it is important to buy only "cold-pressed" as these are not extracted using high temperatures and harmful chemicals which will decrease nutrients and increase rancidity. Highly processed vegetable oils can go rancid easily and can cause increased oxidation stress on the body. It is also important to store vegetables oils and any other unsaturated fat in a cool dark place (ideally the refrigerator) as light also causes them to go rancid.

Most vegetable oils contain high amounts of omega-6 fatty acids. Health experts worry that many people are getting too much omega-6 and not enough omega-3 in their diet, so try to include more omega-3s in your diet from sources like flax oil, walnut oil, hemp oil, and canola oil (as well as fish and fish oil).

My top choices for vegetable oils are extra virgin olive (which doesn't contain tons of omega-3 fatty acids but does contain many antioxidants), flax oil (which contains omega-3 fatty acids and should be kept in the fridge and used only for salad dressings in small amounts and never used for frying), canola oil (has high amounts of omega-3 fatty acids and a high smoke temperature and a long shelf life), avocado oil, and coconut oil.

I like coconut oil even though it is a saturated fat because it contains amazing nutrients. Coconut oil contains a fatty acid found in human breast milk that has strong antifungal and antimicrobial properties. In addition, using coconut oil has been studied with promising evidence indicating it can help reduce symptoms of early dementia and Alzheimer's memory loss. It's also considered to be a great antibacterial and is rich in Vitamins K and E and iron. Research also suggests coconut oil can help with weight management and aid digestion, since it reduces stress on the endocrine system.

Conflicting information leaves us wondering whether we should avoid fat or enjoy it. The main thing we know is that transfat and hydrogenated oil should be avoided at *all* costs. Other fats including monounsaturated (think olives and avocados) and polyunsaturated (think fish and flax) can be eaten regularly and high quality saturated fats (think coconut oil and butter) can be eaten in small amounts. All fats are high in calories but boy are they delicious!

FOOD AND YOU OR YOUR ENVIRONMENT

Is Organic Really Better for You?

While there are many positives to going organic, the main drawback often noted is cost. Many consumers find organic food to be priced higher than conventional food at the supermarket. While this may be true when simply comparing prices in the grocery store or even at a farmer's market, in reality we do "pay" for industrially grown food through subsidies (see Why Do We Need More Local Food? under Food and You or Your Environment, under "L"). But research shows that organic food has far fewer chemical residues and higher nutrients. Is it worth the trade off?

One of the ways that organic gardeners help the soil and eliminate the need for herbicides and insecticides is by rotating crops. Crop rotation is a fundamental organic gardening practice that's been proven effective for thwarting pests and diseases in the vegetable garden. In many ways, alternating crops can actually improve the soil's fertility as well!

A company called Environmental Working Group (EWG) was one of the first to test for toxic substances in human blood and they are working with government bodies to reduce pesticide usage. They were the first to publish the "dirty dozen" list of the 12 most contaminated fruits and vegetables. This list has expanded and includes apples, celery, sweet bell peppers, peaches, strawberries, nectarines, grapes, spinach, lettuce, cucumbers, blueberries, potatoes, green beans, kale, and other greens. They also publish a list of foods that contain fewer pesticide residues so you can buy them "conventionally," meaning you don't have to spend extra to buy organic, including onions, sweet corn, pineapple, avocado, cabbage, sweet peas, asparagus, mango, eggplant, kiwi, cantaloupe, sweet potatoes, grapefruit, watermelon, and mushrooms. This is largely because they have thicker skins that don't absorb as many pesticide toxins.

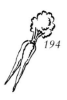

> The United States, the European Union,
> Canada, and Japan have
> comprehensive organic legislation.

If you find buying organic food is too expensive, you may want to try growing your own organic garden. Planting different species in combinations that "work" together or attract "good" bugs will help ensure organic gardening success. Here are some quick tips on plant combinations and which insects to attract that will help to eliminate pests and improve conditions in your organic gardens.

- Mint repels cabbage flies and borage attracts bees and deters cabbage worms. As a bonus its flowers are edible
- Lavender protects from whitefly.
- Basil repels all kinds of flies, including aphids, and attracts bees.
- Marigolds attract bees and beneficial insects.
- Garlic and onions around the border of a garden will deter all sorts of pests.
- Sprinkle cayenne pepper or mix a small amount with water and spray plants to deter small rodents and animals from eating crops.

A question that comes up frequently these days is, "Should I buy organic that comes from a country far away or local food that isn't organic certified?" I believe that if you buy locally and get to know the farmers in your community, they will work hard to produce pesticide-reduced produce that is fresh, full of flavor, and nutrient dense. If you want to include more organic food in your diet, check the dirty dozen guides (Visit Environmental Working Group's website at *www.ewg.org* for more information) for the best options for you.

I personally find organic potatoes and apples just *taste* better and they both contain higher pesticide residues than other foods according to recent research, so buying them might be a good place to start without spending too much on your grocery bill.

HEALTHY YOU

Optimism and Longevity

Can being optimistic affect our health? Yes, not only can positive thinking impact your ability to cope with stress and your immunity, it also has an impact on your overall well-being.

The Mayo Clinic reports a number of health benefits associated with optimism, including a reduced risk of death from cardiovascular problems, less depression, and an increased life-span. While researchers are not entirely clear on why positive thinking benefits health, some suggest that positive people might lead healthier lifestyles. By coping better with stress and avoiding unhealthy behaviors, they are able to improve their health and well-being.[107] Some of longest lived people state that their positive outlook contributed to their long life even though many faced serious life challenges.

A few ways to increase our optimism include thinking proactively when challenges appear and seeing each problem as an opportunity to learn and grow. For those stuck in negative patterns or thoughts, try starting fresh each day with more optimistic thoughts and actions. I have mentioned how foods can affect our mood and influence our thoughts so eating well will help generate more optimistic thoughts along with exercise and sunlight.

Finally we can use the power of humor to build optimism by taking ourselves less seriously. If we make a mistake, be the first to laugh at yourself. A survey sponsored by an international talent agency found that U.S. executives believe that people with a sense of humor do better at their jobs. A whopping 96% of those surveyed said they believed that people with a sense of humor do a better job, so give it a try at work too!

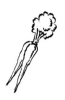

"You are what you eat eats."
Michael Pollan from *In Defense of Food: An Eater's Manifesto*
(1955- , American author, activist, and professor of journalism)

The Great Pumpkin Patch

When I began my vegetable gardening adventure a few years ago, I put compost into the garden in spring and felt quite proud of my rototilling efforts. Later I got busy with work and had no time to weed, let alone water. I didn't realize that all my old pumpkin seeds from my compost would sprout up again!

All of a sudden, it seemed like I had pumpkin vines growing everywhere. For some reason I left it and my cucumbers climbed up the pumpkin vines and the tomatoes did too. It all seemed like an amazing team effort to keep all the various plants growing cooperatively. Of course, I should have plucked out the tiny pumpkin plants right away but the experiment was educational and my sons found it highly entertaining.

We definitely had enough pumpkins for Halloween and pumpkins soup for many months!

REAL "P" FOODS

Pak Choy [*Vegetable*] See "Bok Choy."

Papaya [*Fruit*] Papayas are a source of fiber and carbohydrates. They are high in Vitamin C with small amounts of Vitamins A, E, K and B-complex Vitamins (B9 (folic acid), B2 (riboflavin), and

B5 (pantothenic acid)). Papayas contain minerals potassium, and small amounts of calcium and magnesium, along with antioxidant beta-carotene. They are known as a digestive aid (contains papai) and a beneficial tonic for stomach and intestines. See also Are Rheumatoid Arthritis and Autoimmune Diseases on the Rise? under Food and You or Your Environment, under "R."

Paprika [*Spice*] This versatile spice contains more Vitamin C than any type of citrus. Paprika is also rich in Vitamin A and beta-carotene and contains Vitamins K, E, and B6 (pyridoxine), minerals calcium, zinc, magnesium, phosphorus, potassium, and iron. It possesses detoxifying, anti-inflammatory, and pain relieving properties. It is produced by grinding dried capsicum, or chili pepper, pods. There are different strengths of paprika, such as regular, medium and hot, as well as sweet and smoked. Paprika is used widely throughout Europe in cooking.

Parsley [*Herb*] Parsley is a powerhouse of nutrients including high amounts of Vitamins A, C, and K, and good amounts of E and B-complex Vitamins (B3 (niacin), B2 (riboflavin), B1 (thiamine), B6 (pyridoxine), B5 (pantothenic acid), and B9 (folic acid)). Fresh parsley is high in minerals calcium, potassium, iron, copper, manganese, magnesium, phosphorus, and zinc. It contains good amounts of antioxidants beta-carotene, zeaxanthin, and lutein. Known to reduce blood sugar levels, parsley has antiseptic properties and works as a digestive aid, breathe freshener and diuretic. It is not recommended to eat parsley if pregnant. See "Herbs" for general information. See also Herbaceous Cooking under Healthy You, under "H."

Parsley Root [*Vegetable*] Just as the name suggests, this is the root of the herb parsley plant. This is a variety grown for its large taproot, rather than the leaves (although the leaves are edible too). See "Parsley." See also Root Vegetables under Food for Thought, under "R."

Parsnip [*Vegetable*] Parsnips contain carbohydrates, fiber, Vitamins C, K, E, and B-complex Vitamins (B1 (thiamine), B5 (pantothenic acid), B6 (pyridoxine), B9 (folic acid), and B3 (niacin)), and small levels of minerals manganese, potassium, magnesium, phosphorus, copper, and a little zinc, calcium, selenium, and iron, as well as antioxidants. Part of carrot family, they are great roasted with other root veggies or boiled/mashed and added into mashed carrots. See also Root Vegetables under Food for Thought, under "R."

Passion Fruit [*Fruit*] Passion fruit is high in fiber and carbohydrates and contains high amounts of Vitamins C and A and good amounts of B-complex Vitamins (B2 (riboflavin), B6 (pyridoxine), B3 (niacin) and some B9 (folic acid)). They contain very good amounts of minerals iron, phosphorus, and copper along with some magnesium. Passion fruits are native to subtropical regions of South America and are found in the wild on a fast growing vines.

Peaches [*Fruit*] Peaches are a good source of carbohydrates, fiber and Vitamins C, A and B-complex Vitamins (B3 (niacin), B2 (riboflavin), B1 (thiamine), B6 (pyridoxine), and B9 (folic acid)), along with antioxidants beta-carotene and lutein. They also contain minerals potassium, copper, and some manganese.

Peanuts [*Legume*] Peanuts are high in protein, carbohydrates, fiber, healthy fats, and contain large amounts of Vitamin E and B-complex Vitamins (B3 (niacin), B2 (riboflavin), B1 (thiamine), B5 (pantothenic acid), B6 (pyridoxine), and B9 (folic acid)). Peanuts are a good source of minerals copper, manganese, phosphorus, iron, magnesium, zinc, selenium, and some calcium. Peanuts contain excellent amounts of the antioxidant resveratrol, similarly found in grapes. Peanuts are a legume but are often eaten like a nut. Peanut oil is popular for stir frying and Thai cuisine. See also "Legumes" for general information.

Pears [*Fruit*] Pears contain carbohydrates, fiber, Vitamins C and K, and minerals potassium, copper, and manganese, along with small amounts of antioxidants beta-carotene, lutein, and zeaxanthin. They also possess pectin, which is a water soluble fiber, and boron, which helps the body retain calcium to delay/avoid osteoporosis. Pears helps detox the colon and are a good fruit to have if on the anti-candida diet.

Peas [*Legume*] Peas are an excellent source of carbohydrates, fiber, and protein. Considered one of the most nutritious of the legumes, they also provide a great source of Vitamins A, C, K and B-complex Vitamins (B3 (niacin), B6 (pyridoxine), B2 (riboflavin), B1 (thiamine), and B9 (folic acid)), and very good amounts of minerals copper, iron, manganese, and zinc, and some small amounts of magnesium, potassium, phosphorus, calcium, and selenium. See also "Legumes" for general information.

Pecans [*Nut*] Pecans are rich in protein, carbohydrates, fiber and fatty acids. They are a good source of Vitamin E and B- complex Vitamins (B2 (riboflavin), B3 (niacin), B1 (thiamine), B5 (pantothenic acid), B6 (pyridoxine), B9 (folic acid)), and minerals manganese, potassium, magnesium, phosphorus, copper, and a little calcium, selenium, zinc, and iron. Containing the highest amount of antioxidants of any tree nut, pecans are rich in beta-carotene, lutein, and zeaxanthin. They are great to toast and add to salads. See "Nuts" for general information.

Peppers [*Fruit*] Bell peppers are treated as a vegetable, though they are used as a vegetable, and chili peppers as a spice. Bell peppers contain carbohydrates, fiber, high amounts of Vitamins C, E, A, B-complex Vitamins (B9 (folic acid), B3 (niacin), B2 (riboflavin), B1 (thiamine), and B6 (pyridoxine)), and antioxidants beta-carotene and lutein. They have small amounts of minerals iron, manganese, magnesium, and phosphorus. Red peppers have higher amounts of Vitamin C than oranges! See also "Chili Peppers" and "Hot Peppers."

Perch [*Fish*] Perch is a good source of protein and omega–3 fatty acids. It contains good amounts of B-complex Vitamins (B3 (niacin), B12 (cobalamin), and B6 (pyridoxine)), and minerals manganese, selenium, and phosphorus. (For information on sustainable fish, see "Fish" or visit *www.msc.org/cook-eat-enjoy/fish-to-eat*.)

Persimmon [*Fruit*] Persimmon is a source of fiber, Vitamins C, B6 (pyridoxine), A, and small amounts of Vitamin E. It contains minerals copper and manganese, and good amounts of antioxidants, including beta-carotene, lycopene, lutein, zeaxanthin. These are red or orange when ripe, have a high glucose content, and a balanced protein content. These are used for various medicinal uses.

Pheasant [*Meat*] Pheasant is a good source of lean protein and contains good amounts of minerals phosphorus, selenium and some iron and zinc, along with B-complex Vitamins (B3 (niacin), B6 (pyridoxine), B12 (cobalamin), and B5 (pantothenic acid)). Grown in the wild, they will contain more omega–3 fatty acids.

Phytochemicals. See What Your Body Needs and Why.

Pigeon [*Meat*] Pigeon meat contains protein and high amounts of minerals iron, cooper, phosphorus, potassium, and zinc. It contains many B-complex Vitamins (B3 (niacin), B6 (pyridoxine), B12 (cobalamin), B2 (riboflavin), B1 (thiamine), and B5 (pantothenic acid))

Pigweed. See "Amaranth." See also Dandelions and Other "Weeds" under Food and You or Your Environment, under "D."

Pineapples [*Fruit*] Pineapples are a good source of fiber, and contain Vitamins C, A, B-complex Vitamins (B9 (folic acid), B1 (thiamine), pyridoxine, B2 (riboflavin)), and antioxidant beta-carotene. Pineapples contain high amounts of the mineral manganese, along with some copper and potassium. The enzyme bromelain helps digestion, has anti-inflammatory properties, and can be helpful to reduce symptoms of hay fever or seasonal allergies. See also Are Rheumatoid Arthritis and Autoimmune Diseases on the Rise? under Food and You or Your Environment, under "R."

Pine Nut [*Nut*] Pine nuts are high in protein, fiber, and healthy fats. They contain good amounts of Vitamin E and all B-complex Vitamins. Pine nuts possess healthy amounts of essential minerals like copper, manganese, phosphorus, iron, magnesium, and zinc, and a little selenium. They are one of the richest sources of manganese. See "Nuts" for general information.

Pinto Beans [*Vegetable (Legume)*] Also referred to as Mottled beans, these legumes are an excellent plant source of fiber, carbohydrates, and protein. Pinto beans also contain B-complex Vitamins (B1 (thiamine) and B9 (folic acid)), and minerals manganese, phosphorus, iron, magnesium, potassium, and copper. See also "Legumes" for general information.

Pistachio [*Nut*] Pistachio nuts are high in protein, fiber, and healthy fats. They are high in Vitamins E, A, C, and B-complex Vitamins. Rich in minerals like copper, iron, potassium, calcium, manganese, magnesium, phosphorus, selenium, and zinc, pistachios also contain good amounts of the antioxidant beta-carotene. See "Nuts" for general information.

Plantain [*Fruit*] Plantains contain fiber, carbohydrates, Vitamins A, C and B-complex Vitamins (B6 (pyridoxine), B9 (folic acid), B2 (riboflavin), and B1 (thiamine)), and minerals iron, magnesium, phosphorus, and potassium. Although they look like bananas, they are eaten as vegetables, much like fellow tropical produce potatoes, taro, yam, sweet potatoes, etc. They are one of the staple sources of carbohydrates for larger populations in Asia, Oceania, Africa, and Central Americas.

Plums [*Fruit*] Plums are a source of carbohydrates, fiber, and Vitamins C, A, K and small amounts of B-complex Vitamins (B3 (niacin), B2 (riboflavin), B1 (thiamine), B6 (pyridoxine) and folic acid). They also contain minerals potassium, copper, and manganese, along with antioxidants beta-carotene and lutein.

Pollock [*Fish*] Pollock is a good source of protein and omega-3 fatty acids. It contains good amounts of B-complex Vitamins (B3 (niacin), B12 (cobalamin), and B6 (pyridoxine)), and minerals selenium and phosphorus. (For information on sustainable fish see "Fish" or visit *www.msc.org/cook-eat-enjoy/fish-to-eat*.)

Pomegranate [*Fruit*] Pomegranates contain fiber, carbohydrates, Vitamins A, C, K, E, and small amounts of B-complex Vitamins (B1 (thiamine), B2 (riboflavin), B6 (pyridoxine), B3 (niacin), B5 (pantothenic acid) and B9 (folic acid)). They also have minerals copper, potassium, manganese, and phosphorus. Pomegranate is one of the most extensively cultivated fruits for food, juice, flavoring, and coloring, making it a common ingredient. It is part of a new category of foods often called "super foods." Pomegranates are great for prostrate health.

Pork [*Meat*] Pork contains large amounts of protein, saturated fat, and B-complex Vitamins (B6 (pyridoxine), B12 (cobalamin), B3 (niacin), B2 (riboflavin), B1 (thiamine), and B5 (pantothenic acid)), good amounts of Vitamin C, and high amounts of minerals iron, selenium, phosphorus, zinc, copper, potassium, magnesium, sodium, and some manganese. Pork is a red meat that comes from domesticated pigs. There are two forms of pork, distinguished by their preparation: cured and fresh. Cured pork, such as bacon, hotdogs, or ham, is treated with salt, nitrates, nitrites, and sugar for preservation. Fresh pork receives minimal processing, if any, and includes chops, ribs, and roast. Sausage is not cured, either; it is ground pork, often mixed with spices and herbs, encased in a film made from pig intestine.

Portobello Mushrooms [*Fungi*] Portobello mushrooms contain Vitamins B3 (niacin), B2 (riboflavin), B1 (thiamine), B6 (pyridoxine), B9 (folic acid), B5 (pantothenic acid), and minerals selenium, iron, magnesium, phosphorus, potassium, and manganese. These delicious fungi are really just large crimini mushrooms, or "baby bellas" – same food, just harvested at different times for different sizes and uses. See "Mushrooms" for general information. See also Marvelous Mushrooms – The Magic Food under Food for Thought, under "M."

Potatoes [*Vegetable*] Potatoes contain carbohydrates, fiber, some protein, and good amounts of Vitamin C, B-complex Vitamins (B6 (pyridoxine), B3 (niacin), B9 (folic acid), B1 (thiamine), B5 (pantothenic acid), B2 (riboflavin)) and some Vitamin K. Potatoes also possess good amounts of minerals potassium, magnesium, phosphorus, copper, iron, and some zinc, and antioxidants beta-carotene, zeaxanthin, and quercetin. Some of the popular varieties of potatoes include yellow, red, white, blue, russet, and fingerling. Eat them with the skins on for a nutrient boost. See also "Sweet Potatoes." See also Potatoes – A Staple Worldwide under Food for Thought, below. See also Root Vegetables under Food for Thought, under "R."

Poultry [*Meat*] Most common types of poultry yield similar nutrition. Poultry refers to domestic or wild fowl grown for their meat or eggs and includes chicken, turkey, pheasant, duck, geese, pigeon, emu, ostrich, guinea fowl, and quail. Poultry is the most consumed meat in the world. Duck has the highest nutrients of all poultry. Turkey is high in the amino acid tryptophan, which helps keep us to be calm and relaxed. See also particular species under their specific name.

Prawns [*Shellfish*] Prawns are a shrimp-like shellfish. They contain high amounts of protein and significant amounts of B-complex Vitamins (B12 (cobalamin), B6 (pyridoxine), and B3 (niacin)). Prawns are rich in iron, zinc, selenium, copper, magnesium, and phosphorus. They contain omega-3 fatty acids that support heart health by potentially reducing blood triglyceride level. (For information on sustainable fish see "Fish" or visit *www.msc.org/cook-eat-enjoy/fish-to-eat.*)

Prickly Pear [*Fruit*] Prickly pears, sometimes called cactus fruit, contain fiber, carbohydrates, and good amounts of Vitamin C and some B-complex Vitamins. They also contain good amounts of minerals copper and magnesium and some potassium, calcium, and phosphorus. Prickly pears have a pleasantly sweet tart taste and can range in color from pale green to vibrant red. They are consumed regularly in Mexico and also grown in the United States.

Protein. See What Your Body Needs and Why.

Prunes [*Fruit*] Prunes are dried plums and contain high amounts of fiber, carbohydrates and Vitamins A and K, and B-complex Vitamins (B2 (riboflavin), B6 (pyridoxine), and B3 (niacin), along with small amounts of Vitamins B5 (pantothenic acid) and B1 (thiamine)). Prunes also contain high amounts of minerals potassium, manganese, copper, and magnesium along with small amounts of phosphorus, iron, and calcium. Because of a false perception that prunes are used only for relief of constipation, many of today's distributors have stopped using the word "prune" on packaging labels and call them "dried plums" instead. Prunes and other dried fruit contain more sugar and less water content but prunes are still a fairly low Glycemic Index (GI) food because of the high fiber content. See also "Plums."

Pulses [*Vegetable (Legume)*] The seeds of leguminous plants are known as legumes or pulses. Pulses are the main source of protein for vegetarians. See "Legumes" for nutrients and information.

Pumpkin [*Fruit*] Part of gourd family, pumpkins are technically a fruit, although they are generally regarded as a vegetable, except when thinking about that favorite fall pie. Pumpkins contain carbohydrates, fiber, huge amounts of Vitamin A along with Vitamins C, E, and some B-complex (B2 (riboflavin), B9 (folic acid), B3 (niacin), B6 (pyridoxine), B1 (thiamine) and B5 (pantothenic acid)). They also possess minerals potassium, copper, iron, phosphorus, and zinc (a cup will provide a day's worth), as well as the antioxidant beta-carotene. Known as an immunity booster, pureed pumpkin is great added to smoothies, baking, or morning oatmeal, and roasted pumpkin can be added to salads or stir-fry.

Pumpkin Seeds [*Seed*] Pumpkin seeds are a rich source of mega-3 fatty acids and protein as well as excellent amounts of Vitamin B3 (niacin) and minerals iron, zinc, and selenium. They also contain the health promoting amino acid tryptophan, which is converted to GABA (gamma-aminobutyric acid) in the brain, which relieves anxiety and promotes creation of the chemical serotonin, which makes us feel calm and happy. See also The Stress'll Kill Ya under Food and You or Your Environment, under "S."

Purslane [*Vegetable*] Purslane contains more omega-3 fatty acids than any other plant and is a good source of Vitamins A, C, B-complex Vitamins (B2 (riboflavin), B3 (niacin), and B6 (pyridoxine)), minerals iron, magnesium, copper, potassium, and manganese with some calcium and phosphorus, and antioxidants. It is known as weed in North America but grown for food in India. Purslane was said to be Gandhi's favorite food. See Dandelions and Other "Weeds" under Food for Thought, under "D."

FOOD FOR THOUGHT

Potatoes – A Staple Worldwide

Potatoes are America's favorite vegetable. U.S. consumers eat about 130 pounds of potatoes per person each year, including French fried, baked, and mashed. Around the world, potatoes are one of the staple crops and are believed to have been initially grown in Peru. In fact, the word "potato" comes from the Spanish word "*patata*."

Potatoes are the roots of the potato plant. The plant produces flowers but the "seed" comes from the "eyes" of old potatoes. If you store a potato too long you will see some growths sprouting from it; these are the eyes. New crops are grown by cutting up old potatoes, with each chunk including at least one eye, and planting these chunks in the soil.

Sometimes called "spuds" after a spade-like tool that is used to dig them out of the earth, potatoes are harvested in the fall in most of North America, but can be left in the soil through the winter. Unlike some other vegetables that can be eaten raw, potatoes require cooking to eat, although Scarlett O'Hara was known to eat them raw. Potatoes contain many phytochemicals. An analysis of 100 wild and commercially grown potatoes has turned up 60 different phytochemicals and vitamins. Among them are Vitamins C, B9 (folic acid), flavonoids, and kukoamines. (The last two compounds may help lower blood pressure.) Potatoes also contain the powerful antioxidant quercetin (although at lower levels than onions).[108]

> In 1995 potatoes became first vegetable to be grown in space.

Yams and sweet potatoes are close relatives and contain higher amounts of many nutrients. The yam is a root vegetable that gets confused very often with a sweet potato. They're actually not even part of the same family and, when most people think of sweet potatoes, they're actually thinking of yams.

Yams have a purplish skin and an orange inside and can weigh up to 150 pounds. Originating in Africa and Asia, they're starchy but have a sugary flavor and are good for roasting. Sweet potatoes have their origins in South America. Peruvian sweet potato remnants have been found dating as far back as 8,000 BC. They can be grown in poor soils with little fertilizer. Because they are sown by vine cuttings rather than seeds, sweet potatoes are relatively easy to plant. Other tubers eaten regularly in South America include mashua, ulloco, and oca, which have been eaten for thousands of years and are still important staple crops to many who live there. Of course potatoes have been a staple in other countries for centuries as well. The Great Famine in Ireland between 1845 and 1852 was caused by a potato disease known as potato blight. The shortage of potatoes, which was the primary food source, led to the death of around 1 million people and many other fled overseas.

Potatoes are easy to include in meals. Sweet potatoes and yams are more nutrient rich and lower on the GI scale (meaning they don't affect our blood sugar levels) than regular potatoes so try to include them more often as a substitute. I bake cut sweet potatoes with cayenne in coconut oil for 25 minutes and have a delicious side dish with very little effort!

By far the most common way potatoes are consumed is as potato chips, which I myself even find too tempting to resist at times. If you have a craving for this high fat high, salty food, try switching to brands with fewer ingredients and less additives and try to take a small handful or two and then close the bag and put it far away so you don't eat it all!

FOOD AND YOU OR YOUR ENVIRONMENT

Can the Right Foods Increase Productivity, Energy, and Prosperity?

How would you like to wake up refreshed and ready to give it your all every day? How about getting to work and being productive and energetic all day long? Does this sound like a dream to you? Well it is actually very possible and could help you productivity and work fulfillment soar.

You guessed it! Food is the answer. The right kind of food, eaten in the right amount, and at the right time of day can dramatically increase your energy, productivity, and success.

Working 12-14-hour days will leave you exhausted, dissatisfied, and take a toll physically, mentally, and emotionally. This leads to lower levels of engagement at work, higher levels of anxiety and distraction, higher turnover rates, and soaring medical costs, just to stay on the insane treadmill. Many executives are at a breaking point and wondering if there is a better way?

I believe we need to start focusing on managing our energy not our time. Time is a fixed resource that can be wasted, depleted, or misused but energy can be renewed. Energy in physics is capacity to work and it comes from four sources in humans: emotions, mind, body, and spirit. In each area energy can be expanded and renewed regularly by practicing specific habits daily.

To effectively reenergize their employees, organizations need to shift emphasis from getting more out of people to investing more in them so they stay motivated and bring their A-game to the workplace. Individuals need to recognize the cost of energy-depleting behaviors and take responsibility for changing them. One of the best ways to recharge our energy is with the food choices we make every day.

One thing many of us do every day is drink coffee in the morning to kick start the day and get energized. Caffeine in moderation has some positive health benefits as it contains antioxidants (go for organic, shade grown, and grind your own beans for maximum flavor), but too much will dehydrate you, affect your digestion, and cause your energy levels to actually drop. So some is okay but no more than three 8-ounce cups a day is recommended by some experts. Caffeine is a stimulant that competes with adenosine, a chemical that helps induce sleep. So, the more caffeine you drink, the less adenosine is available for making you tired, and your sleep may suffer. Caffeine takes about 12 hours to be fully removed from your system.

The great habit to develop to become energized all day is to drink filtered water. This is particularly important to boost energy after exercise, when your body has lost fluid through sweat. Water-rich foods like fruit, soup, salad, etc., also count toward fluid intake. Coffee and tea are diuretics so do not count toward fluid intake. In fact, many suggest that you should drink two glasses of water for every coffee you consume. The sugar in soda and sodium in sports drinks also make them poor choices for hydration benefits.

> Increasing productivity and prosperity – can it be as easy as drinking more water?

Water regulates your body temperature, transports nutrients throughout your body, and carries waste away. Unfortunately, you cannot depend on thirst as an indicator of your fluid needs and you could be mildly dehydrated without knowing it. Fatigue is one symptom of mild dehydration. You should get in the habit of consuming fluids regularly, even if you're not active. Alcoholic drinks will cause further dehydration and also affect the quality of sleep so save that glass of wine for weekends or special occasions and don't make it into an everyday habit. Even a 2% drop in hydration levels can dramatically reduce physical performance in athletes according to recent research.[109] The same thing could happen with your work performance if you let yourself get dehydrated.

Below are some other great food and health tips to increase your productivity and energy.

- **Eat Antioxidant-rich Foods:** Colorful fruits and vegetables are rich in nutrients, especially antioxidants, which will keep your liver functioning well and your body rid of free radicals that cause fatigue and lead to disease. The dark greens of collards, Swiss chard, spinach, and other leafy vegetables supply generous servings of Vitamins A and C, calcium, iron, fiber, and protein.
- **Eat Some Protein but Not Too Much:** A small amount of protein with each meal, especially breakfast, will get your day off

right. Protein takes longer to digest and keeps you feeling full longer. High quality protein at breakfast, like free-range eggs, high protein grains, such as steel-cut oats, mixed with quinoa or yogurt are my favorites to start a busy day. Eating protein also stops cravings and keeps us from reaching for sugary carbohydrates or treats that will cause blood sugar fluctuations and ultimately weight gain.

• **Eat Smaller Meals Often:** This refuels your body throughout the day and evens out energy and blood sugar levels, so there are very few ups and downs. It is also important to not skip meals as that will definitely lead to fatigue.

• **Avoid Refined Foods and Sugar:** When you eat a refined sweet food, you get a spike in blood sugar, which gives you an initial burst of energy. But then you experience a rapid drop in blood sugar that leaves you feeling tired. If you repeat this during the day you end up exhausted. Complex carbohydrates in whole grains, vegetables, and legumes are the fuel of choice because they digest more slowly and provide a steady supply of energy for the body and also provide vitamins and minerals to keep us healthy.

• **Check your Iron Levels:** Iron-deficiency anemia is one of the most common nutritional deficiencies in North America. Iron is essential for producing hemoglobin, the main component of red blood cells. Hemoglobin carries oxygen to your body's cells where it is used to produce energy and perform essential metabolic functions. If your iron stores are low, your red blood cells can't supply as much oxygen to the cells. The consequences of iron deficiency are fatigue, low energy, and difficulty in concentrating. The best food sources are red meats, organ meats, iron-fortified cereal products, whole-grain or enriched breads, dried fruits, green leafy vegetables, beans, nuts and seeds, and blackstrap molasses.

- **Check Thyroid Function:** A low functioning thyroid (hypothyroid) can affect metabolism and energy levels. Thyroid function is improved with iodine-rich foods like sea vegetables and selenium-rich foods like Brazil nuts.

Our physical body needs to be recharged regularly as well to function at its best. Moderate exercise can help. Even walking briskly for 2-3 hours a week will reduce the chance of coronary artery disease by 68% and taking time to go for a brisk 10-minute walk at work will increase energy for hours. Stress and strong negative emotions, like anxiety, fear, and anger, can deplete our energy. Chronic stress and stress-induced sleep deprivation, or insomnia, will cause rapid changes in our energy levels. Some ways to reduce stress include visualization, meditation, laughter, and taking time to talk about stress with a counselor. At the office, working to fuel positive emotions in yourself and others by expressing appreciation for others in specific and detailed ways will increase energy levels as will looking at upsetting situations as learning opportunities instead of failures or catastrophes.

Eating better, staying hydrated, getting exercise, and reducing and managing stress will help you think more clearly and thrive in your work environment. This could set you up for a work promotion or help you successfully complete an important life project. Good Luck!

HEALTHY YOU

Pain Management

Many of us, as we age, are dealing with some chronic pain or discomfort which isn't fun and can affect our sleep quality and our vitality. Prescriptions for pain have soared in recent decades and pain-killers can greatly improve the quality of life for the 30 million Americans who suffer from chronic pain.

Americans are using more pain-killers than ever, and this increases the risk and incidents of pain-killer abuse. The U.S. is the world's largest consumer of pain-killers, using 71% of the world's oxycodone and 99% of the world's hydrocodone, or Vicodin. In 1991 there were 40 million prescriptions for pain-killers worldwide, but by 2001, there were 180 million prescriptions, most of them in the U.S.110

What other options are there?

Some people have reported pain relief combining medication with alternative treatments like massage, acupuncture, meditation, tai chi, yoga, hypnotherapy, physiotherapy, and chiropractic. Others have tried using some natural supplements and anti-inflammatory herbs like devil's claw, cayenne, turmeric, butterbur, magnesium, rosemary, arnica, and white willow bark. It is critical to check with your doctor or health-care provider before trying anything new to treat your pain as prescription drugs have side effects. Eating a healthy diet with anti-inflammatory herbs and spices will help to lower pain and increase mobility and mood.

"Trees that are slow to grow bear the best fruit."
Molière
(1622-1673, French playwright)

Real Men Don't Eat Quiche!

Back in the mid-80s, a friend of mine was living with her boyfriend and was trying to become a more accomplished cook. She served a healthy and French-inspired meal of Quiche Lorraine and Frisee Salad to her partner. His unfeeling retort was, "Real men don't eat quiche!"

Well, men who don't eat quiche are missing out on some great nutrition and taste. A blend of eggs and cream, quiche also contains almost any variety of vegetables, meats, and cheese. As a dish it has high amounts of protein, calcium, and vitamins and minerals. Eggs are a good post-workout food and will aid in muscle rebuilding.

The next week she served egg-and-bacon pie and he gobbled it up.

REAL "Q" FOODS

Quail [*Meat*] Quail meat (and eggs) contain protein, iron, selenium, and Vitamins B12 (cobalamin), B2 (riboflavin) along with small amounts of Vitamins A and B9 (folic acid).

Quince [*Fruit*] Quince has good amounts of carbohydrates, fiber, and Vitamin C, and small amounts of minerals potassium, copper, and iron. It looks like a short green pear with a soft and fuzzy skin. Grown like an apple or pear, it has a long history of use throughout Asia and Europe. The medicinal effects come from quince seeds, which when soaked in water are used to soothe inflamed skin and taken internally to relieve digestive discomfort.

Quinoa [*Grain*] Quinoa is high in carbohydrates, fiber, and protein. It contains good amounts of Vitamin E and B-complex Vitamins (B9 (folic acid), B6 (pyridoxine), B2 (riboflavin), B1 (thiamine), B3 (niacin), and B5 (pantothenic acid)) along with minerals manganese, magnesium, phosphorus, copper, potassium, iron, zinc, and calcium. Quinoa is lower in sodium compared to wheat, barley, and corn. Quinoa also contains high amounts of antioxidant phytonutrients, including quercetin and kaempferol. In fact, the concentration of these two flavonoids in quinoa can sometimes be greater than their concentration in high-flavonoid power berries like cranberry. In comparison to cereal grasses like wheat, quinoa is higher in protein and fat and can provide valuable amounts of heart-healthy fats in the form of oleic acid. Quinoa can also provide small amounts of the omega-3 fatty acid, alpha-linolenic acid (ALA).[111] A relative of Swiss chard and beets, quinoa is not considered a "true" grain and is gluten free. See also "Grains" for general information. See also Quinoa: Super Food under Food for Thought, below.

FOOD FOR THOUGHT

Quinoa: Super Food

The Food and Agricultural Organization of the United Nations (FAO) officially declared that the year 2013 be recognized as "The International Year of the Quinoa" due to its explosive growth in popularity.

Quinoa (pronounced keen-wah) is extremely high in protein compared to other cereal grains and is considered a complete protein because it contains all eight of the essential amino acids we need for tissue development. This makes it the top recommended grain for vegetarians. Gluten free, it also appeals to those who now follow a low-gluten or gluten-free diet.

> "Quinoa was to ancient Andean societies
> what wine was to the Greeks, wheat to
> the Romans, cotton to the Arabs."
> – Alexander von Humboldt

Technically, quinoa is a seed, not a grain, and originated in the Andes mountain region of South America, where it was cultivated as long as 5,000 years ago and was regarded as a sacred food by the Incas. To this day, most of the quinoa in the world comes from the Andean regions of Peru and Bolivia. The high protein content of quinoa puts it in high demand in North America and other rich countries, but for many other countries, often poorer ones, it is a staple. Local prices of quinoa have shot up, as *Globe & Mail* columnist Joanna Blythman writes, "In Lima, quinoa now costs more than chicken." To meet growing demand, local farmers are growing more of this crop in order to prevent shortages or high prices in countries where this crop is in high demand.

There are a few different varieties of quinoa, but the most common type is white quinoa, which has a light, fluffy texture and a slightly nutty flavor. Red quinoa has a more pronounced nutty flavor, and black quinoa is a little crunchier.[112]

If you can cook rice, you can cook quinoa – it's incredibly easy. Combine 1 cup quinoa with 2 cups water (or broth) in a medium saucepan (or think 1:2 ratio when cooking). Bring to a boil, then reduce heat to low, cover, and simmer until most of the liquid has been absorbed, about 15 to 20 minutes. Fluff with a fork before serving. As a base for curries, stir-fries, or tomato sauce, it becomes a nutrient-dense alternative to rice and pasta. Ground quinoa is now available at many stores and can be used as a great protein boost in baking, rather than tired and unsubstantial white flour. Remember that quinoa needs to be rinsed thoroughly before you cook it, because the grains are naturally coated with a bitter tasting substance that discourages birds from eating it.

Farmers across the world are starting to grow more quinoa as a lucrative alternative crop because is it a hardy plant and doesn't suffer from the same diseases that affect cereals, so it is good insurance to diversify and the prices are good. You can even try growing it in your own backyard garden and will be surprised how easy it is.

FOOD AND YOU OR YOUR ENVIRONMENT

Questioning Your Calories?

Today North Americans consume more food and calories than they did 50 years ago. Between 1970 and 2000, our daily caloric intake increased by almost 25%, averaging just under 3,000 calories/day. In the late 1800s average consumption was 5 pounds of sugar a year per person; today the figure has increased to an average of 135 pounds annually, including sucrose (table sugar) and high fructose corn syrup. That's the equivalent of 2-3 pounds of sugar each week![113]

Today we often eat on the go – while listening to the radio, talking, watching TV, or trying to navigate through traffic. Fewer people are stopping to quietly appreciate the nourishment in front of them and question the process that brought the food to their plates. A shocking 20 % of food consumed in the U.S. is eaten in the car while rushing from event to event.

> **Consider how and what you are eating is affecting your health.**

According to the U.S. National Center for Health Statistics, an astounding 62% of adult Americans were overweight in 2000, up from 46% in 1980. Twenty-seven percent of adults were so far overweight that they were classified as obese (meaning at least 30 pounds above their healthy weight) and that is twice the percentage classified in 1960. An upward trend for obese children is also occurring in the U.S. and around the world. Multiple factors can account for weight gain, including diet, lack of exercise, and genetic factors to name a few.

Obesity-related costs place a huge burden on the U.S. economy and direct health costs attributable to obesity were estimated at $52 billion in 1995 and $75 billion in 2003.[114] Just north of the border, we find similar statistics, but most alarming is the impact on our children. The number of obese kids in Canada has tripled in the past 15 years (Tremblay & Willms, 2000) and obesity alone cost Canadian heath care an estimated $1.8 billion in 1997 (Birmingham et al, 1999). Consider the facts below:

- Less than one-third of Americans eat more than one fruit per day. Only about 25% of U.S. adults, and fewer children, eat the recommended five or more servings of fruits and vegetables each day, while in Canada only 14% of 9 to 12 year-olds eat four or more vegetable and fruit servings daily (Heart & Stroke Foundation of Canada, 2002).
- One in four Americans consumes fast food daily. There are almost 50,000 fast food chain restaurants in the United States. Americans spend over $100 billion on fast food every year. Further, 75% of Canada's 7- to 9-year-olds buy food at a convenience stores two or more times a week (e.g., chips, sweetened beverages, chocolate, and pizza).
- In 2000, Americans ate 52 teaspoons of added sugar every day. America's consumption of corn sweeteners (i.e., high fructose

corn syrup) has gone up eight times since the 1950s. (See Mountains of Corn under Food for Thought, under "C.")

- In 2001, Americans spent only 10% of their disposable income on food. In 1991, it was 11.6%. In 1971, it was 13.4%. Type 2 diabetes – once believed to affect only adults – is now being diagnosed among young people.

What can we do to stop these trends? Making sure we take time to cook with whole ingredients and educate our children on the importance of proper nutrition will make a significant impact. If we all question the food and life habits we have formed and work to instill better ones in our children (and ourselves) we can start to beat obesity numbers down and improve health and life quality for many. Patience, commitment, and daily movement will spur change as well. It is not easy to change, but for those who persist, they will be richly rewarded.

HEALTHY YOU

Quiet It Down – Things Are Too Noisy

Traffic, TVs, video games, music, phones ringing, cell phones dinging … it's full on all the time. Noise especially over 30 decibels is associated with high blood pressure, anxiety, and stress.

There's a lot of great research showing that quiet time is very beneficial to your health. Taking time in your busy day to "chill out" can lower blood pressure, boost your immune system, and make you happy, because periods of rest or silence boost your brain chemistry and help you focus better too.

Creating quiet time in your day takes planning but is worth the investment. It's like recharging your batteries and will give you more energy and peace of mind too.[115] If we are not careful, we can easily speed through life, not savoring moments and feeling constantly stressed out and unfulfilled. Books on meditation and mindfulness are increasing in popularity because we've come to realize the benefits of slowing down for a moment to feel truly alive and live more joyfully.

But how can you carve out more me time to relax, be quiet, and just breathe? Try the following tips.

- Start your day with a one-minute silent gratitude exercise to quietly tap into all the good things in your life.
- Do housework less often. Perfection is nice but health is nicer. Use the time for a quiet activity instead, like reading a good book or doing yoga.
- Schedule set times for email, texts, Facebook, etc., so they don't take over your day.
- Turn an unused room into a relaxing space with candles and plants, and use it for meditation or mindfulness.
- Get outside and practice visualization or mantras to quiet the mind. I like to take 3 minutes to do deep breathing each day as I visualize a relaxing scene like a lake or being in the mountains.

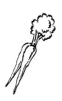

*"We reap what we sow. We are the makers of our own fate.
The wind is blowing; those vessels whose sails are unfurled
catch it, and go forward on their way, but those which
have their sails furled do not catch the wind. Is that
the fault of the wind? We make our own destiny."*
Swami Vivekananda
(1863-1902, Indian Hindu monk and key figure in the introduction
of the Indian philosophies of Vedanta and Yoga to the Western World)

A Rainbow of Raspberries

As a child, I used to look forward to spending summer vacation up at our cottage. Every year, would look forward to picking raspberries in August after a bountiful July blueberry season.

One of my best friends and I would spend hours carefully picking raspberries, so as not to get too badly scratched by the canes. We'd take our haul back to the cottage to make jam and pies for everyone to enjoy.

We loved the sweet flavor, but we didn't realize we were eating a Power Food. Raspberries along with many other berries (blueberries, blackberries, cranberries, strawberries) are packed with nutrients and a variety of antioxidants that may help to prevent some forms of cancer and many other ailments.

Back then we picked red raspberries but today they come in a rainbow of colors – red, purple, gold, or black. We even have some bushes in our backyard and my boys eat them regularly.

REAL "R" FOODS

Rabbit [*Meat*] Rabbit meat is high in protein and low in fat and sodium. It contains Vitamins B2 (riboflavin), and B12 (cobalamin), and minerals iron, calcium, phosphorus, selenium, copper, and zinc. Rabbit meat is almost cholesterol free and the sodium content is comparatively less than other meats. Rabbits reproduce quickly making them one of the most productive domestic livestock animals out there. Rabbit meat does not have a strong flavor and is comparable to chicken.

Radicchio [*Vegetable*] Radicchio contains fiber, carbohydrates, huge amounts of Vitamin K, and some Vitamin E, C, and B5 (pantothenic acid). It also has high amounts of the mineral copper, along with small amounts of iron, manganese, zinc, and phosphorus. Like other chicory class of vegetables, radicchio is very low in calories and contains high amounts antioxidants such as zeaxanthin, and lutein. See "Lettuce" for general nutrients.

Radish [*Vegetable*] Radish contains carbohydrates, fiber, some Vitamins C, E, B9 (folic acid), B6 (pyridoxine), and small amounts of minerals copper, iron, magnesium, and manganese. Radishes are very good for the liver due to their detoxification properties. Both radish roots and green tops can be eaten. They're great to eat raw with dips and add to salads. See also Root Vegetables under Food for Thought, below.

Raisins [*Fruit*] Raisins are dried grapes. They contain good amounts of carbohydrates, fiber, Vitamin C and B-complex Vitamins (B1 (thiamine), B6 (pyridoxine), B2 (riboflavin), B5 (pantothenic acid), and B9 (folic acid)). Raisins are a great source of minerals iron, potassium, calcium, manganese, magnesium, copper, fluoride, and zinc. Like their original fruit, grapes, raisins contain the antioxidant resveratrol known for anti-inflammatory, antimicrobial properties and to reduce the risk of stroke.

Rapadura [*Sweetener*] Rapadura is an unrefined sugar whose process keeps nutrients within the final sugar product. The pure juice is extracted from the sugarcane using a press, which is then evaporated over low heats, and finally ground to produce a grainy sugar. It is produced organically, so does not contain chemicals or anticaking agents. Rapadura has a molasses-like taste not found with processed sugar. See "Sugar" for general information. See also Sugar – A Diet No No under Food for Thought, under "S."

Rapeseed [*Vegetable*] Rapeseed contains fiber and huge amounts of Vitamins E and K, and some iron. It is commonly used for a cooking oil and is very low in saturated fats. It contains both omega-6 and omega-3 fatty acids, but also contains compounds that make it difficult for humans and animals to digest. Rapeseed is a member of the brassica and cruciferous family, which include mustard, cabbage, and turnips, and is a major oil-yielding crop, ranking third after soybeans and palm. Canola is an improved-variety of rapeseed developed in Canada in the 1970s that is easier for both humans and animals to consume. See What Foods Fight or Help Prevent Cancer? under Food and You or Your Environment, under "C."

Rapini [*Vegetable*] Rapini contains carbohydrates, fiber, and Vitamins A, C, B9 (folic acid), and lots of Vitamin K. It also has minerals, potassium, iron, and calcium, and antioxidant properties. Rapini is best cooked as it has a slightly bitter taste. Rapini is also known as "broccoli rabe" and is one of the most popular greens in Italy. It is part of the cruciferous vegetable family, which means it also contains sulfur, which has a specific compound called methyl solfonyl methane (MSM) that assists detoxification of the liver. See What Foods Fight or Help Prevent Cancer? under Food and You or Your Environment, under "C."

Raspberries [*Fruit*] Raspberries contain carbohydrates, fiber, Vitamins C, and K, and small amounts of Vitamin E and B-complex Vitamins (B6 (pyridoxine), B3 (niacin), B2 (riboflavin), and B9 (folic acid)). They contain small amounts of minerals manganese, copper, iron, potassium, and magnesium. Fresh raspberries have twice as much fiber as blueberries and when frozen they contain double the Vitamin C of frozen blueberries. Raspberries contain large amounts of antioxidants that protect against cancer, inflammation, aging, and neurodegenerative diseases. More specifically, they contain ellagic acid, a powerful antioxidant thought to inhibit cancer-cell formation, and anthocyanin (blue-red pigments found in blueberries too) that offer protection against hypertension and have also been linked to an increase in neuronal signaling in brain centers and have been shown to improve memory function.[116] See also "Berries" for general information.

Raw Sugar [*Sweetener*] Raw sugar is cane sugar that has been minimally processed. Raw sugar has a higher molasses content than table sugar, which gives it additional flavor and crunchiness. Products like rapadura and sucanat are also made from raw sugar.[117] See also Sugar – A Diet No No under Food for Thought, under "S."

Red Currant [*Fruit*] These berries are high in fiber, Vitamin C, and minerals iron and potassium. These are small round red or white berries that are used in making jams, tarts, and salads. See also "Currants."

Red Jostaberries. See "Red Currant."

Red Looseleaf Lettuce [*Vegetable*] Red looseleaf lettuce contains fiber, high amounts of Vitamins A and K, small amounts of Vitamins C and B9 (folic acid) and other B-complex Vitamins. It has small amounts of manganese, iron, and potassium and high amounts of antioxidants like beta-carotene and zeaxanthin. A group of scientists from Spain found that the red-leafed lettuce varieties (red oak leaf and lollo rosso) had the highest antioxidant activity among the tested varieties.[118] See also "Lettuce" for general nutrients.

Reishi. See "Ganoderma."

Rhubarb [*Vegetable*] Rhubarb stalks are rich in carbohydrates, fiber, Vitamins K, A, B-complex Vitamins (B9 (folic acid), B2 (riboflavin), B3 (niacin), B6 (pyridoxine), B1 (thiamine), and B5 (pantothenic acid)), and small amounts of beta-carotene. They contain good amounts of calcium along with other minerals iron, copper, potassium, and phosphorus. Rhubarb is rich in antioxidants. A perennial plant that is easy to grow, it will last 10-15 years once established. Leaves are not recommended for eating due to their high content of oxalic acid, which reduces mineral absorption.

Rice [*Grain*] This grain comes in many varieties (there are 4,000 worldwide), but white and brown are the most common. White and brown rice are the same grain, but white rice has had the husk removed. What difference does that make? Brown rice has 6 times as much Vitamin B1 (thiamine), 3 times as much B2 (riboflavin), 5 times as much B3 (niacin) and 2 times as much B6 (pyridoxine) and B9 (folic acid) as white rice. It also contains carbohydrates, fiber, protein, Vitamins A, C, and minerals calcium, iron, magnesium, manganese, and zinc, all of which occur in greatly reduced quantities in white rice. As a cereal grain, it is the most widely consumed staple food for a large part of the world's population, especially in Asia. It is the most important agricultural commodity after sugarcane and corn, according to data of the Food and Agriculture Organization of the United Nations Statistics Division (FAOSTAT 2012). Varieties are many, including white, brown, jasmine, basmati, arborio, etc. Rice is gluten free and used as a substitute for many wheat noodles in many recipes for those who are wheat sensitive. Some issues around arsenic levels in rice have been reported so buying organic rice may be worthwhile. See also "Grains" for general information, and specific varieties for any significant differences in nutritional content.

Rocket. See "Arugula."

Roe [*Fish*] Roe are fish eggs and contain protein, omega-3 fatty acids, Vitamin B12 (cobalamin) and some of Vitamins B2 (riboflavin) and E. Roe also contains minerals selenium and phosphorus. (For information on sustainable fish see "Fish" or visit *www.msc.org/cook-eat-enjoy/fish-to-eat*.)

Romaine Lettuce [*Vegetable*] Romaine lettuce contains fiber and high amounts of Vitamins K, A, and B9 (folic acid). It contains some Vitamin C and small amounts of minerals manganese and potassium. Romaine lettuce will keep for 5-7 days. All types of lettuce should be stored away from ethylene-producing fruits like apples, bananas, and pears as these fruits will cause lettuce leaves to brown. See also "Lettuce" for general nutrients. See also Are Rheumatoid Arthritis and Autoimmune Diseases on the Rise? under Food and You or Your Environment, below.

Romanesco [*Vegetable*] Romanesco contains carbohydrates, fiber, protein, and Vitamins A, C, K, and B-complex Vitamins (B2 (riboflavin), B3 (niacin), B5 (pantothenic acid), B6 (pyridoxine), and B9 (folic acid)). It has minerals manganese, magnesium, phosphorus, potassium, and contains the amino acid tryptophan, and carotenoid antioxidants. Romanesco resembles a cauliflower, but is of a light green color and the bud is uniquely shaped.

Rosemary [*Herb*] Rosemary, is a perennial herb that can be used both as a fresh green, a dried herb, an extract, and as a tea. It contains fiber, high amounts of Vitamins A, C, and B-complex Vitamins (B9 (folic acid), B6 (pyridoxine), B2 (riboflavin), B5 (pantothenic acid), B3 (niacin)), has high amounts of iron, and good amounts of minerals calcium, manganese, magnesium, copper, zinc, and potassium. Rosemary is known for antibacterial, anti-inflammatory and contains antioxidants believed to reduce inflammation, help memory, lower risk of strokes and Alzheimer's disease, lower blood sugar, and ease arthritis pain. Rosemary can ease digestion, and stimulate appetite and the liver to work more efficiently at eliminating toxins. Rosemary oil can be used externally to to treat bites and stings and soothe gout and rheumatism. Rosemary tea is considered good for colds. See "Herbs" for general information. See also What Foods Fight or Help Prevent Cancer? under Food and You or Your Environment, under "C" and also Herbaceous Cooking under Healthy You, under "H."

Rutabaga [*Vegetable*] Rutabagas contain carbohydrates, fiber, Vitamin C and B-complex Vitamins (B6 (pyridoxine), B1 (thiamine), B3 (niacin), and B9 (folic acid)), and minerals manganese, magnesium, phosphorus, potassium, and some calcium. Whether you call it rutabaga, swede, turnip or yellow turnip, it is a root vegetable that originated as a cross between the cabbage and the turnip. See What Foods Fight or Help Prevent Cancer? under Food and You or Your Environment, under "C" and also Root Vegetables under Food for Thought, below.

Rye [*Grain*] Rye contains carbohydrates, fiber, protein, Vitamins A, E, K and B-complex Vitamins (B1 (thiamine), B2 (riboflavin), B3 (niacin), B6 (pyridoxine), B9 (folic acid)) and choline. It also has minerals magnesium, calcium, copper, and selenium along with small amounts of iron, zinc, and manganese. Rye products generally have a lower Glycemic Index (GI) than products made from wheat and most other grains, making them healthy for diabetics. It is also known to aid digestion. Long seen as a weed, rye eventually gained respect for its ability to grow in areas too wet or cold for other grains. It is a traditional part of cuisine in Northern Europe and Russia. See also "Grains" for general information.

FOOD FOR THOUGHT

Root Vegetables[119]

Did you know that many of our favorite vegetables grow underground and are called root vegetables? The various underground parts of the plant include tubers, taproots, rhizomes, corms, and bulbs. The term "root vegetable" describes plants where the underground portions are consumed, but their nutritional value might also include edible stalks and greens as with turnips and celery for example.

> **Root vegetables in root cellars
> roo-duce waste!**

Many root vegetables are nutritionally rich and some starchy varieties form important staples in many diets and communities across the world, especially in colder climates where weather conditions limit the growth of other cereals like rice, corn and wheat. Because roots act as energy storage centers for plants root vegetables are typically high in nutritional value.

There is a long list of edible root vegetables.

- **Corms and Bulbs:** fennel, garlic, onions, shallots
- **Rhizomes:** arrowroot, ginger, ginseng
- **Taproots:** beets, burdock root, carrot, celeriac, jicama, parsley root, parsnip, radish, rutabaga, turnip
- **Tuberous Roots:** cassava, sweet potato, yam
- **Tubers:** black cumin, Jerusalem artichoke, mashua, potato, turmeric, ulluco

Since the Iron Age, people have used the natural coolness of the earth to preserve root vegetables. They discovered that they could create root cellars to shelter food from unseasonable temperatures as well as natural disasters like tornados. Although refrigeration made root cellars obsolete, people are again using them to become more self-sufficient.

Learning how to store root vegetables is very easy and the benefits include saving money, reducing food miles, reducing waste and packaging, eating healthier food, and feeling good about having a good supply of high quality local food on hand throughout the winter. Most roots will store simply in dirt or sand for 3-5 months or more with proper care.[120]

Did you know that?

- Originally, wild carrot varieties ranged in color from white to purple. In the 1600s, Dutch agriculturalists developed carrots that emphasized orange tints and phased out purple.
- The average American eats 126 pounds of potatoes per year and fresh potatoes have more potassium than bananas, spinach, or broccoli and are full of fiber and Vitamin C.
- Fresh beets are very high in Vitamin B9 (folic acid), which is good for pregnant women and brain health. The greens attached to the beets are also tasty, and can be sautéed with garlic and some olive oil and be eaten just like spinach, or used in soups to provide some extra texture and nutrition.
- Turnip is gaining popularity as a respected root vegetable. Try blending some into your next batch of mashed potatoes for added flavor and Vitamin C.[121]

Root vegetables are part of many delicious recipes and a favorite at my dinner table. Check out the recipes section for some great root vegetable soups and dishes.

FOOD AND YOU OR YOUR ENVIRONMENT

Are Rheumatoid Arthritis and Autoimmune Diseases on the Rise?

Do you know anyone suffering from an autoimmune disease today? The word "auto" is Greek for self. The immune system is a complex network of molecules built to defend the body against pathogens and eliminate infections caused by bacteria, viruses, or other microbes. If a person has an autoimmune disease, the immune system mistakenly attacks itself for a variety of complicated reasons causing chronic inflammation and disease.[122]

There are over a hundred autoimmune diseases, including type 1 diabetes, rheumatoid arthritis, Graves' disease, celiac disease, scleroderma, multiple sclerosis (MS), lupus, Addison's, Crohn's, polymyositis, and psoriasis to name a few. Nearly 24 million Americans are suffering from an autoimmune disease and autoimmune diseases are the third leading cause of social security disability payments behind heart disease and cancer. There are 50 known autoimmune diseases affecting two million Canadians, according to Dr. Edward Keystone, at Mt. Sinai Hospital in Toronto. Autoimmunity disproportionately affects women; ratios vary by disease, but overall, almost 80% of people with autoimmune disorders are female [123] Canada has highest rate of MS in the world and cases have tripled over the past 60 years; celiac disease rates have tripled in last 25 years in western countries; and diabetes is now being called an autoimmune disease and is predicted to effect one in three by 2020.

Do you remember hearing anything about autoimmune diseases a decade ago? So what has changed? During this same time period there has been a massive increase in the cases of allergies and a huge increase in the rates of obesity. Is there a connection? Some people believe that there is a link between allergies and autoimmune disease. Getting tested for food allergies can help greatly to reduce symptoms of inflammation when food sensitivities are identified and irritating foods are eliminated from the diet. More than three-quarters of the body's immune cells are in the gastrointestinal tract and those trillions of gut bacteria are believed to influence autoimmune diseases.

Other experts have pointed the finger at the overuse of antibiotics that can lead to antibiotic resistance and depletion of healthy gut flora. When employed properly antibiotics save lives but when overused they impact our gut bacteria and increase our susceptibility to disease by reducing our immune response. Some even attribute the rise in autoimmune disorders to a lack of Vitamin D, from reduced exposure to sunlight. Researchers found Vitamin D deficiency in a large number of studies of patients with autoimmune disease and supplementation has shown to be helpful. According to Harvard School of Public Health, one billion individuals suffer a

Vitamin D deficiency worldwide.[124] For some people genetics plays a role but no one can say for sure why we are seeing so many people suffer with the chronic pain associated with these diseases.

Many researchers are starting to wonder if our diet plays a contributing role in the increase of autoimmune diseases. The typical Western diet is high in processed foods, refined starches, added sugars, and animal fats, which are highly acidic and prone to causing inflammation in our bodies as well as depleting minerals, according to a 2006 paper in the *Journal of the American College of Cardiology*. Studies show that autoimmune patients do much better if they follow "the autoimmune diet," which means consuming foods that are anti-inflammatory

> A Mediterranean diet and other adjustments to diet have been found to reduce the pain of those suffering with autoimmune diseases.

If you or someone you know suffers from an autoimmune disease it may be worthwhile to work with a doctor who is open to treating you not just with drugs but with dietary changes as well. A study showed that, by adjusting to a Mediterranean diet, patients with rheumatoid arthritis could obtain a reduction in inflammatory activity, an increase in physical function, and improved vitality. These findings support the daily intake of monounsaturated fatty acids, as a component of the Mediterranean diet, and suggests that monounsaturated fatty acids might actually be suppressing autoimmune disease activity.[125]

Below are some foods that have been successfully studied to help reduce the pain caused by inflammation associated with autoimmune diseases.

- **Extra Virgin Olive and Avocado Oil:** These monounsaturated oils contain Vitamin E that helps to fight free radicals and also help to lubricate joints and prevent constipation.

- **Kefir:** Fermented dairy products like kefir contain probiotics that boost our healthy bacteria and digestion and Vitamin D that assists in immune response. They also contain high amounts of calcium and magnesium that help support joint health.
- **Mushrooms:** Mushrooms, like shiitake, maitake, enoki, oyster and others, have incredible immune-boosting and immune-stabilizing effects and are used to help both underactive and overactive immune systems worldwide.
- **Papaya and Pineapple:** Papaya contains papain and pineapple contains bromelain, both enzymes that help digestion and reduce inflammation.
- **Romaine Lettuce:** Leafy green vegetables, like romaine lettuce, contain vitamins, folic acid, and the minerals manganese and chromium that will help alkalinize the body and regulate blood sugar. Leafy greens contain high amounts of water that helps flush toxins and other irritants out of the system, which cause inflammation.[126] They are also low in calories so can help in shedding weight that may be putting pressure on joints.
- **Spices –Turmeric, Ginger and Cayenne:** Turmeric contains curcumin, a substance that actively reduces inflammation. Ginger and cayenne work in a similar way to lower inflammation.
- **Tart Cherries and Blueberries:** Tart cherries have an active ingredient, cyaniding, which might be ten times stronger than aspirin in fighting inflammation without the risk of side effects. The proanthocyanins in blueberries naturally reduce inflammation.
- **Wild-caught Fish:** Fish has high amounts of Omega-3 fatty acids, which fight inflammation naturally.

As well as eating foods that will help reduce inflammation, those who suffer from autoimmune diseases might benefit from avoiding processed foods, trans fats, sugar, excessive amounts of meat, and gluten. In some cases, it is believed that some foods from the nightshade family, including tomatoes, potatoes, eggplant, and peppers, contain a chemical that can trigger joint pain in some people with autoimmune disease although the evidence is sparse and widely debated.

Autoimmune diseases cause daily discomfort and pain that can increase stress levels. Reducing stress can help reduce inflammation in the body. Keeping a healthy body weight will reduce pressure on joints and daily movement and stretching can help to relieve stiffness. Some naturopaths have had success with helping reduce pain using supplements like white willow bark, devil's claw, boswellia, omega-3s, gamma linolenic acid, flax/hemp/evening primrose oil, burdock, and probiotics. Always check with your doctor or health-care provider before adding supplements to your pain management program.

HEALTHY YOU

Reduce Food Waste

Consumers in North America and Europe waste about 209-253 pounds of food per person every year. The USDA says the average person in the U.S. eats 4.7 pounds of food per day. So that means the amount of food we each waste in the U.S. per year would feed us for about 1.5-2 months (44 to 54 days to be exact).127 Globally, one-third of the food produced for human consumption is lost, about 1.3 billion tons. There are simple ways to avoid food waste, including learning about proper food storage, freezing, and cellaring techniques.

- Buy seasonal fruit and vegetables, buy only what you need or freeze and preserve extra amounts to use during winter months.
- Eat more whole food without wrappers or plastic to reduce waste and increase nutrients.

- When selecting vegetables for storage, discard any spoiled produce. Also, when using vegetables from storage, check over the produce and discard any showing signs of rot as they will spoil other adjacent pieces.
- Practice proper storage techniques for fruit and vegetables to extend freshness. To extend storage life, do not wash produce until you are ready to eat it and store fruits and vegetables separately. Fruits like low moisture; berries need to be refrigerated but melons and avocados can soften on the counter and be moved to the fridge when ripe. Buy bananas green and let them ripen to use when you want them. Vegetables stay fresh in general in a moist environment in the crisper drawer of your fridge but too much moisture can cause brown spots to appear. Store tomatoes on the counter and potatoes, onions, and, hard shell squashes in a cool, dry, well-aired cupboard or kitchen pantry.

And if all else fails and you still have food going bad, divert organic waste to your composter. Composting is easy; you need to remember to alternate brown material, like leaves and dirt, with green material, like fruit and veggie peelings. Add a bit of water and turn occasionally to create "black gold" for your garden.

Reducing food waste keeps your food bill and bank account fitter, the environment heathier, and ensures you eat the freshest food possible!

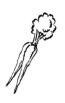

Some Like It Hot

I love to cook with spices and have been known to make things a bit hot. I love the heat!

Did you know that the best way to "cool" your mouth from a spicy dish is not water? Drink milk or eat a bit of bread.

Although, too much spice can take away from natural flavor, most spices are easy to use and will not only make things more delicious but boost the nutrition factor as well. Spices are in themselves a power food and we should all incorporate them more often into our daily cooking and food preparation.

Below are some interesting trivia points about spices.[128]

- Christopher Columbus mistakenly discovered allspice as well as America in 1492.
- The spice known as cinnamon is actually bark from a cinnamon tree.
- The Indonesians use cloves to make aroma cigarettes called "kreteks."
- Cumin is an ancient Egyptian spice.
- The nutmeg spice is harvested from the center seeds of the fruit from the nutmeg tree.
- Paprika is produced by grinding dried capsicum pods.

REAL "S" FOODS

Saffron [*Spice*] Saffron is high in protein and a good source of fiber. It has high amounts of Vitamins C, A, B-complex Vitamins (B6 (pyridoxine), B2 (riboflavin), B9 (folic acid), and B3 (niacin)), and the mineral manganese, along with very good amounts of iron, magnesium, phosphorus, copper, potassium, calcium, selenium, and zinc. It contains some antioxidants and is used as an antiseptic, antidepressant, anticancer, digestive, sleep, and arthritis aid. Saffron is known to lower bad cholesterol and promote total well-being. Saffron contains a carotenoid compound that gives the spice its characteristic golden-yellow color. It is commonly used in dishes like biryani, risotto, and paella. See "Spices" for general information and cooking suggestions.

Sage [*Herb*] This herb is a perennial that has been used in traditional European and Chinese medicines for thousands of year. Sage's plant parts have many notable plant-derived chemical compounds, essential oils, minerals, and vitamins that are known to have disease-preventing and health-promoting properties, including Vitamins A, C, and B-complex Vitamins (B9 (folic acid), B6 (pyridoxine), and B2 (riboflavin)) as well as minerals potassium, zinc, calcium, manganese, copper, and magnesium. Sage is known for antifungal, antiallergic, anti-inflammatory, and menopausal benefits. See also Menopause – Can Food Help the Transition? under Food and You or Your Environment, under "M."

Salad Rocket. See "Arugula."

Salmon [*Fish*] Salmon is an excellent source of protein and omega-3 fatty acids. Salmon is rich in Vitamins D, E, and B-complex Vitamins (B12 (cobalamin), B3 (niacin), B1 (thiamine), B2 (riboflavin), B5 (pantothenic acid), B6 (pyridoxine), and choline) along with minerals selenium, phosphorus, potassium, magnesium, copper, and manganese. Some salmon is healthier for you than others, including wild Alaskan or Pacific salmon, which has fewer contaminants like mercury and higher populations for sustainability. (For information on sustainable fish see "Fish" or visit *www.msc.org/cook-eat-enjoy/fish-to-eat.*) See also What's to be Done about the Rise in Heart Disease? under Food and You or Your Environment, under "H."

Salmonberries [*Fruit*] The ripe fruit has a sweet taste and is yellow to orange-red in color. They are made into jams, candies, jellies, and wines. The Native Americans eat these along with half-dried salmon roe, hence the name. Salmonberries are also called thimbleberries. See "Berries" for nutrients and information.

Sapodilla/Sapote [*Fruit*] This tropical fruit is a good source of fiber, Vitamins C, A, and B-complex Vitamins (B9 (folic acid), B3 (niacin), and B5 (pantothenic acid)), and minerals potassium, copper, and iron. It is rich in the antioxidant tannin, a polyphenol that neutralizes acids, giving it beneficial anti-inflammatory, antiviral, and antibacterial properties.

Sardines. See "Fish" For nutrients and information. See also Can Certain Foods Make Us More Intelligent? under Food and You or Your Environment, under "I."

Saskatoon Berries [*Fruit*] These berries are rich in Vitamin C, minerals manganese, magnesium, iron, calcium, potassium, and copper, and the antioxidant beta-carotene. They are native to Canada and are quite similar to blueberries in appearance. See also "Berries" for general information.

Savory [*Herb*] Winter Savory is a perennial herb and summer savory is annual herb. Both are rich sources of fiber, carbohydrates, Vitamins A, C, and B-complex Vitamins (B6 (pyridoxine), B3 (niacin), and B1 (thiamine)), and minerals potassium, iron, calcium magnesium, manganese, zinc, and selenium. It contains the essential oil thymol that has been scientifically found to have antiseptic and antifungal properties, and a compound that inhibits growth of bacteria like E. coli. Savory relieves gas and diarrhea and stimulates appetite. See "Herbs" for general information. See also Herbaceous Cooking under Healthy You, under "H."

Scallions [*Vegetable*] Scallions contain some carbohydrates, fiber, and Vitamins A, C, K, and E along with B-complex Vitamins (B9 (folic acid), B2 (riboflavin), and B1 (thiamine)). As for minerals, they possess good amounts of iron and some copper, calcium, manganese, and magnesium. They also contain with antioxidant beta-carotene. Like onions, shallots, and leeks, scallions are antiviral, antifungal, and antibacterial.

Scallops [*Shellfish*] These sweet treats from the sea are high in protein, omega-3 fatty acids, and minerals magnesium, potassium, selenium, copper, zinc, iron, phosphorus, and calcium. Scallops also contain Vitamins A, E, and B-complex Vitamins (B6 (pyridoxine), B12 (cobalamin), B3 (niacin), B1 (thiamine), B2 (riboflavin), and B9 (folic acid)). (For information on sustainable fish see "Fish" or visit *www.msc.org/cook-eat-enjoy/fish-to-eat*.) See also "Shellfish" for general information.

Scotch Thistle. See "Milk Thistle."

Sea-buckthorn Berries [*Fruit*] These are grape-sized orange berries that are found in the Himalayas. These are rich in antioxidants and vitamins that help in weight loss and aid against dementia. See "Berries" for nutrients and information.

Sea Urchin [*Shellfish*] Sea Urchin is a good source of protein and omega-3 fatty acids. It contains good amounts of B-complex Vitamins (B3 (niacin), B12 (cobalamin) and B6 (pyridoxine)), and minerals selenium and phosphorus. (For information on sustainable fish see "Fish" or visit *www.msc.org/cook-eat-enjoy/fish-to-eat*.)

Seaweed [*Sea Vegetable*] All seaweed types contain iodine, which is used in making thyroid hormones, necessary for maintaining normal metabolism in all cells of the body. Almost all types contain good amounts of Vitamins A and some B-complex Vitamins (B1 (thiamine), B2 (riboflavin), B6 (pyridoxine) and B12 (cobalamin)).

In fact, seaweed is one of the few vegetables that contains B12, making it ideal for vegetarians. It also provides good amounts of fiber, carbohydrates, and protein. Seaweed has almost as much protein as legumes. Seaweed contains good amounts of minerals potassium, magnesium, manganese, iron, calcium, phosphorus, copper, zinc, and iodine. Most seaweeds contain algin, a fiber molecule that binds minerals. In the body, algin can attract toxic metals in the digestive tract, including lead, arsenic, and mercury, and take them out of the body, so it is known as a great way to cleanse the body and blood.[129]

Types of seaweed include agar-agar, dulse, hijiki, kelp, kombu, nori, purple laver, sea lettuce (ulva), and wakame, to name a few. Each type of seaweed is rich in its own unique set of nutrients.

- Dulse is very high in Vitamins B6 (pyridoxine) and B12 (cobalamin).
- Hijiki is high in calcium and fiber.
- Kelp is high in Vitamins K, B9 (folic acid), and minerals magnesium, calcium, and iodine.
- Nori has the highest amount of protein compared to the other types.
- Sea Lettuce, or ulva, is very high in iron.
- Wakame has the highest amount of calcium.

Although more scientific research is needed, seaweed has also been used in some parts of the world to cure arthritis, skin conditions, tuberculosis, colds, and the flu. It has even been considered an alternative medicine as a treatment for cancer.[130] See also What Foods Fight or Help Prevent Cancer? under Food and You or Your Environment, under "C" and also Kelp to the Rescue under Healthy You under "K."

Sesame Seeds [*Seed*] Sesame seeds are high in B-complex Vitamins (B1 (thiamine), B3 (niacin), B6 (pyridoxine), B9 (folic acid) and

B2 (riboflavin)) and contain huge amounts of minerals copper, iron, calcium, manganese, magnesium, phosphorus, selenium, and zinc. They are a great source of mono–unsaturated omega-6 fatty acid, oleic acid, and contain carbohydrates and fiber. Sesame seeds are the highest non-dairy source of calcium. Tahini is ground sesame seeds.

Seed [*Classification*] A seed is an embryonic plant enclosed in a protective outer covering called the seed coat, usually with some stored food. It grows into a plant. Seeds provide protection and a food source for the embryonic plant and can be eaten as a food source or carried on the wind to a new location for greater distribution. Most people think of sunflower seeds, chia and flax as seeds but really all legumes, nuts and cereals are also technically seeds. Currently garden enthusiasts are starting to protect heirloom or heritage seeds (heirloom seeds are old, open-pollinated, and have a reputation for being high quality and easy to grow) to protect biodiversity. See also specific varieties for nutrients and information.

Serrano Peppers [*Vegetable*] Serrano peppers contain fiber, carbohydrates, Vitamins C, A, K, and B-complex Vitamins (B6 (pyridoxine), B3 (niacin), B9 (folic acid), B2 (riboflavin)) along with minerals manganese, potassium, magnesium, copper, and phosphorus. See also "Hot Peppers."

Shallots [*Vegetable*] Shallots contain good amounts of carbohydrates, fiber, Vitamins A, C, and B-complex Vitamins (B9 (folic acid), B1 (thiamine), B5 (pantothenic acid) and high amounts of B6 (pyridoxine)). Shallots possess minerals iron, copper, manganese, phosphorus, potassium, and some magnesium and zinc. Shallots have a unique active ingredient fructo-oligosaccharides, a prebiotic. Some researchers have chosen prebiotics as a new area in food and nutrition research as they take center stage for their potential to promote gut health by encouraging the growth and function of "good" bacteria that live in our digestive tract. Shallots are more subtle in flavor than onions.[131] See also Root Vegetables under Food for Thought, under "R."

Shellfish [*Classification*] Shellfish is a type of fish that have an exoskeleton and includes mollusks and crustaceans. Most shellfish are found in salt water but some are land dwellers, like crabs. Popular mollusks include clams, mussels, oysters, winkles, and scallops. Popular crustaceans eaten are shrimp, lobster, crayfish, and crabs. Most shellfish eat a diet composed primarily of phytoplankton and zooplankton. Shellfish are among the most common food allergens. See also particular species under their specific name.

Shiitake Mushroom [*Fungi*] Shiitake mushrooms contain fiber, carbohydrates, and a small amount of protein. They have a huge amount of Vitamin B5 (pantothenic acid) along with Vitamins B2 (riboflavin), B6 (pyridoxine), B3 (niacin), B9 (folic acid), and some Vitamin D. Shiitakes are high in the mineral selenium and have good amounts of minerals copper, magnesium, phosphorus, and potassium, and some zinc. Native to China, they've been used as a symbol of longevity in Asian countries due to their health-promoting properties. They contain an active compound called lentinan, which not only helps to boost the immune system, but also promotes anticancer activity.[132] See "Mushrooms" for general information. What Foods Fight or Help Prevent Cancer? under Food and You or Your Environment, under "C" and also Marvelous Mushrooms – The Magic Food under Food for Thought, under "M" and also Are Rheumatoid Arthritis and Autoimmune Diseases on the Rise? under Food and You or Your Environment, under "R."

Shrimp [*Shellfish*] Shrimp are high in lean protein and omega-3 fatty acids, and minerals iron and selenium, along with Vitamin B12 (cobalamin). Shrimps are considered low in mercury contamination but there are issues in some parts of the world with shrimp farming and sustainability. (For information on sustainable fish see "Fish" or visit *www.msc.org/cook-eat-enjoy/fish-to-eat.*) See also "Shellfish" for general information.

Snow Peas [*Legume*] Snow peas contain carbohydrates, fiber, and some protein. They are rich in Vitamins C, K, and A and have some B-complex Vitamins (B1 (thiamine), B6 (pyridoxine), B5 (pantothenic acid), and B9 (folic acid)). A source of minerals iron, manganese, copper, and magnesium, they also contain the antioxidant beta-carotene. Eat them raw dipped in hummus, diced up and added to salads, or use whole in stir-fry.

Sorghum [*Grain*] Sorghum is a gluten-free grain with good amounts of protein compared to other grains. It is rich in carbohydrates and fiber with Vitamin K and B-complex Vitamins (B2 (riboflavin), B3 (niacin), B1 (thiamine), B9 (folic acid), B6 (pyridoxine)) and minerals iron, potassium, phosphorus, and a small amount of calcium. Sorghum ranks as the fifth in the world as the most important crop due to its many nutritional benefits and its drought-resistant quality.[133] Believed to have originated in Africa, sorghum can be eaten like popcorn, cooked into porridge, ground into flour for baked goods, or even brewed into beer. See also "Grains" for general information.

Sorrel [*Vegetable*] Sorrel is a spring green that has high amounts of fiber, Vitamins C and A, along with good amounts of minerals iron, calcium, potassium, and magnesium. Its leaves are rich in antioxidants and believed to have diuretic properties. Sorrel does contain high amounts of a substance called "oxalic acid" that binds with calcium, reducing its absorption, so include more calcium-rich foods when eating it to ensure adequate daily intake.

Soybeans [*Vegetable (Legume)*] High in protein and containing all the essential amino acids, this legume is a source of carbohydrates, fiber, Vitamin K, B-complex Vitamins (B9 (folic acid), B2 (riboflavin), and B1 (thiamine), B6 (pyridoxine)) along with minerals iron, calcium, magnesium, phosphorus, potassium, copper, manganese, and selenium. Soy is best digested when used in a fermented form, such as soy sauce, tempeh, miso, or tamari, to aid digestion and absorption because it contains properties that make it difficult to digest on its own and will bind with other minerals to impair proper absorption. Soybeans are a complete protein source so are good for vegetarian diets, although buying organic is important. Soy has been shown to relieve certain menopausal symptoms as it contains "plant estrogens" that may act like estrogen in the body. Soy also contains a powerful isoflavone known as genistein that has powerful antioxidant properties. Try using tempeh in chili or stir-fry for meatless meals. See also "Legumes" for general information.

Spaghetti Squash [*Vegetable*] Spaghetti squash contains fiber, carbohydrates, Vitamin C, and B-complex Vitamins (B6 (pyridoxine), B3 (niacin) and B5 (pantothenic acid)) along with very small amounts of minerals manganese, potassium, magnesium, calcium, and iron. Spaghetti squash can be served like pasta with sauce and parmesan as a lower-calorie equivalent and is easy to prepare. See also "Squash" for general information.

Spelt [*Grain*] Spelt is a good source of carbohydrates, fiber, Vitamins E and B3 (niacin), and minerals calcium, magnesium, selenium, zinc, iron, and copper. Spelt contains more fiber and protein than wheat, but is much lower in gluten, making it a good substitute for those with sensitivities. (There are reports that some people sensitive to wheat can tolerate spelt, but no medical studies have confirmed this finding.) Spelt flour is an ancient grain that has lately made a comeback in North America. Spelt's husks protect it from pollutants and insects, which mean growers can avoid using pesticides, unlike other grains.[134] Spelt tastes similar to wheat so try it next time you bake for variety! See also "Grains" for general information.

Spices [*Classification*] A spice is the dried seed, fruit, bark, or vegetative substance of a plant primarily used for flavoring, coloring, or preserving food. Spices are distinguished from herbs, the leafy green of the plant (see also "Herbs"). A spice may have an extra use, usually medicinal, religious, cosmetic, or as a vegetable. Many spices have antimicrobial properties.

Spices contain a large amount of plant-derived chemical compounds that are known to have disease-preventing and health-promoting properties. They have been in use since ancient times for their anti-inflammatory, carminative (meaning it is soothing to the gastrointestinal tract and reduces bloating or flatulence), and anticancer properties. Spices are noted for the high amount of antioxidants they contain. Spices may also increase digestion power by stimulating gastrointestinal enzyme secretions. Curcumin may reduce tendinitis. Turmeric has been shown to help prevent breast cancer by inhibiting growth of cells that fuel tumor growth. Saffron has been shown to be a natural aphrodisiac according to scientists at the University of Guelph. Coriander seed oil has the ability to kill strains of bad bacteria, including E. coli and salmonella. Black pepper has been shown to block the formation of fat cells.

On the other hand, some spices, like cloves, can be toxic in large amounts. Most spices are so high in nutrients that you only need to consume a small amount to gain the benefit – an amazing thing.

Below is a general guide to using spices more often in your kitchen.

- **Beans (dried)**: cumin, cayenne, chili, onion powder, pepper
- **Beef**: chili, curry, cumin, garlic, mustard, onion powder, pepper
- **Chicken and Poultry**: allspice, cinnamon, curry, fennel, garlic, ginger, mustard, onion powder, paprika, saffron
- **Eggs**: chili, curry, fennel, ginger, lemon peel, onion powder, paprika, pepper

- **Fish:** anise, cayenne, celery seed, curry, fennel, garlic, ginger, lemon peel, mustard, onion powder, saffron
- **Potatoes:** caraway, cayenne, celery seed, coriander, garlic, onion powder, paprika, poppy seed
- **Salad Dressings:** celery seed, fennel, garlic, horseradish, mustard, paprika, pepper, saffron
- **Soups:** chili, cumin, fennel, garlic, onion powder, pepper
- **Desserts:** allspice, anise, cardamom, cinnamon, cloves, ginger, lemon peel, nutmeg, orange peel, vanilla, carob
- **Tomatoes:** celery seed, cayenne, cinnamon, chili, curry, fennel, garlic, ginger, onion powder, paprika

See also specific varieties for nutrients and information. What Foods Fight or Help Prevent Cancer? under Food and You or Your Environment, under "C" and also Herbaceous Cooking under Healthy You, under "H."

Spinach [*Vegetable*] Spinach is a powerhouse of nutrients. It contains carbohydrates, fiber, high amounts of Vitamins K, A, C, E and B-complex Vitamins (B9 (folic acid), B2 (riboflavin), B6 (pyridoxine), B1 (thiamine), and B3 (niacin)), and good amounts of minerals manganese, iron, magnesium, copper, calcium, potassium, and zinc. It also contains many antioxidants, including lutein and beta-carotene. It also has small amounts of protein. Spinach is part of a family of plants that includes beets, chard, spinach, and quinoa and that is showing an increasing number of health benefits not readily available from other food families. It is considered a power food but contains a substance called oxalic acid that can effect absorption of minerals. To neutralize the oxalic acid, steam it briefly and then discard the water before sautéing. See also What's to be Done about the Rise in Heart Disease? under Food and You or Your Environment, under "H."

Spirulina [*Sea Vegetable (dried)*] A planktonic blue-green algae-like organism, spirulina has a brilliant blue/green pigment. It has very high amounts of protein and is a powerhouse of over 100 nutrients. It is high in Vitamins A, C, E, and B-complex Vitamins (B1 (thiamine), B2 (riboflavin), B3 (niacin), B6 (pyridoxine), and B9 (folic acid)), and very high in minerals iron, copper, magnesium, manganese, calcium, phosphorus, selenium, and zinc. Spirulina has more antioxidants than almost any other food. In the U.S., NASA has chosen to use it for astronaut's food in space, and even plan to grow and harvest it in space stations in the near future.[135] Spirulina is great for detoxing the blood and supporting the liver and immune system. Spirulina was used as a food source by the Aztecs until the sixteenth century. It lives in salt water and warm alkaline volcanic lakes in the hot regions of the world. Spirulina is often bought in powder form and added to smoothies, and tastes good.

Sprouts [*Vegetable*) Sprouts are the young plants of a variety of vegetables, with the most common being alfalfa, mung beans, radish, broccoli, peas, garbanzo beans, lentils, and fenugreek. They are considered a power food because of their nutrient and enzyme content. They contain good amounts of Vitamins C, A, and B-complex Vitamins, carbohydrates, fiber (depending on the type of grain or vegetable sprouted), and minerals iron, calcium, phosphorus, and sulfur. Sprouts are best eaten raw. According to research undertaken at the University of Minnesota, sprouting increases the total nutrient density of a food. These studies also confirmed a significant increase in enzymes, which means the nutrients are easier to digest and absorb. Try growing your own sprouts (kits are inexpensive and easy to use) to add to salads or sandwiches.

Squash [*Vegetable*] Squash contains high amounts of carbohydrates, fiber, Vitamin A and good amounts of Vitamins C, E, and B-complex (B6 (pyridoxine), B3 (niacin), B5 (pantothenic acid) and B9 (folic acid)), and minerals iron, magnesium, copper, and potassium, and some calcium and phosphorus. Squash has high amounts of antioxidants beta-carotene and lutein. See also specific varieties for nutrients and information.

Squid [*Shellfish*] Usually referred to as calamari on restaurant menus, squid is high in protein, omega-3 fatty acids, Vitamins B12 (cobalamin) and B3 (niacin), and minerals phosphorus, zinc, copper, and selenium. (For information on sustainable fish see "Fish" or visit *www.msc.org/cook-eat-enjoy/fish-to-eat.*)

Star Fruit [*Fruit*] Star fruit contains carbohydrates, fiber, Vitamin C and small amount of B-complex Vitamins (B9 (folic acid) and B5 (pantothenic acid)), along with minerals copper and potassium.

Stevia [*Sweetener*] Stevia is a small, sweet-leaf herb found in South American countries and it contains fiber, carbohydrates, a small amount of protein and Vitamins A and C along with minerals iron, phosphorus, calcium, potassium, sodium, and magnesium, and zinc in small amounts. However, in the form generally marketed to the public, these nutrients do not appear. Stevia may offer several health benefits. It doesn't trigger an insulin response and so can be used as a sweetener by diabetics. Also, it is a natural, low-calorie sweetener which may help reduce dependence on high calorie sugar, fructose, and corn syrup. Stevia does not cause cavities. See "Sugar" for general information. See also Sugar – A Diet No No under Food for Thought, below.

Strawberries [*Fruit*] Strawberries have carbohydrates and fiber, are high in Vitamin C, and some of Vitamins K, E, B9 (folic acid), and B6 (pyridoxine). They contain good amounts of manganese and some potassium and magnesium along with antioxidants such as lutein, zeaxanthin, and beta-carotene in small amounts. Strawberries are the only fruit whose seeds grow on the outside and are a perennial plant. See also "Berries" for general information.

Sucanat [*Sweetener*] Sucanat contains small amounts of Vitamins A, and B-complex, and minerals potassium, calcium, magnesium, and phosphorus. Sucanat is dehydrated cane juice, which is similar to rapadura in that it is a combination of molasses and sugar, but sucanat is dehydrated, while rapadura is evaporated. See "Sugar" for general information. See also Sugar – A Diet No No under Food for Thought, below.

Suet [*Fat*] Suet is the hard animal fat found around the kidneys of beef. It contains a high amount of fatty acids and some protein. Suet is used by traditional cooks for its flavor.

Sugar [*Classification*] Sugar is a sweetener. Refined sugar has almost no nutrients and rapadura or organic whole cane sugar contain very small amounts of Vitamins A and B-complex and minerals potassium, magnesium, calcium, and phosphorus. See also particular sweeteners under their specific names. See also Sugar – A Diet No No under Food for Thought, below.

Sugarberries [*Fruit*] These have a large seed covered by a hardened fruit wall. They turn reddish or purplish when they become ripe. These are as sweet as dates but have a very thin fleshy layer. These are mostly enjoyed by birds. See "Berries" for nutrients and information.

Sunchoke. See "Jerusalem Artichoke."

Sunflower Seeds [*Seed*] Sunflower seeds are high in protein and omega-6 fatty acids. They also contain carbohydrates, fiber, high amounts of Vitamins E, B-complex Vitamins (B6 (pyridoxine), B1 (thiamine), B9 (folic acid), B3 (niacin), B2 (riboflavin)), and are an excellent source of minerals copper, phosphorus, selenium, manganese, magnesium, iron, zinc, and potassium. Sunflower seeds contain antioxidants that help reduce blood sugar levels and beneficial tryptophan that is a natural mood lifter and calming agent. Sunflower seeds should be stored in the fridge to avoid rancidity. See also What's to be Done about the Rise in Heart

Disease? under Food and You or Your Environment, under "H."

Swede [*Vegetable*] Swedes are similar to rutabagas and turnip in nutrients and a popular root vegetable. Swedes are the traditional accompaniment to haggis, a traditional Scottish dish, where they are known as neeps. Over-sized swedes tend to be woody and tough so choose smaller ones, with smooth skin if possible. See "Rutabaga" for nutritional information.

Sweet Dumpling Squash. See "Squash" for nutrients and information.

Sweet Pitayas. See "Dragon Fruit."

Sweet Potatoes [*Vegetable*] Sweet potatoes contain high amounts of carbohydrates, fiber, Vitamin A, and E, and good amounts of B-complex Vitamins (B5 (pantothenic acid), B6 (pyridoxine), B1 (thiamine), and B2 (riboflavin)), and minerals manganese, potassium, magnesium, phosphorus, and some iron. They have very high amounts of the antioxidant beta-carotene. Great baked with almond butter and cinnamon as toppings! See also Potatoes – A Staple Worldwide under Food for Thought, under "P," Root Vegetables under Food for Thought, under "R" and also The Stress'll Kill Ya under Food and You or Your Environment, below.

Swiss Chard [*Vegetable*] Swiss chard has high amounts of carbohydrates, fiber, Vitamins K, A, C, E, and some B-complex Vitamins (B9 (folic acid), B6 (pyridoxine), and B2 (riboflavin)). It also has high amounts of minerals iron, magnesium, copper, manganese, phosphorus, and zinc, and antioxidants beta-carotene and lutein. Swiss chard, along with kale, mustard greens, and collard greens, is one of several leafy green vegetables often referred to as "greens." Swiss chard is part of the chenopod family, which includes beets, spinach, and quinoa. This family shows an increasing number of health benefits not readily available from other food families. It is considered a power food but contains a substance called oxalic acid that can affect absorption of minerals.

To neutralize the oxalic acid, steam it briefly and then discard the water before sautéing.

FOOD FOR THOUGHT

Sugar – A Diet No No

Sugar can be made from many plant sources, including sugarcane, sugar beets, and corn. Sugar can also from trees, such as maple, palm coconut, nutmeg, and birch.

> **Did you know that there are over 50 different names for sugar?**

Sugar comes in various degrees of processing and it is worth paying attention to this because refined sugar has no nutrients whereas other types of sugar retain some small amounts of vitamins and minerals and don't affect your blood sugar in the same way or as quickly. Here's a list of the more common sugars, listed from most to least processed, to help you evaluate which one you would like to try.

1. **White Sugar:** There is virtually no nutritional value to white sugar. It is the most heavily processed and refined of the sweeteners and the most popular type sold in stores.
2. **Brown Sugar:** Many people think brown sugar is a better alternative to white sugar but it is just white sugar mixed with molasses. While molasses has some nutrients, the amount used for brown sugar is only for coloring and flavoring so does not add nutritional value.
3. **Raw Sugar:** Also referred to as "sugar in the raw" and turbinado, many people opt for this sweetener as it "sounds" less processed and more natural. But it is still a refined sugar, but has undergone one less step than the white sugar process and retains more molasses.
4. **Rapadura:** Rapadura is less processed than white, brown, or raw

sugar, as the pure juice is extracted from sugarcane using a press. It is then evaporated over low heat without removing the nutrient-rich molasses. It is produced organically and is also known as "organic whole cane sugar." Because it is dehydrated at a low heat, most vitamins and minerals have been retained.

5. **Sucanat:** Sucanat is whole, unrefined cane sugar. It's made by simply crushing freshly cut sugarcane, extracting the juice, and heating it in a large vat. Once the juice is reduced to a rich, dark syrup, it is hand paddled. Nothing is added or taken out so more nutrients are retained.

6. **Corn:** Today much of the sugar we eat is in the form of high fructose corn syrup (HFCS). HFCS is added to many processed foods that we find in the grocery store, including ketchup, chicken nuggets, and granola bars.

7. **Agave Nectar:** Sometimes called agave syrup, it is most often produced from the blue agaves that thrive in the volcanic soils of southern Mexico. Agaves are large, spikey plants that resemble cactus or yuccas in both form and habitat, but they are actually succulents similar to aloe vera. You need to be aware of the source of agave as many on the market are highly processed, which increases the amount of fructose in the sugar. Raw agave nectar is a natural sweetener and does have small amounts of vitamins and minerals.

8. **Honey:** This sweetener is a sugar from bees. See "Honey" for the nutritional details, but it is a pretty good choice, especially when used in raw liquid form as it has both nutrients and medicinal properties and tastes delicious to most.

9. **Stevia:** Stevia leaves contain 100 vital nutrients, and can a have taste profile 30 times sweeter than sugar. Many people believe that stevia is the healthiest sweetener. It is tasty, nutritious, may have health benefits, both internally and topically, and appears to be safe for people of all ages.[136] Stevia was originally discov-

ered more than 1,500 years ago growing in clumps of two or three plants along the edges of the rain forests of Paraguay by the native Guarani people and has been used ever since. It also doesn't trigger an insulin response and so can be used as a sweetener by diabetics and is a low-calorie choice for those who are trying to lose weight.

10. **Xylitol:** Xylitol is a sugar alcohol that naturally occurs in the fibers of certain fruits and vegetables but for commercial purposes it's most often extracted from the bark of birch trees. One teaspoon of xylitol has 10 calories, compared to sugar, which has 15 calories. However, the sugar alcohols in xylitol don't have much impact on your blood sugar levels so they are also considered safe for diabetics. It contains only trace amounts of vitamins and minerals, but it aids in the absorption of calcium and B vitamins in your body. It can be highly toxic to dogs and other animals.

Eating too many foods with high sugar content can lead to high blood sugar, causing the body to store fat. Over long periods of time this additional body fat can cause more serious health issues. Some foods we consider to be healthy have high sugar content, like concentrated orange juice, fruit-based yogurts, and even whole wheat bread, so it is a good idea to watch your intake

A simple way to avoid high blood sugar spikes is to combine high carbohydrate dishes with low carbohydrate ones and add protein and healthy fats to reduce the blood sugar roller-coaster affect. For example, an easy morning switch is to serve multigrain bread with a fruit/vegetable blended juice and nuts or seeds or eggs or plain yogurt.

Fat was once considered the enemy by leading nutritionists but new research shows that consuming moderate amounts of healthy fats, can help maintain health and weight. More and more sugar is implicated in obesity and diseases and the evidence is powerful enough to pay attention to when making choices. Consider the below facts.

- Refined sugar has *no* vitamins, *no* minerals, *no* enzymes, *no* fiber, *and no* fat. Everything beneficial is removed during the processing except empty calories that cause the body stress.
- Refined sugar makes the digestive system acidic, causing vitamins and minerals to leach from the body, especially calcium from the bones and teeth. It also depletes potassium and magnesium which are both essential for cardiac health.
- Sugar suppresses the immune system causing stress on the pancreas, inhibits blood flow and affects aging.
- Sugar is highly addictive. It releases an opiate-like substance that activates the brains' reward system.

If you love sugar, cut down and start switching from white refined sugar to more natural kinds like honey, agave, or maple syrup to sweeten recipes or food, or consider stevia and xylitol for coffee and tea. Gradually cut back more and more and you will find that you don't miss it! Instead you will start tasting the natural sweetness of real foods like fruits and even sweet vegetables. You'll find the sugar you once loved is not as tasty as the real stuff!

FOOD AND YOU OR YOUR ENVIRONMENT

The Stress'll Kill Ya

Life goes faster and faster and the pace can lead to burn-out or long-term anxiety. The statistics on burn-out, depression, anxiety, and other stress-related mental illnesses are staggering in North America. Almost one in five of us is medicated for anxiety and Paxil and Zoloft (two of the more popular anti-anxiety medications) ranked in the top ten prescribed medications in the U.S. in recent years.[137]

Deadlines, competing demands, responsibilities, and fear about work or relationships can cause stress overload. The body is built for life or death situations with the so called "flight or fight" response. But today, instead of running from the saber tooth tiger, we are running from a feeling of panic that we won't make a work deadline or get through traffic to pick up our kids. When we are in high-stress mode, stress hormones like adrenaline and cortisol flood our bodies and shut down digestion. Over prolonged periods this can have a big impact on our health.

Too much stress will actually cause our performance at work and home to plummet and our health to suffer. Can eating food reduce stress? Well, yes it can! There are definitely stress-busting foods out there and eating them regularly will help you cope during high-stress times.

> Adding stress-busting foods to your diet can be one of the weapons in your arsenal to conquer today's level of stress!

Reach for the below foods to combat stress.

- **Alfalfa Sprouts:** Alfalfa sprouts and other raw sprouts like radish, pea, mung bean, and broccoli are loaded with magnesium, which is a calming mineral. Magnesium helps to regulate blood pressure to keep us calm so reach for it regularly and even more when you are stressed out and put them in sandwiches and salads.
- **Camomile Tea:** Don't overdo it with caffeine or sugar when you are stressed out. Although you may feel a boost initially, it will eventually lead to a deeper energy crash as they dehydrate the body, stimulate stress hormones, and make it more difficult to cope. Reach for filtered water or chamomile tea instead, which will help calm and balance mood and energy. A study

from the University of Pennsylvania tested chamomile supplements on 57 participants with generalized anxiety disorder for 8 weeks, and found it led to a significant drop in anxiety symptoms.[138]

- **Camu Camu Berries:** Camu Camu Berries contain the highest known amount of Vitamin C of any food. Vitamin C is a powerful antioxidant that helps to reduce physical and mental fatigue from stress and improve immune function because this nutrient is stress sensitive and can be depleted quickly under stress. High dietary intake of Vitamin C may help reduce the effects of chronic stress by inhibiting the release of stress hormones, thus preventing these hormones from dampening the immune response.

- **Oysters:** Oysters, and other tasty shellfish like clams and crabs, contain high amounts of the mineral zinc, which is necessary for the synthesis of serotonin and helps support the immune system. Zinc is believed to support our adrenal glands that produce our stress hormones, adrenaline, cortisol, DHEA, and norepinephrine, which get taxed after repeated and chronic stress. Most think of oysters as an aphrodisiac and maybe that is because they help relax us and boost our mood.

- **Pumpkin Seeds:** Pumpkin seeds and other trytophan-rich nuts and seeds help you here. Pistachios, walnuts, pumpkin seeds, and sunflower seeds contain tryptophan, an amino acid that helps create serotonin, a calming chemical in the brain.

- **Sweet Potatoes:** Sweet potatoes can be great for reducing stress-because they satisfy the urge you get for carbohydrates and sweets when you are under a great deal of stress. They are packed full of beta-carotene and other vitamins, and the fiber helps your body to process the carbohydrates in a slow and steady way that doesn't impact blood sugar. They also are loaded with B-complex Vitamins that help boosts levels of serotonin, and can cut levels of cortisol and adrenaline. Other good stress-busting carbs include brown rice, oatmeal, and quinoa.

Any food with magnesium, Vitamin B12 (cobalamin) (and other B-complex Vitamins), zinc, and high in antioxidants can be beneficial for helping you deal with stress.

There are also herbal supplements like peppermint, lavender, passionflower, and ginseng that may be useful for reducing stress. A new class of herbs known as the "adaptogen" are being used with some promise to lower stress. According to herbalist David Winston, adaptogens help safeguard the body's energy resources from becoming depleted and mitigate the impact of stress and oxidation and support our adrenal glands, which handle our stress hormones. Adaptogenic herbal remedies include ashwagandha, holy basil, rhodiola, licorice, and astragalus.[139] Always check with your doctor or health-care provider if your stress levels are high and ensure any natural treatment doesn't interfere with current medications and check for any other underlying health issues.

Other ways to reduce stress include exercise, yoga, meditation, spending time in nature, talking to a compassionate friend or counselor, volunteering for those in need, and laughing or watching a funny movie or show. Learning stress management techniques doesn't mean the stress will go away! It just means that we learn to handle each difficult situation better. Eating stress-busting foods and taking care of your body will definitely help you manage your stress more effectively so you can feel more confident in your daily lives and work.

HEALTHY YOU

To Sleep, Perchance to Dream

Sleep is critical to health. Without it, our bodies and cells do not have enough time to repair daily tissue damage or regenerate. Chronic sleep deprivation can lead to elevated levels of cortisol that can cause elevated stress, persistent fatigue, potential blood sugar issues, or lead to more serious problems.

Most of us need to aim for 7-8 hours of high quality sleep each night. One food that might help with sleep is tart cherry juice. Scientists found that taking tart cherry juice for two weeks helped increase sleep time by almost an hour and a half each night in adults with insomnia. Cherry juice has been known to contain the naturally-occurring hormone melatonin, which is frequently used in supplement form as a sleep aid.[140] Other suggestions for a super sleep include:

- Taking your minerals at night as they are relaxing to the body and help induce sleep. Magnesium at night is a great sleep aid.
- Developing a good bedtime routine and aim to go to bed at the same time every day.
- Keeping electronics away from the bed and stop working or working out at least 2 hours before bed if possible. Cover alarm clocks.
- Having the room dark and cool to maximize quality and quantity of sleep.

*"Women are like tea bags. They do not know how strong
they are until they get into hot water."*

Eleanor Roosevelt

(1884-1962, American politician)

Tantalizing Tomatoes Look like Hearts

I have always been fascinated by food I have to admit. But one day I stumbled on a great article about how many foods are actually shaped like the organs they help keep healthy. I found that incredibly cool!

For example, tomatoes contain lycopene in large quantities, which is an antioxidant that protects the heart and DNA. Have you ever noticed that solid flesh dividing up the pulp and seeds inside a tomato look like the four chambers of the human heart? Or that a carrot slice looks like the human eye and contains loads of Vitamin A that is important to eye health. And this odd phenomenon goes on. Onions look like cells and contain a sulfur compound that clears free radicals from cells; walnuts look like a tiny brain and contain omega-3 fatty acids that support our brain health.

It is reassuring to know that nature has made it easy to find nourishing foods to help us keep healthy!

REAL "T" FOODS

Tahini/Sesame Seed Paste [*Seed*] Like garbanzo beans, tahini is also high in protein. Apart from that, it is a great source of calcium and iron. Tahini consists primarily of ground sesame seeds, which may be hulled or unhulled. It's an essential ingredient in Middle Eastern dishes such as hummus, and used as a common table condiment. See "Sesame Seed."

Tallow [*Fat*] Beef and mutton fat is called tallow and contains high amounts of saturated fat and some Vitamin E. Small amounts of saturated fat from grass-fed animals is a healthier choice than saturated fat from grain-fed animals. Saturated fat is high in calories and should be consumed only in small amounts.

Tangerines [*Fruit*] This citrus fruit contain carbohydrates, fiber and is high in Vitamins C, A, and some B-complex Vitamins. Tangerines contain minerals copper, calcium, and magnesium, and several antioxidants, including beta-carotene, lutein, and zeaxanthin.

Taro [*Vegetable*] Taro contains fiber, carbohydrates, and Vitamins E, C and B-complex Vitamins (B6 (pyridoxine), B1 (thiamine), B5 (pantothenic acid), and some B9 (folic acid)) along with some minerals copper, magnesium, iron, and calcium. Taro also contains the antioxidant beta-carotene. The part of the plant eaten is the corm (or tuber), which grows to the size of a turnip. It is eaten like a potato and is popular in South America and Africa.

Tarragon [*Herb*] Tarragon contains high amounts of Vitamins A, C, B-complex Vitamins (B2 (riboflavin), B6 (pyridoxine), B9 (folic acid), B3 (niacin), and B1 (thiamine)), and minerals calcium, iron, magnesium, manganese, copper, potassium, and zinc. It has good amounts of fiber and is known for its ability to stimulate appetite. See "Herbs" for general information. See also Herbaceous Cooking under Healthy You, under "H."

Tatsoi [*Vegetable*] Tatsoi, or spoon mustard, contains fiber and huge amounts of Vitamins C and A. It also contains good amounts of Vitamin B9 (folic acid) and some B6 (pyridoxine), B2 (riboflavin) and B1 (thiamine) along with minerals calcium, iron, and potassium. Tatsoi contains more Vitamin C than oranges, as much calcium as milk, and is packed with the antioxidant beta-carotene and other carotenoids. See "Lettuce" for general nutrients. See What Foods Fight or Help Prevent Cancer? under Food and You or Your Environment, under "C."

Tea [*Herb*] True tea is made from cured leaves of the tea plant, an evergreen that grows mainly in tropical and subtropical climates. Tea is a source of carotene, a precursor to Vitamins A, C, B-complex Vitamins (B1 (thiamine), B2 (riboflavin), B6 (pyridoxine), B9 (folic acid), and B5 (pantothenic acid)), and minerals manganese, potassium, and fluoride. Black, green, and white tea contains theanine (like caffeine), but herbal teas, which come from the dried leaves of other plants, do not contain theanine. Green tea contains the highest level of polyphenols (flavonoids), which are known for their antioxidant activity. In the processing of black teas another antioxidant is formed – theaflavin. The polyphenols in tea possess 20-30 times the antioxidant potency of Vitamins C and E. Kombucha is a fermented tea. See Tea, The Drink of Emperors, under Food for Thought, below. See also How Can We Hold onto Yesterday's Memories? under Food and You or Your Environment, under "Y."

Teff [*Grain*] Tiny yet packed with nutrients, teff is an ancient grain. It has over twice the iron of other grains, and three times the calcium. Teff has high amounts of carbohydrates, fiber, B-complex Vitamins (B6 (pyridoxine), B2 (riboflavin), B1 (thiamine), B3 (niacin), B5 (pantothenic acid)), and small amounts of Vitamin K. It has huge amounts of minerals manganese, calcium, iron, magnesium, phosphorus, potassium, copper, zinc, and selenium. In addition, teff has high amounts of protein along with omega-3 fat acids and it is gluten free. Native to Ethiopia where it provides one quarter of the total cereal production, teff is an easy-to-grow type of millet largely unknown outside of Ethiopia, India, and Australia. It can be cooked as porridge, added to baked goods, or even made into "teff polenta." Try adding a tablespoon to your smoothie or cereal. See also "Grains" for general information.

Tempeh [*Fermented Food*] Because tempeh is fermented, it has increased enzymes and nutrients. Tempeh is high in protein and contains all essential amino acids. It is a source of carbohydrates, fiber, Vitamin K, and B-complex Vitamins (B9 (folic acid), B2 (riboflavin), B1 (thiamine), B6 (pyridoxine)), and minerals iron, calcium, magnesium, phosphorus, potassium, copper, manganese, and selenium. It is considered healthier than tofu because it is made from the whole soybean whereas tofu is made by discarding the nutrient rich "whey." The process of making tempeh also breaks down hard-to-digest proteins, making it easier for humans to digest nutrients and removes enzyme inhibitors which reduce absorption. Tempeh originated in Indonesia thousands of years ago and is made from cracked, cooked soybeans, mixed with a grain such as millet, rice, or barley along with beneficial bacteria to give it a meaty taste and firm chewy texture. Tempeh can be stir-fried, sauteed, baked, microwaved, and stewed. Choose tempeh over tofu for added nutrients, enzymes, and better digestion. See also Kefir, Kimchee, Kombucha, and Vitamin K! under Food for Thought, under "K," Menopause – Can Food Help the Transition? under Food and You or Your Environment, under "M," and also Understanding Ancient Foods Today under Food for Thought, under "U."

Thimbleberries [*Fruit*] The thimble-like shape of these fruits give them their name. They have a beautiful red color when they become ripe. These are fleshy fruits that are so delicate that they may break in your hand when picked from the plant. See "Berries" for nutrients and information.

Thyme [*Herb*] Thyme is a perennial herb that is rich is volatile oils, Vitamins A, C, K, and minerals calcium, iron (1 cup of thyme tea has about 19% of your daily recommended amount of iron, although I wouldn't recommend eating that amount), and manganese. Thyme contains antioxidants and has been used since ancient times for medicinal and culinary reasons. Thyme is believed to promote digestion, relieve symptoms of a cough, cold, and upper respiratory infections, and work as an antispasmodic to relieve intestinal cramping. What Foods Fight or Help Prevent Cancer? under Food and You or Your Environment, under "C" and also "Herbs" for general information. See also Herbaceous Cooking under Healthy You, under "H."

Tilapia [*Fish*] Tilapia is high in protein and a good source of omega-3 fatty acids. It contains good amounts of Vitamin B12 (cobalamin) and some B3 (niacin), and minerals selenium and phosphorus. (For information on sustainable fish see "Fish" or visit *www.msc.org/cook-eat-enjoy/fish-to-eat.*)

Tofu [*Vegetable*] Tofu is often regarded as a "whole" food but in fact is a processed food. Also known as bean curd, it is made by coagulating soy milk and then pressing the resulting curds into soft white blocks. It is high in protein and contains all essential amino acids. A source of carbohydrates, fiber, Vitamin K and B-complex Vitamins (B9 (folic acid), B2 (riboflavin), B1 (thiamine), B6 (pyridoxine)), it also contains minerals iron, calcium, magnesium, phosphorus, potassium, copper, manganese, and selenium. Tofu offers a complete protein as it has all the essential amino acids but it made using high pressure and chemical solvents that decrease its nutrient values. It can also be difficult to digest and contains properties that can cause it to bind with other minerals, causing fewer nutrients to be absorbed. Tofu can cause digestive discomfort.

Tomatoes [*Fruit*] Tomatoes have carbohydrates, fiber, and good amounts of Vitamins C and A and moderate amounts of B-complex Vitamins. They contain good amounts of the mineral potassium and some manganese along with several antioxidant compounds, including lycopene (when tomatoes are cooked the lycopene content is increased), beta-carotene, and zeaxanthin. Usually thought of as a vegetable, tomatoes are, in fact, a fruit. See also What's to be Done about the Rise in Heart Disease? under Food and You or Your Environment, under "H."

Triticale [*Grain*] Triticale is a power food that contains high amounts of carbohydrates and good amounts of protein and Vitamin E. It has huge amounts of B-complex Vitamins (B1 (thiamine), B9 (folic acid), B5 (pantothenic acid), B3 (niacin), B2 (riboflavin), and B6 (pyridoxine)), and the mineral manganese along with very good amounts of minerals magnesium, phosphorus, copper, zinc, iron, potassium, and calcium. A hybrid of durum wheat and rye, it's been grown commercially for only 35 years. Today about 80% of the world's triticale is grown in Europe. It grows easily without commercial fertilizers and pesticides and is very hardy, growing well even in poor soils, making it ideal for organic and sustainable farming. Triticale has a delicious wheat-like flavor. Rolled triticale can be eaten like oatmeal and triticale flour can be used in baking instead of whole wheat for added nutrients. See also "Grains" for general information.

Trout [*Fish*] Trout is high in protein and omega-3 fatty acids. It is a great source of B-complex Vitamins (B12 (cobalamin), B6 (pyridoxine), B1 (thiamine), B2 (riboflavin), and B3 (niacin)) and minerals magnesium, phosphorus, selenium, copper, iron, and potassium. (For information on sustainable fish see "Fish" or visit *www.msc.org/cook-eat-enjoy/fish-to-eat.*)

Tuber. See Potatoes – A Staple Worldwide under Food for Thought, under "P" and also Root Vegetables under Food for Thought, under "R."

Tuna [*Fish*] Tuna is high in protein and omega-3 fatty acids. It is a great source of Vitamin A and B-complex Vitamins (B12 (cobalamin), B6 (pyridoxine), B3 (niacin), B2 (riboflavin), B1 (thiamine), and B5 (pantothenic acid)). It contains good amounts of minerals selenium, phosphorus, and magnesium, and some potassium and iron. (For information on sustainable fish see "Fish" or visit *www.msc.org/cook-eat-enjoy/fish-to-eat.*)

Turban Squash. See "Squash" for nutrients and information.

Turbinado [*Sugar (Natural)*] Turbinado sugar contains minerals potassium and some small amounts of magnesium and calcium. It is produced by pressing fresh sugarcane to remove its nutrient-rich juice. See "Sugar" for general information. See also Sugar – A Diet No No under Food for Thought, under "S."

Turkey [*Meat*] Turkey is a good, lean source of protein and most turkey contains some omega-3 fatty acids, especially pasture-raised turkey. It contains good amounts of B-complex Vitamins (B1 (thiamine), B2 (riboflavin), B6 (pyridoxine), and B12 (cobalamin)), and minerals iron, potassium, phosphorus selenium, and zinc. Turkey contains good amounts of the amino acid tryptophan that helps create serotonin in the body and has a calming effect. This is why we like to nap after a big holiday turkey dinner! See also Happiness and Foods that Create Bliss under Food for Thought, under "H."

Turmeric [*Spice*] Turmeric is a powerhouse of nutrients. It has huge amounts of fiber and is high in protein. It has good amounts of Vitamins C, E, K, B-complex Vitamins (B6 (pyridoxine), B2 (riboflavin), B3 (niacin), and B9 (folic acid)), large amounts of minerals iron, manganese, copper, and magnesium, and good amounts of phosphorus, potassium, zinc, and calcium. Curcumin, along with other antioxidants, has been found to have antiamyloid and anti-inflammatory properties, making turmeric effective in preventing, or at least delaying the onset, of Alzheimer's disease. It has been in use for a very long time as an important ingredient in traditional Chinese and Ayurvedic (tra-

ditional Indian) medicines for its antimicrobial, anti-inflammatory, carminative, and antiflatulent properties. See "Spices" for
general information and cooking suggestions. See also What
Foods Fight or Help Prevent Cancer? under Food and You or
Your Environment, under "C," Root Vegetables under Food for
Thought, under "R," Are Rheumatoid Arthritis and Autoimmune Diseases on the Rise? under Food and You or Your Environment, under "R," and also How Can We Hold onto
Yesterday's Memories? under Food and You or Your Environment, under "Y."

Turnips [*Vegetable*] Turnips contain carbohydrates, fiber, are high in
Vitamins C and B6 (B6 (pyridoxine)) and have small amounts
of other B-complex Vitamins, and minerals copper, manganese,
calcium, and iron. The greens contain antioxidant compounds
and additional minerals. Often confused with rutabaga, it is generally accepted that turnip and cabbage were crossed to produce
rutabaga. See What Foods Fight or Help Prevent Cancer? under
Food and You or Your Environment, under "C" and also Root
Vegetables under Food for Thought, under "R."

Tuscan Cabbage. See "Kale." See What Foods Fight or Help Prevent
Cancer? under Food and You or Your Environment, under "C."

FOOD FOR THOUGHT

Tea, the Drink of Emperors

Did you know?

- Legend has it that tea was discovered by Chinese Emperor Shen
  Nung in 2737 BC. A tea leaf accidentally fell into his bowl of
  hot water, and the rest is history.
- Tea bags were invented in America in the early 1800s. Now 96%
  of tea served around the world is made using tea bags.

- There are four major tea types – black, green, white, and oolong. Darjeeling is known as the premium of black teas.
- For centuries tea was used only as a medicine. It took almost 3,000 years for it to become an everyday drink.
- Iced tea was invented at the 1904 St. Louis World's Fair.
- Tea used to be very expensive. It was kept in a locked tea chest in the parlor.
- High Tea was created during the Victoria era, when it was eaten with the evening meal and served at a high dining table. Low Tea was created to allow for a light snack before dinner and was served in sitting rooms at the low tables near chairs and sofas.

Throughout history, tea has been associated with cultural traditions and historical events. Most of us remember learning about the Boston Tea Party where massive amounts of tea were thrown into the Boston harbor to protest taxes imposed by the British in 1773. This event is believed to have been a spark which ignited the American Revolutionary War a few years later.

But tea also has a rich history of health benefits. Tea has been around for more than 2,000 years in Asia and Russia and has been used both medicinally and as a popular drink but didn't gain prominence in the West until recently.

Green tea, black tea, oolong tea, and white tea are true teas and they all come from the same tea plant. The leaves are simply processed differently. Green tea leaves are not fermented; they are withered and steamed. Black tea and oolong tea leaves undergo a crushing and fermenting process. White tea is neither cured nor fermented.

In general green, white, and black teas have the highest amount of antioxidants, but they are different from the antioxidants found in fruit and vegetables, making them a good compliment to your diet. Kombucha is a probiotic beverage that is made from sweetened tea that's been fermented by a symbiotic colony of bacteria and yeast and is known to improve digestion and fight candida (harmful yeast) overgrowth.

> **Tea is soothing and delicious –**
> **and good for you too.**

The number of herbal and fruit teas is almost endless, with peppermint, chamomile, and ginger being the most popular for their calming and digestive benefits. Many are known for medicinal qualities as well like aiding digestion and sleep.

Tea is gaining ground over coffee. Consumption of tea is being studied for its reported benefits on enhancing immune function, lowering LDL cholesterol levels, increasing HDL cholesterol levels, reducing blood pressure, thinning the blood, reducing the risk of a heart attack, lowering the risk of stroke, reducing the risk of cancer, aiding digestion, preventing dental cavities and gingivitis, and the list goes on. In a study involving bladder cancer cells, green tea extract seemed to make the cancer cells behave oddly. Another study found that men who drank oolong tea plus green tea extract lost more weight and total body fat, compared with men who drank plain oolong tea. Also, the green tea drinkers had lower LDL cholesterol and improved prostate function. There's also evidence that tea extracts applied to the skin (in a lotion) can block sun damage that leads to skin cancer. In moderation caffeine can be a benefit as it stimulates the metabolism, increasing brain function and alertness. All this research seems to suggest that it might be good to add tea to your beverage of choice list.[141]

Below is an antioxidant powerhouse tea recipe:

Somalian Tea
1 tea bag, regular black tea
4 cardamom seeds, crushed
1/2 teaspoon clove, crushed

1 tablespoon honey or sugar

1 1/2 cups water, boiling

1 tablespoon milk

Directions: Add tea bag, cardamom seeds, cloves, and honey/ sugar to a large mug. Add boiling water. Stir well. Add the milk to another mug then strain tea into that mug. Stir and serve.

Make time for a relaxing cup of tea!

FOOD AND YOU OR YOUR ENVIRONMENT

Why We Need to Nourish … the Topsoil?

What is soil? It's not just dirt. It is needed to feed the plants we grow all around the world.

Soil is a mixture of minerals, air, water, sand, silt, and clay mixed with organic matter such as roots, decaying plant parts, fungi, earthworms, bacteria, and microorganisms. An acre of healthy topsoil can contain 900 pounds of earthworms, 2,400 pounds of fungi, 1,500 pounds of bacteria, 133 pounds of protozoa, and 890 pounds of arthropods and algae.

Topsoil is the uppermost layer of soil. It is defined as the top 2 inches of soil but can vary from 2 inches to several feet deep and is where nutrients from organic matter are found. It is generally darker in color than the subsoil below and often referred to as "Black Gold."[142] Of all soil, topsoil is the richest source of nutrients that sustains plant, animal, and human life.

> An investment in soil preservation is an investment in continuing our rich food supply.

It takes about 500 years for a single inch of topsoil to be created in nature and much less time for soil erosion to occur.[143] Jamie Lee Curtis narrated a documentary, *Dirt*, about our ever-decreasing topsoil and demonstrated how people all over the world are learning to preserve the soil that all life depends on to exist and thrive. Soil depletion occurs when the components that contribute to fertility are removed and not replaced and the conditions that support soil's fertility are not maintained. This results in poor crop yields. In agriculture, depletion can be due to excessively intense cultivation, fertilization or chemical usage, monocropping and inadequate soil management. According to ScienceDaily LLC, soil's organic matter represents the largest fraction of earthbound carbon in the biosphere. This means that climatic change can be slowed down with proper management of the soil. Climate protection and topsoil preservation are intimately connected.

While soil erosion is a serious issue, the good news is that innovative people are using nature to find solutions. Deep-rooted perennial plants, flowers, trees, shrubs, and grasses provide natural mechanisms for preserving a soil environment's structure and composition. Grass is one of our most amazing topsoil preservers and forms a symbiotic relationship with soil to help retain topsoil material and buffer the impact of wind and rain that can cause erosion.[144] For larger farms, planting a wood lot beside the crops can have the same impact. Mulching and no-till farming are also used more extensively in agriculture with success. With research, improved best practices for soil management, and good old composting, farmers are starting to better manage the soil which supports our food supply. Dirt isn't just dirt anymore when you realize the complexity of the life teaming in each and every handful – or shovel full – out there!

HEALTHY YOU

Tender Loving Touch

I don't need to promote having more sex like I do eating more vegetables which is a relief.

Sex is great for our health in many surprising ways, including improved immune response, lowered blood pressure, lowered risk of heart attack, and reduced chances of getting prostate cancer according to research. Sex can even help with pain management. "Orgasm can block pain," says Barry R. Komisaruk, PhD, a distinguished professor at Rutgers University. It releases a hormone that helps raise your pain threshold. And sex can also improve the quality of our sleep. "After orgasm, the hormone prolactin is released, which is responsible for the feelings of relaxation and sleepiness," according to Sheenie Ambardar, MD.[145]

And tender loving touch and physical closeness with your partner can soothe stress and anxiety. Touching and hugging releases the body's natural "feel good" hormone dopamine and increases our brain's pleasure and reward systems. This boosts our self-esteem and happiness which is also great for our health.

Remember to take time for physical tenderness with your loved one even if you have to leave the laundry, dishes, and bills for another day!

$\mathcal{U}$

*"If you give a man a fish you feed him for a day.
If you teach a man to fish you feed him for a lifetime."*
Chinese Proverb

Bread on the Run – Unleavened

When I was a little girl, I went to Sunday school to learn the bible stories. One spring Sunday morning, we had a hands-on lesson to teach us about Passover, a Jewish festival that commemorates the Exodus. In their haste to escape slavery in Egypt, the Israelites did not have time to allow their bread to rise – unleavened bread.

Since then I have learned that many cultures have unleavened bread in their cuisines.

- Matzo – Jewish
- Tortilla – Mesoamerican/Mexican
- Roti – South Asian

Unleavened bread simply refers to bread made from grains, but without yeast, baking powder, baking soda, or other leavening agents. It contains similar nutrients to leavened bread, depending on the flour used.

Unleavened breads are generally flat breads; however, not all flat breads are unleavened.

REAL "U" FOODS

Udo [*Vegetable*] Udo contains fiber, carbohydrates, and Vitamins C, A, K, and B-complex Vitamins. It contains minerals manganese, copper, and some iron. Udo is a Japanese vegetable and a member of the ginseng family. It has asparagus-like stalks and a flavor similar to fennel. It can be lightly cooked in soups or other dishes and it is also added raw to salads.

Ugli Fruit [*Fruit*] Ugli fruit contains carbohydrates, fiber, Vitamin C, beta-carotene, and potassium. This citrus fruit also has quercetin and other powerful antioxidant compounds. With its unsightly appearance, rough, wrinkled, greenish-yellow rind, wrapped loosely around the orange pulpy citrus inside, it comes by its name honestly, but the taste is beautiful.

Ulluco [*Vegetable*] Ulluco is a popular South American tuber vegetable that resembles a small potato. This tuber contains carbohydrates, fiber, protein, calcium, Vitamin C, and beta-carotene. The leaves are also edible and a spoonful has almost as many nutrients as spinach. The most widely recognized and commercially viable of the tubers, ulluco is popular for its taste. It is easy to grow, frost resistant, and moderately drought resistant, although the plant prefers soils that are rich in organic matter. Ulluco tubers come in a variety of colors and shapes. Because of their high water content, they are most suitable for boiling, and the soft, shiny skins need no peeling before eating. See also Root Vegetables under Food for Thought, under "R."

FOOD FOR THOUGHT

Understanding Ancient Foods Today

Did you know that the great ancient civilizations, like Egypt, Asia, India and Greece, all recorded their observations on the positive effects of plants and foods on health, as well as their healing virtues? The importance of a good diet in maintaining health was, in fact, the foundation of all medical treatment until the beginning of the twentieth century.

A lot of the recently hyped "power foods" that provide enormous nutrients and have high levels of antioxidants were eaten regularly by ancient civilizations, such as the Romans, Aztecs, and Ancient Asian cultures. Below are some of the super foods eaten by ancient civilizations that we have newly rediscovered today.

Acai and Camu Camu Berries

Acai berry was introduced to the western world in the 1990s, but it has existed for thousands of years. Indigenous to the rain forest, the acai (pronounced ah-sigh-ee) was used by Amazonian tribes to prevent and to cure various ailments. Acai berries contain 30 times more antioxidants than a glass of red wine, 10 times more than red grapes, and twice as many as blueberries. Acai berries are rich in fiber and in oleic acid, a heart-healthy monounsaturated fat shown to lower LDL cholesterol while raising HDL cholesterol and improving circulation. It also prevents the oxidation of LDL cholesterol which results in arteriosclerosis. (See also "Acai Berry" for all nutrients.) Camu camu berries are another one of the new "old" power berries being promoted by health experts! They too are grown in the rain forests of the Amazon and contain the highest natural Vitamin C content of any plant in the world.[146]

Black Rice

Brown rice is better for us than white rice, as it contains more fiber, vitamins, and minerals. But what is black rice? Black rice was revered in ancient China as it was thought to ensure a long and healthy life. During the years when China was ruled by an emperor, black rice was dubbed as the "Forbidden Rice." It was cultivated in very small amounts because it was only for the emperor's consumption. Black rice is abundant in anthocyanin, found in deep red, blue, or purple colored foods, which is a potent antioxidant, riding the body of harmful free radicals that can cause accelerated aging and cancer. In fact, a study published in the *International Journal of Oncology* (in December 2009)[147] revealed that anthocyanin might inhibit the growth and, in some cases, destroy human colon cancer cells. While many fruits such as blueberries are revered for their high anthocyanin content, a tablespoon of black rice has more antioxidants than a similar amount of blueberries, as well as having less sugar and more fiber.[148] See also "Grains" for general information, and "Rice."

> A number of these ancient super foods were reserved for royalty and the wealthy, but today they are available to all.

Chia and Hemp Seeds

Chia seeds are indigenous to South and Central America and were once considered a staple food item among the Aztecs, Incas, and Mayans. If you have ever seen a chia seed you will know they are incredibly tiny so it is hard to believe that they were used as an energy source by Aztec warriors. A small amount of chia seeds was believed to sustain a warrior for an entire day as they are high in protein, fiber, phosphorus, calcium, and manganese, as well as omega-3 fatty acids, which lower LDL (bad) cholesterol while raising HDL (good) cholesterol, reduce inflammation and aid in proper brain function. While walnuts, flax seeds, and cold-water fish are celebrated for their high omega-3 content, chia is truly amazing in its quantity. Chia seeds have 8 times more of this essential fatty acid than salmon and are one of the richest sources of omega-3 on the planet. Chia seed can absorb more than 12 times its weight in water which was key for helping Aztec warriors prolong hydration during battles. (See "Chia Seeds" for all nutrients.)

Hemp is one of the oldest crops in the world. The hemp plant has been used for fuel, fiber, and medicine for over 5,000 years. The earliest recorded use of hemp by ancient civilizations dates to 8000 BC in Europe and Asia. In ancient China, hemp seeds provided cooking oil until the introduction of sesame oil during the Han period. Hemp seeds contain protein, fiber, essential fatty acids, antioxidants, amino acids, vitamins, and minerals and are easily digestible, gluten free, and tasty, too. (See "Hemp" for all nutrients.)

Cinnamon

In 1492, Columbus sailed the ocean blue; he was seeking a new spice trade route. Among these prized spices was cinnamon. Its benefits have been documented as early as 2700 BCE throughout China, Europe, and Egypt. In the time of ancient Rome, cinnamon was actually valued more than gold and it was used to treat an array of illnesses and their symptoms, including inflammation, poisonous bites, colds, the flu, and other respiratory infections. While many ancient civilizations used this spice for its medicinal properties, today it has scientifically been proven that cinnamon offers many health benefits. Cinnamon contains many potent antioxidant compounds, as well as possessing antimicrobial activity, so it may help to reduce the risk of food-borne diseases caused by bacteria. Cinnamaldehyde, the organic compound that gives cinnamon its flavor and fragrance, helps to prevent unwanted clumping of blood platelets as well as acting as an anti-inflammatory. The medicinal use of cinnamon gaining the most attention these days concerns blood sugar stabilization. Multiple studies have shown that cinnamon may help control and lower blood glucose levels, which is important for people who have type II diabetes or who are prone to the disease. (See "Cinnamon" for all nutrients.)

Dark Chocolate

The history of chocolate began in South and Central America and the Amazon regions. Chocolate was considered a divine gift, a form of currency, a source of power, and a health food by people of ancient cultures. The Mayans were the first chocolate lovers and treasured cacao for its energy and mood-enhancing properties. Cacao was used in ceremonies, burials, and a drink made with a coarse paste, spices and chilies, and hot water. The Aztecs prized the cacao bean as well and reserved the bean for the rich nobles.[149] Cacao beans are so nutrient-dense that scientists haven't even begun to identify all the benefits in the little bean. The highest nutrients are found only in raw cacao beans or nibs (or really, really dark chocolate) and they have high amounts of minerals, vitamins, and tons of antioxidants that are great for your heart and skin. They also contain the amino acid tryptophan, which makes the neurotransmitter known as serotonin that promotes positive feelings. (See "Cacao" for all nutrients.)

Fermented Vegetables

People in ancient civilizations, from Mongolian nomads to Babylonian royalty to Asiatics ate fermented beans and vegetables to stop gastrointestinal problems; and Russian and Mongolian military troops campaigning across vast distances ate sauerkraut for scurvy prevention, and against diarrhea that occurred with the pathogen exposure and hygiene of the travel. Fermented vegetables are a high source of Vitamin C and can be stored for long periods of time without refrigeration. Dishes of vegetables are nutritious in themselves, but when fermented also contain beneficial bacteria that aid our digestion and health. [150] Kimchee (fermented cabbage and spices) was recently named by *Health Magazine* as one of the world's healthiest foods. Like other fermented vegetable dishes, it is loaded with nutrients and is an enzyme-rich probiotic and digestive aid. Probiotic-rich foods supply the body with "good bacteria" and are also believed to help prevent "leaky gut" and boost immunity. In Russia, a lacto-fermented beverage called "kvass" has long been made from beets and during war times was used against infections and disease. Ancient Iraqis and Egyptians made similar drinks. Fungus-fermented teas have been used throughout Russia, China, Japan, Poland, Bulgaria, Germany, and Southeast Asia (called "chainyi grib" in Russia and "kombucha" in Asia, which means "mushroom"). Australian Aborigines lacto-fermented legumes to make a bubbly, sour drink, and South American indigenous people fermented several drinks they say prevented digestive problems including diarrhea. (See also Kefir, Kimchee, Kombucha, and Vitamin K under Food for Thought, under "K.")

Ancient civilizations didn't have over-the-counter or prescription medications so they had to incorporate the right foods into their diet to maximize their energy, vitality, and immunity. Maybe we should incorporate more of these powerful ancient foods into our daily diets as well!

FOOD AND YOU OR YOUR ENVIRONMENT

Urban Green Roofs and Urban Gardens – Will they Offset Shrinking Farm Land?

As the population grows, urban communities have less space to grow food. To offset the lack of land for growing food and the decreasing amount of park and green space, urban gardens are becoming increasingly popular.

Urban rooftop gardens and green roofs help reduce environmental problems encountered with dense urban populations and encourage sustainable development – conserving energy and water, improving air and water quality, assisting in storm water management, absorbing solar radiation, becoming a source of local food production, providing habitat restoration, and creating natural relaxation retreats.[151]

Chicago is one of the leading U.S. cities for rooftop gardens but even they have a fraction of the green roofs they have in European countries like Germany. In Germany, experts say, 15-20% of the flat roofs in the entire country are green and the total is measured in billions of square feet. Local governments in Germany have regulatory incentives for building green roofs, including a "rain tax," which charges property owners for impervious surfaces that lead to rainwater runoff and fill up local storm sewers.[152]

**Look up. Look way up –
to find your fruits and veggies!**

Growing food in urban gardens is becoming a healthy lifeline for many urban poor who have limited access to freshly grown food. All over the world innovative non-profit organizations are teaching people to grow their own food so they can eat more nutritiously. They have garden facilities that provide access to healthy vegetables and fruit, bake ovens, and cooking classes along with greenhouses, education on food systems and urban agriculture, and access to community gardens.

In his book, *The Good Food Revolution,* Will Allen describes his incredible efforts to create urban gardens for low-income youth in the U.S. His company operates greenhouses in impoverished areas of the U.S. where grocery stores are often non-existent and delivers workshops for kids. He developed creative ways to increase his output by growing vegetables vertically up trellises and supporting or hanging them from baskets to increase the amount and varieties of vegetables. He also developed a business using vermiculture (composting using worms) by taking local food scraps from stores that would otherwise end up in landfill sites, and adding worms to create a rich fertilizer that he can sell for a nice profit. He also grows some of his vegetables hydroponically (or without soil).

Many communities around the world are committed to investing in the development of educational urban gardens for school children as well. Teaching children how to grow and eat quality food, is a great idea and one that is growing in popularity everywhere. With community gardens, urban gardens, and urban green roofs becoming the norm there is a real opportunity to improve food access for those in need and teach others about the importance of nutrition for good health!

HEALTHY YOU

Uncooked! Eating Food in the Raw

Not everybody is the same. Even if you do not have allergies or sensitivities, everyone's system operates a little differently. That's one reason many nutritionists vary their recommendations of food and diets after an individual assessment. But what we all recommend consistently is incorporating some raw fruit and vegetables into your diet (unless you have a diagnosed digestive issue that forbids it).

Raw foods, especially sprouts, contain incredible amounts of nutrients and enzymes that we need to properly digest and metabolize food. When we cook foods, we destroy some of the enzymes, vitamins, and minerals necessary for good health. If we eat too much overcooked, microwaved, and processes foods, it can deplete our enzyme reserves and clog our colons, which may lead to health issues. Many cultures incorporate some raw, enzyme-rich foods into their cuisines, from raw salads and fruits to raw animal protein, such as sushi.

Although there are some people who eat a high amount of their food raw, I believe that balance is important in everything and we need both raw, detoxifying foods and warm, cooked foods as well. Try to eat some raw foods every day for added fiber, enzymes, and antioxidants!

*"A spoonful of honey will catch more flies
than a gallon of vinegar."*
Benjamin Franklin
(1705-1790, American polymath and
founding father of the United States)

Venison Versus Bambi Guilt

A few years ago, I traveled to see a dear friend in Western Canada and brought my family. We stayed locally and enjoyed skiing and living in the mountains.

One night we all met for dinner at her house and she served the most delicious hamburgers I had eaten in years. After we had finished enjoying a great meal, she asked if I noticed a difference in the taste of the meat. She explained that her husband had gone hunting and brought back a delicious deer. It dawned on me suddenly that we were eating venison which until then I hadn't tried because of what I call my "Bambi Guilt!"

She explained that the deer population was too high and not only is culling a good idea, but wild deer, or venison, is a highly nutritious and antibiotic- and hormone-free lean source of protein.

REAL "V" FOODS

Veal [*Meat*] Veal provides Vitamins A and B12 (cobalamin) and very
good amounts of some other B-complex Vitamins (B2 (riboflavin),
B5 (pantothenic acid), B6 (pyridoxine), B3 (niacin), and B1 (thi-

amine)). It has good amounts of minerals copper, zinc, phosphorus, iron, and selenium, and some manganese. Veal comes from a young cow fed a specific diet, including large quantities of milk in a restricted pen.

Vegemite [*Yeast*] Vegemite is a highly nutritious yeast extract, with some of the highest levels of B-complex Vitamins of any food per serving, including B1 (thiamine), B2 (riboflavin), B3 (niacin), and B9 (folic acid). Vegemite also contains trace amounts of the minerals iron, potassium, zinc, and selenium. Aussies and Kiwis are very proud of their unique creation.

Vegetables [*Classification*] All vegetables contain varying amounts of vitamins and minerals along with antioxidants and fiber that are needed by the body for many functions and overall health. The Latin word for vegetable is "*vegetare*" and means to enliven or animate, fitting given the importance of vegetables in our diet for health benefits and vitality! Vegetables are alkalizing to the body and anti-inflammatory. Some of the main types of vegetable families include allium (chives, garlic, leek, onion, and shallot), brassica and cruciferous (bok choy, broccoli, Brussels sprouts, cabbage, cauliflower, collard greens, kohlrabi, mustard greens, rapini, rutabaga, turnip, etc.), gourd (squash, pumpkin, zucchini), grass (wheatgrass, bamboo), legumes (beans, lentils, soy) and nightshade (peppers, tomatoes, potatoes). See particular species under their specific name.

Vegetable Marrow. See "Zucchini."

Venison [*Meat*] Venison meat comes from a deer and is high in protein and has good amounts of B-complex Vitamins (B2 (riboflavin), B3 (niacin), B6 (pyridoxine), B12 (cobalamin), B5 (pantothenic acid), B1 (thiamine)), and minerals zinc, phosphorus, iron, and selenium and some potassium. Being game (or wild meat) venison is known to be a healthier choice because it is grass fed and pasture raised without hormones or antibiotics and has low is saturated fat.

Vinegar [*Fermented Food*) Vinegar contains the nutrients of the ingredients used in the fermentation process. Apple cider vinegar, for example, contains Vitamins A, and C, minerals potassium, boron, iron, and calcium, beta-carotene, and pectin. Vinegar is known for its antibacterial, antibiotic, and antifungal properties. Vinegar is made by a chemical change called fermentation. During fermentation, the sugar in wine or juice is changed into alcohol and gas. As the gas evaporates, it leaves only the alcohol and fruit flavor. The next step is called oxidation, when the oxygen in air mixes with the vinegar bacteria in the alcohol or juice to change it into vinegar. See Incredible Vinegar – Live Longer! under Food for Thought, below. See also Kefir, Kimchee, Kombucha, and Vitamin K! under Food for Thought, under "K."

Vitamins. See What Your Body Needs and Why.

Vongole. See "Clam."

FOOD FOR THOUGHT

Incredible Vinegar – Live Longer!

Vinegar has been made and used for thousands of years for both medicinal and culinary purposes. It is mentioned in the bible for its soothing and healing properties and traces of it have been found in Egyptian urns dating from around 3000 BC. The ancient Greeks, Romans, and Chinese used it thousands of years ago to preserve food and as a condiment or seasoning in recipes.

In more recent times (1864), Louis Pasteur showed that vinegar results from a natural fermentation process. It was used to treat wounds on battlefields in World War I. Vinegar has several medical benefits from relieving indigestion to purifying and revitalizing our bodies to fighting against bacteria and fungi to relieving headaches.

Vinegar derives from the Old French
"vin aigre," which translates as "sour wine."

A new review article reports on recent studies showing different types of vinegars that may benefit human health. They have therapeutic properties that include beneficial effects on cardiovascular health and blood pressure, antibacterial activity, reduction in the effects of diabetes, and increased vigor after exercise. In addition, a few studies showed that people who consumed certain types of vinegar daily may have a decreased appetite.

Cal Orey, in her book *The Healing Powers of Vinegar*, outlines the health benefits of raw, unpasteurized apple cider vinegar for weight management, digestion, high blood pressure, high cholesterol, osteoporosis, memory, and overall health and vitality.

All types of cooking vinegar enhance the flavor of dishes and below are the main five types of vinegar and their uses

1. **Fruit Vinegar:** This type of vinegar is made from mixed fruit by alcoholic fermentation. Fruit vinegar is made with apples, oranges, pineapples, blackberries, blueberries, and bananas. Apple cider vinegar is the most commonly used vinegar and it is made by alcoholic fermentation with apple juice. It is perfect as a seasoning in all types of salads and sauces. Raw apple cider vinegar (traditionally fermented without pasteurization or distillation) retains the most nutrients and can be found in most stores.

2. **Wine Vinegar/Balsamic, Red and White:** This is a product made by alcoholic fermentation and acidification of grape juice. It is widely used in Italy and France. It is also called red wine vinegar, sherry vinegar, white wine vinegar, or balsamic vinegar Balsamic of Modena is the most expensive because it is aged the longest time. Red and white wine vinegars are everyday vinegars. They are good

for salad dressings and marinades. Red wine vinegar is best used with heartier flavors and foods, like beef, pork, and vegetables.

3. **Rice Vinegar:** Widely used in Asian countries where there is an abundance of rice crops, the flavor of rice vinegar is mild and slightly sweet. Its color varies depending on which grain is used, black rice, white rice, or red yeast rice. Rice vinegar is the mildest of all, with much less acidity than other vinegars. It's often used in Asian or Chinese cooking.

4. **Malt Vinegar:** Used mostly for sprinkling on fish and chips, this vinegar is made from barley.

5. **Herb Flavored Vinegars:** This type of vinegar comes with addition of various herbs. Flavored vinegar are often blended with thyme, basil, tarragon, and rosemary. It can also be combined with sugar or honey.

All vinegars should be stored tightly closed in a cool, dark place. They will last for about 1–3 years after opening; after that time, the flavors will diminish.[153]

Besides being good for our health, vinegar can help with the environment as well. Vinegar has been widely acclaimed as a natural and "green" household cleaner. Below are several favorite vinegar cleaning "recipes" you can try.

- **Microwave Oven:** Mix together 2 tablespoons of lemon juice or vinegar and 2 cups of water in a 4-cup glass microwave-safe bowl. Microwave on high for 2-3 minutes. Carefully remove the bowl and wipe the microwave with paper towels.
- **Sluggish Drains:** Pour 1/2 cup baking soda down the drain. Add 1/2 cup white vinegar and cover the drain. Let this mixture foam for a few minutes, then pour 8 cups of boiling water down the drain to flush it. Do not use this combination after using any commercial drain opener or cleaner.

- **Coffee Maker:** Every few months fill the water reservoir with equal parts white vinegar and water and put it through the brew cycle. Then use clean fresh water and run the brew cycle three times

Make a habit of incorporating vinegar into your diet and try the different types to find the ones you like best. They bring flavor to dishes and will help with your digestion and vitality and even cleaning your household too!

FOOD AND YOUR ENVIRONMENT

Do We Need Vitamin Supplements?

Vitamins and dietary supplements are non-drug and non-hormone based products that can be consumed orally in the form of pills, powders, liquids, or by intravenous injection (common with B12 (cobalamin) shots). Their function is to supplement the diet, giving consumer's added nutrition in their diet, including amino and fatty acids, vitamins, minerals, and fiber. The global vitamin and supplement market is worth $68 billion according to research from Euromonitor.[154]

Some medical professionals believe that vitamins are vital and others think they are completely unnecessary as long as you eat a balanced diet. Like a lot of food topics, it can get confusing. The reality is that many of us do not have time to eat a perfect diet or have extra stress or health issues in our lives that affect our ability to utilize the nutrients we ingest or create a need for more nutrients to off-set system imbalances. Chronic stress/sickness, smoking, or limited diets will deplete nutrients and pregnancy calls for extra nutrients for the growing fetus. Also, food transported long distances, the current norm in our food system, loses nutrients during the trip and in storage, which can mean we consume fewer nutrients in certain foods.

The most important supplements depend on your own health and needs. Some health-care professionals agree that taking a high quality fish oil or krill oil supplement for omega-3 fatty acids and a good probiotic supplement and vitamin D is a good idea to boost our immune system and support brain and heart health. Others think magnesium is key. In her book *The Magnesium Miracle*, Carolyn Dean, M.D., N.D.,[155] writes that she believes a large percentage of the population is deficient in magnesium, which together with calcium, Vitamins D and K is responsible for bone health and also many nerve, muscle, heart and enzyme functions in the body. She talks about how some people take too much calcium but forget about magnesium which creates system imbalances as calcium and magnesium work together.

There is also a debate over the pros and cons of synthetic vitamins versus natural ones.[156] The largest vitamin suppliers in the world are BASF, Pfizer, and DSM. More than 50% of the vitamins we consume, whether in supplements or a box of cereal, come from China and are synthetically manufactured.

You might assume that Vitamin C comes from an orange and Vitamin A from a carrot, but that is incorrect. Vitamin C starts with corn and then undergoes a complex, multi-step bacterial and chemical process. Vitamin A comes from acetylene gas, a chemical derived from petroleum refining.[157] Food-based supplements are gaining in popularity and some people choose to buy organic vitamins instead because they believe our bodies utilize the natural form much better. (I like food-sourced vitamins like the ones from New Chapter, Garden of Life, and Mega Food made with organic dehydrated fruits and vegetables.[158])

> The first step should be to get your nutrition from natural, whole foods; supplements can be added if needed – but check with your doctor.

Whether you decide to add supplements or not, it is important to check with your doctor for any interactions with existing medication and focus first on a variety of fruits, vegetables, probiotic foods, and omega-3 fatty acids every day to meet nutritional requirements. Remember vitamins are stimulating and best taken in the morning, while minerals are relaxing and best taken at night.

Below are some guidelines on using supplements in their various forms.

- **Tablets:** This is the most common way to take supplements. They have a longer shelf life. Fillers and binders are used to make them more stable; some could be natural and others artificial. Some of the chemical coatings of the tablets can cause trouble for some sensitive patients.
- **Capsules:** Easier to swallow, capsules *may* work better than tablets for those with digestion issues. You can open the capsule and sprinkle the contents over food/liquid. Most capsules are made from beef or pork gelatin (derived from the collagen inside animal skins and bones). Gelatin is readily digested and absorbed, and extends the shelf life to 5 years. Vegetarian capsules are available and usually made from soy, but you may see "cellulose" on the ingredient list.
- **Powdered:** This form is easily absorbed, and a good alternative if you can't swallow or have weak digestion.
- **Liquid:** This is the best form to take, and is most often used for infants and children. Taken this way adults will get the same advantages as from powered supplements. Watch for food dyes and artificial sweeteners.
- **Injections:** B12 (cobalamin) shots are often injected. An injection of Vitamin K is given at birth. Vitamin C may be administered in this form as part of a heavy metal chelation or cancer therapy.

Some people decide to take supplements and others choose not to spend the money when they can focus on high quality food instead. The choice is individual and depends on many personal and health factors.

HEALTHY YOU

Visualize to Actualize!

Many of us often set health goals in January, in the form on New Year's resolutions. Some of us want to lose 10-15 pounds, others want to work out more, and some want to reduce their stress or spend more time with their families to have a better work/life balance. We all have areas that we want to improve for greater health and visualization is a powerful tool to create a new and improved reality.

Visualization is creating positive pictures in the mind of a desired outcome in the future – like the new you 15 pounds lighter. Even though it takes time to achieve your dreams, visualizing success will help you get there. Our minds are not aware of the difference between visualization and actually doing or having something. This means that the brain will respond in a way similar to if the experience was real! This can really work to inspire you to follow through on goal setting with positive action steps.

If you want to try a visualization exercise, it is best to put yourself in a calm state for the best outcome. Hey, even if you feel a bit silly at first, visualizing positive and successful outcomes boosts your mood, lowers your stress and makes you feel more confident in your life. Give it a try!

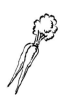

W

"Water is the driving force of all nature."
Leonardo da Vinci
(1452-1519, Italian polymath)

You Can Lead a Horse to It

I have always been a bit of a hydration enthusiast. My friends would say that my one addiction is water!

They always ask, "How can you enjoy drinking water so much? It's so boring and you have to go to the bathroom all the time." These are common objections that people make when nutritionists, trainers, or doctors suggest they drink more water.

I remember traveling in Europe once with friends and visiting an Island off of the coast of Ireland. The tour guide said that there is very little fresh water on the island and at that moment, I clutched my water bottle tightly while my friends laughed heartily knowing I wouldn't be sharing my supply with them that day!

But water is an incredible drink and can be spruced up with added slices of lemons or limes. Water is the preferred beverage in my household and we are all grateful for the clean water we are lucky to drink every day. Research shows that even a 2% drop in hydration levels significantly affects our ability to perform tasks and maintain energy levels!

REAL "W" FOODS

Walnuts [*Nut*] Walnuts are high in protein, carbohydrates, fiber, and omega-3 fatty acids. They are an excellent source of Vitamin E, B-complex Vitamins (B1 (thiamine), B6 (pyridoxine), B2 (riboflavin), B5 (pantothenic acid) and B9 (folic acid)) and minerals manganese, phosphorus, zinc, magnesium, copper, iron, selenium, potassium, and calcium. Walnuts are a rich source of the powerful antioxidant glutathione. See "Nuts" for general information. See also Can Certain Foods Make Us More Intelligent? under Food and You or Your Environment, under "I."

Wasabi [*Vegetable*] Wasabi a good source of fiber, Vitamins C, B-complex (B6 (pyridoxine), B2 (riboflavin), B1 (thiamine), B9 (folic acid)), and minerals calcium, magnesium, potassium, manganese, zinc, phosphorus, and copper, and some iron. The wasabi plant is a member of the cruciferous family. It is the grated rhizome of this plant that provides the fiery hot flavor that quickly turns into a lingering sweet taste. Wasabi is a staple condiment in Japanese cuisine, served with sushi or noodles.

Water. See What Your Body Needs and Why.

Watercress [*Vegetable*] Watercress is high in carbohydrates, fiber, B-complex Vitamins (B2 (riboflavin), B3 (niacin), B6 (pyridoxine), B1 (thiamine) and B5 (pantothenic acid)) and is also an excellent source of Vitamins A, C, K, and E, and flavonoid antioxidants like beta-carotene, lutein, and zeaxanthin. It is also good source of minerals like copper, calcium, potassium, magnesium, manganese, and phosphorus. Noted for its peppery or tangy flavor, it is aquatic or semi-aquatic and part of the brassica family. See What Foods Fight or Help Prevent Cancer? under Food and You or Your Environment, under "C."

Watermelon [*Fruit*] Watermelon is high in carbohydrates, fiber, a good source of Vitamins A and C, and some B-complex Vitamins (B6 (pyridoxine), B1 (thiamine)). Watermelon also contains minerals magnesium, potassium, and manganese along with numerous antioxidants, including beta-carotene, lycopene, lutein, and zeaxanthin, which prevent free radicals from causing cell damage and possibly even cancer, asthma, and arthritis. See also What's to be Done about the Rise in Heart Disease? under Food and You or Your Environment, under "H."

West Indian Cherry. See "Acerola."

Wheat [*Grain*] Whole grain wheat contains carbohydrates, fiber, B-complex Vitamins (B1 (thiamine), B3 (niacin), B6 (pyridoxine), B9 (folic acid), B5 (pantothenic acid)), and minerals iron, magnesium, phosphorus, potassium, zinc, copper, manganese, selenium along with small amounts of protein. Two main varieties of wheat are widely eaten. Durum wheat is made into pasta, while bread wheat is used for most other wheat foods. Bread wheat is described as "hard" or "soft" according to its protein content; as "winter" or "spring" according to when it's sown; and as "red" or "white" according to color of the kernels. Hard wheat has more protein, including more gluten, and is used for bread, while soft wheat creates "cake flour" with lower protein. Wheat is the most popular grain we eat because it contains large amounts of gluten, a stretchy protein that enables bakers to create satisfying breads. Look for whole grain whole wheat in the ingredient list for the best quality and nutrient-dense bread. Red Fife wheat is another variety worth checking out. See also "Grains" for general information.[159]

Wheatgrass [*Vegetable*] Wheatgrass is an incredible power food that contains good amounts of Vitamins C, A, and K, and large amounts of B-complex Vitamins (B6 (pyridoxine), B2 (riboflavin), B3 (niacin), B1 (thiamin), and B5 (pantothenic acid)). Wheatgrass also contains large amounts of minerals zinc, manganese, and copper along with some iron and selenium. It also has large amounts of chlorophyll, and is thought to have a wide variety of health-promoting properties like increasing red blood cell count; cleansing the blood, organs and gastrointestinal tract; simulating metabolism. Wheatgrass can be found in the frozen food section of some health stores and can be added to smoothies for a nutrient supercharge.

Whey [*Dairy*] A by-product of cheese-making process, whey is a very good source of Vitamin B2 (riboflavin), calcium, phosphorus, and protein, and a good source of Vitamins B1 (thiamine), B12 (cobalamin), B5 (pantothenic acid), and minerals magnesium, potassium, zinc, and selenium. Whey is the liquid that is left behind after the first stages when making cheese. High in protein, whey is often processed into more concentrated forms, such as whey protein, whey protein isolates, whey protein concentrate, and whey protein hydrolysate and hydrolyzed protein.[160] See also Happiness and Foods that Create Bliss under Food for Thought, under "H."

White Beans. See "Navy Beans."

White Button Mushroom [*Fungi*] White button mushrooms contain some fiber and protein along with B-complex Vitamins (B2 (riboflavin), B3 (niacin) and B5 (pantothenic acid)) and some minerals copper, selenium, potassium, and phosphorus. Button mushrooms are the most consumed mushrooms in the United States, accounting for 90% of mushroom intake, according to the United States Department of Agriculture. The June 2007 issue of the *Journal of Nutrition* reports that eating button mushrooms can boost the immune system by increasing the activity of natural killer cells.[161] Like other mushrooms they have been studied for their many health boosting benefits. See "Mushrooms" for general information. See also Marvelous Mushrooms – The Magic Food under Food for Thought, under "M."

White Sugar [*Sweetener*] White sugar contains carbohydrates but no vitamins or minerals. All nutrients are removed during processing leaving only sugar. See "Sugar" for general information. See also Sugar – A Diet No No under Food for Thought, under "S."

Whortleberries. See "Huckleberries."

Wild Pork. See "Boar."

Wild Rice [*Grain*] Wild rice is highly nutritious with good amounts of B-complex Vitamins (B1 (thiamine), B2 (riboflavin), B3 (niacin), B9 (folic acid)), and minerals potassium, phosphorus, zinc, and magnesium, along with more protein than wheat. Wild rice has twice the protein and fiber of brown rice, but less iron and calcium. It is gluten free. The strong flavor and high price of wild rice mean that it is most often consumed in a blend with other types of rice or other grains. See also "Grains" for general information.

Wineberries [*Fruit*] These are red or orange in color and become ripe around summer or early autumn. Contrary to the name, these are not fit to make wines due to their tartness. See "Berries" for nutrients and information.

Winkles. See "Shellfish" for nutrients and information.

FOOD FOR THOUGHT

Water – The Source of Life!

Did you know that the human body is anywhere from 55% to 78% water, depending on body size. A rule of thumb, two-thirds of the body consists of water, and it is the main component of our brains, blood, muscle, and bones. We need it to maintain high levels of energy and to flush out toxins from our bodies. But is water quality an issue?

Many people worry about whether water supplies are being depleted as well and this can be worrisome because without water, there is no life. The world's population is growing by about 80 million people each year and freshwater withdrawals have more than tripled over the past 50 years. Author Robert Glennon,[162] in his book *Unquenchable*, describes some of the water shortage disputes that have been occurring in the U.S. and the innovative ways that people have worked together to reduce water wastage. Additionally, smart organizations are coming up with amazing ways to improve water quality, reduce water usage, and recycle water. At the local level, politicians are starting to include bans on bottled water as it takes approximately 5 liters of water to produce a 1-litre water bottle – and we drink over 28,000,000,000 bottles of water each year, of which 86% of the empty bottles end up as garbage or in our oceans and leach a harmful toxic chemical called BPA. In addition, tests consistently show that tap water may be equal or sometimes better in quality than bottled water so many people are switching back to filtered tap water instead.

Below are some easy ideas everyone can use to conserve water in their households.

1. Avoid buying water in plastic bottles. Use your own stainless steel or glass container and water supply. Buy a filter if you are worried about water quality as excellent ones are available at a reasonable price.
2. Install efficient fixtures in bathrooms, kitchens, and other areas where water is required. A faucet that leaks 1 drip per second wastes 3,000 gallons of water a year!
3. Run your clothes washer and dishwasher only when they are full. You can save up to 1,000 gallons a month. And check out Energy Star products for their reduced water usage as well as energy efficiency.
4. All types of gray water can be reused. Gray water gets its name from its cloudy appearance and from its status as being between fresh, potable water (known as "white water") and sewage water ("black water"). In a household, gray water is the leftover water from cooking, baths, showers, hand basins, and washing machines and it can be used to water plants instead of being dumped. You can also collect water from your roof in rain barrels to water your garden.
5. Shower 1-2 times less each week. Research shows that washing your hair less can help it look healthier and will increase the

longevity of any color treatments as well which is an added bonus!

> Aim for 6-8 cups of filtered water (or watery fruits and vegetables) every day and enjoy more health with it.

If we conserve or recycle our household water usage, we will have more for agriculture and to drink which is vital to every function in our bodies. To say water is important is a major understatement! Yes, I love drinking water, so I take protecting it seriously

FOOD AND YOU OR YOUR ENVIRONMENT

Wheat Sensitivity and Celiac Disease? What's Up?

Can you imagine life without a slice of toast, a muffin, or a piece of birthday cake? To most people that answer is no!

People with celiac disease are unable to eat foods that contain the protein gluten, which is found in wheat and certain other gluten-containing grains. With this disease, gluten sets off an autoimmune reaction that causes the destruction of the villi in the small intestine (small finger-like projections that protrude to increase surface area for absorption to help us digest food). Celiac sufferers produce antibodies that attack the gluten, but the same antibodies also attack the intestine, causing damage and illness.

> For many wheat is delicious and a dietary staple; for others it makes life very difficult and painful.

Celiac suffers experience a range of symptoms, including growth problems for children, decreased appetite and failure to gain weight, chronic diarrhea or constipation, vomiting, abdominal bloating and pain, and fatigue. New research now also refers to celiac disease as a major risk factor for infertility for both men and women.

Gluten can be found in wheat, rye, barley, bulgur, bran, couscous, durum, farina, farro, kamut, malt, matzo flour, traditional pasta, panko, seitan, semolina, spelt, triticale, udon, and wheat/wheat bran.[163] It is also found in many personal care products and foods, such as canned soups and ice cream, as it acts a thickener. Grains without gluten include amaranth, arrowroot, buckwheat, garbanzo bean flour, corn, flax, flours from nuts/beans/seeds, millet, potato starch or flour, oats (for some, oats also cause problems), quinoa, rice, sago, sorghum, tapioca, teff, and wild rice.

In the past many people made grains easier to digest by using fermentation techniques, like those employed in making sourdough bread. Some gluten-sensitive people claim to have no digestive issues eating sourdough bread as the glutens are partially digested by the active fermentation agent before they are consumed. Sprouting, soaking, and genuine sourdough leavening "pre-digests" grains, allowing the nutrients to be more easily assimilated and metabolized.

William Davis, M.D., of *Wheat Belly* fame,[164] provides readers with an education on the production of modern wheat and how cross-breeding has increased gluten amounts significantly. He believes, based on his research with many patients, that gluten has become more difficult for many people to digest today, even if they are not gluten sensitive. He examines decades of clinical research and the positive results achieved by eliminating gluten from the diet with patients suffering from a range of health issues, including diabetes, rheumatoid arthritis, dementia, and obesity.

No one knows for sure why there is a large increase in the number of cases of people diagnosed with celiac disease or gluten sensitivity. If you have no issues digesting wheat then enjoy it in moderation but try to incorporate other grains into your diet as well for variety and health. If you suspect that wheat or gluten is making you ill or causing bloating, fatigue, or rashes, then visit your doctor to get tested for wheat sensitivities or intolerances, as there are a range of blood tests available to easily test for intolerances.

HEALTHY YOU

What Is Healthy Weight?

Traditionally there has been only one way to assess your weight: the scale. But the amount you weigh doesn't necessarily tell the whole story. Today, there are other methods of self-assessment.

MEASURE YOUR WAIST: A large waistline may be a greater risk to your heart health than extra weight on the hips and thighs. Inhale and exhale, letting out all the air in your lungs. Breathe normally. Place the tape around your waist, between the bottom of your ribs and the top of your hipbones. Hold the tape firmly but don't press in.

If you're a man and your waist measures more than 40 inches (102 cm) or a woman measuring more than 35 inches (88 cm), you are at increased risk of developing health problems.

BODY MASS INDEX (BMI): The BMI is a ratio of your height and weight. It applies to those between the ages of 18 through 65, except if you're pregnant, breastfeeding, or very muscular. Use a BMI chart, easily found on the Internet. If your BMI is:

- between 18.5 and 24.9, you're at lowest risk of developing health problems.
- between 25 and 29.9, you're considered overweight.
- 30 or more, you're considered obese.

Of course, when our pants feel one size too small they are also telling us we have overindulged! Maintaining a healthy weight involves eating well, being physically active, and staying committed to long-term weight stability. It is worth the investment initially to form good habits but they will become your new normal over time and make you feel great.

*"As long as you have food in your mouth,
you have solved all questions for the time being."*
Franz Kafka
(1883-1924, German writer)

Xtra, Xtra!

When I think of X and food, the things that come to mind are Xtra helpings, Xtra large portion sizes, Xtra delicious and Xtra pounds!

As a child, I had a large appetite and ate a lot of junk food that never filled me up. I would sneak a bag of cookies form the cupboard and eat them all! Little did I know then, but my body was craving real food. The processed food, although high in calories, was not satisfying my nutritional needs.

Learning to catch ourselves and change our habits can make a huge difference in our health. For me, I learned to go out for a walk or exercise or drink a glass of water when I had the urge to eat unhealthy foods and then I stopped craving them altogether.

Now, my healthy habits are part of who I am and even in the most stressful situations, I will reach for the foods that really help ... real whole foods.

REAL "X" FOODS

Xylitol [*Sweetener*] Xylitol contains only trace amounts of vitamins and minerals, but it aids in the absorption of calcium and B vitamins in your body. It is a sweetener made from birch bark extract and tastes sweet but doesn't cause tooth decay due to its molecular structure. Xylitol doesn't cause a spike in blood sugar but is best used in small amounts for those who have blood sugar imbalances. Like chocolate, xylitol may be safe for humans but isn't safe for dogs or other animals. See "Sugar." See also Sugar – A Diet No No under Food for Thought, under "S."

Xylocarp [*Fruit Subcategory*] Xylocarp is a hard and woody fruit. A coconut is an example of this.

FOOD FOR THOUGHT

Xpensive or Cheap? What's Our Food Cost?

I know many of us can all get touchy about the price of food. Most of us don't think about quality at all but get steaming mad about price. But is the low-cost of processed food really cheap?

Processing by big firms is very profitable with high margins and few competitors. That is why grain and meat, not fruits and vegetables, remain the foundation of a cheap food diet. Grains (mostly corn and soy) are converted into cheap meat by feeding them to livestock. And grains can be stretched so that four cents of corn provides four dollars of cornflakes. How can you add value to a delicious carrot?

> Is the cost of our current food system breaking the bank and our health?

Fruit and vegetables should be the foundation of a healthy diet but require no extra processing so they get left out of many advertising campaigns, and left off many plates. Food processing is the second largest manufacturing industry in Canada, after transportation equipment. The food industry employs approximately 258,000 people. In 2011, sales of food processing products were valued at $83.7 billion.

But is all this processed food is good for us? Even a small reduction of processed food would make a significant difference in our health if it is exchanged for fruits and vegetables, fresh herbs and spices, or higher quality free-range meat. I have to admit, that even I find it hard to resist corn chips once in a while. The key is to eat processed foods *occasionally* and keep junk food to an absolute minimum. Your body will thank you.

Below is a list of countries and the percentage of their total household income that is spent on food.

- U.S.: 5.8%
- U.K.: 8.7%
- France: 13.9%
- Japan: 14.3%
- South Africa: 21.4%
- Chile: 23.7%
- Mexico: 24.5%
- India: 33.4%
- Vietnam: 39.7%
- Egypt: 41.5%
- Azerbaijan: 51.6%[165]

When you factor in transportation, taxpayer subsidies to large agribusinesses, the cost of adding large amounts of antibiotics to feed, and growing list of people who become ill and in need of medical assistance as a result of poor diet, I wonder if it might be worth it to consider spending more on food to make sure we are getting quality and variety from our local farmers and grocery stores. Someone once said that if you don't want to be living junk lives, you have to stop eating junk food. Why not pay just a little bit more for quality and health at the same time!

FOOD AND YOU OR YOUR ENVIRONMENT

Xtra Uses for Crops

We have already spoken about how important crops are for a source of food and we have learned about how different plants have been used over history for natural remedies. So what else are crops used for?

Biofuel

Biofuel has become popular, but is it a good and sustainable source of energy?

According to Wayne Roberts,[166] biofuel production all started with the Arab oil crisis in the 1970s. When oil prices rose, Henry Kissinger, who was Secretary of State at the time, countered by focusing on a food strategy. Food became the U.S. checkmate to the strategic power of Arab oil.

Biofuel became a natural result of excess food production and a desire to be self-reliant. But biofuels seem to be using up food that could be fed to people instead and the energy used to make biofuels is exceeding the energy created. The rain forest, which we all know is important for climate stabilization, is being cut down to grow corn, soy, and biofuel crops. Developing countries that rely on corn as a staple, like Guatemala, are struggling to feed their populations because of the record high corn prices. And Guatemala isn't an isolated case.[167]

> The idea of alternative fuels is a good one, and scientists are starting to find better non-food crops for achieving fuel independence.

Some scientists are discovering that perennial crops like the grass miscanthus and switch grass, have high yields and are starting to grow them as an eventual alternative to corn in producing ethanol.

As a bonus, miscanthus is also a nitrogen fixer, in other words, it reduces the amount of nitrogen that escapes into the environment.[168] In addition, the University of California Davis Study recently found that grape pomace (the mashed up skins and stems left over from the wine and grape juice making process) could be used as an efficient source for biofuel.[169] Scientists are also excited about micro-algal fuels that are considered renewable since they are powered by sunlight. President Barack Obama, speaking in February at the University of Miami, advocated for investments in algae fuel development, saying they could replace up to 17% of the oil the United States now imports for transportation. This is very exciting news and doesn't impact our food sources to manufacture.[170]

Clothing
Linen is made from flax/linseed fibers and the crop is naturally pesticide resistant. Some people who want natural fibers are switching to hemp clothing as it is also a naturally hardy crop and also less water intensive than cotton.

We all know that cotton is grown to make cotton clothing. Most cotton is a Genetically Modified Organism (GMO) crop that uses a huge amounts of pesticide. Organic cotton is starting to become more popular but the cost is still too high for most to afford. Some consumers have put pressure on companies to do better with chemical usage and now you will find some clothes labeled "better cotton" as the farmers have made a significant effort to grow cotton with fewer pesticides, which is good news for those who love to wear organic cotton

More than 50% of our clothing is still made using crude oil, including polyester, nylon, and acrylic, with nylon being the worst for greenhouse gases like nitrous oxide.[171] Many companies outsource clothing manufacturing to developing countries to make low cost/low quality clothing for mass consumption but are starting to watch to ensure better treatment for workers following the 2013 tragedy in Bangladesh.

Plants are also used in clothing production for buttons, darning balls, rope, latex, components of leather, needles, pins, starch, stuffing, weaving, and a long list of other clothing-related items. The list of extra uses for crops goes on and on.

Crops are also used for a variety of other products that we use every day, including paper, dyes, soap, corks, oils for lamps, waxes, insulation, plaster, roofing, thatching, compost, fertilizer, green manure, potash, alcohol, biomass, charcoal, kindling, wax, wick, cosmetics, hair products, soap, toothpaste, fire retardant, bedding, incense, brushes, string, gum, containers, brooms, musical instruments, adhesive, jewelry, furniture, basketry, preservatives, sandpaper, wood, etc.[172]

Next time you drive along a country road and see a farmer's field, you can now imagine more than the food on your plate. Plants are truly incredible and offer us almost limitless gifts in return for sun, soil, and water!

HEALTHY YOU

Living in the Xpress Lane

We live in a world of constant stimulation and speed – emails, texts, TV, video games, and large workloads. Constantly being rushed means we stop living in the moment and are always constantly feeling harassed and stressed. This causes our stress hormone cortisol to soar, which affects our blood sugar levels, concentration, and lowers our ability to make the happy hormones, dopamine and serotonin.

According to studies published in the Harvard Business Review, hurrying to meet deadlines at work or constant multitasking will not only kill employees' creativity but also reduce their productivity and increases the odds that your work will be sloppy or have mistakes.

Mindfully slowing down can benefit our lives physically, emotionally, mentally, and spiritually and we might just accomplish more in the end.

Here are some quick tips to help you along the slow path to health.

1. **Eat Slower:** Digestion begins in the mouth as saliva secretes enzymes that signal the digestion process. Eating slower improves digestion, reduces bloating and gas, boosts digestive enzymes along with putting us in a more relaxed state of mind. Eat with family or friends and truly enjoy your food and a great conversation.

2. **Move Slower:** Living at a frenetic tempo leads you to breathe more shallowly, depriving your brain and body of oxygen, leading to exhaustion and anxiety. Accidents associated with rushing or texting while driving are scary and it isn't worth it. When you feel yourself starting to go at warp speed, try deep breathing exercises to keep your cool. Even romantic moments with your loved one are best when we take time to be fully engaged.

3. **Take Time to Listen and Be in the Present**: When we are rushing we are not living in the moment or even listening to others as we are so freaked out about our next to-do on our long list. Learning to take time to observe the moment you are in now, including how it looks, feels, and smells, and awakening all our senses will bring us more joy and possibly success as well. When listening to others, slow down and listen to the words they are saying as well as what is being conveyed by their facial gestures and movements. This will boost your communication skills and lead to happier relationships and a greater feeling of calm and inner peace.

y

"Nature does not hurry, yet everything is accomplished."

Lao-Tzu

(Zhou Dynasty, Chinese philosopher and poet)

Yucca or Yuca?

A friend of mine was relating a recent adventure to Peru, covering all the details she could remember while huffing and puffing up the Inca trail to Machu Picchu. She was especially enthusiastic about the porters, who took very good care of them and fed them very well. When she finished the hike a porter suggested she find a Peruvian restaurant to try Yuca Fries, a local delicacy.

She found a restaurant after an extensive search and as she was reviewing the menu, she noticed that it was listed a Yucca instead of Yuca Fries. Yucca with two "c" s is an inedible, ornamental plant. The edible variety is yuca with one "c." In fact, its proper name is cassava, but the root is often commonly called yuca.

Well, two "c" or one "c", apparently what she ate was simply delish and well worth the effort to find a local restaurant.

REAL "Y" FOODS

Yak [*Dairy*] Yak butter is made from the milk of the domesticated yak. Whole yak's milk has about twice the fat content of whole cow's milk, producing a butter with a texture closer to cheese. It contains a higher amount of calcium than cow's milk too, but has similar nutrients to cow's milk. It is a staple food item and trade item for herding communities in Central Asia and the Tibetan Plateau.

Yak [*Meat*] Yak meat is high in lean protein and contains omega-3 fatty acids as yaks are pasture-raised. Yak meat contains B-complex Vitamins (B6 (pyridoxine) and B12 (cobalamin)), and minerals iron, calcium, and phosphorus. Yaks have very lean meat because, like bison, their fat is a separate layer outside the muscles that is easy to separate (unlike beef where the fat is marbled with muscle). Yak meat has twice the protein and half the fat of skinless chicken breast. The fat that yak meat does contain, like any grass-fed meat, has very high percentages of omega-3 fatty acids and conjugated linoleic acids (good fats). Yaks are exclusively grass fed (and are very efficient food processors – a yak eats only about one-third of what a cow eats) and very disease resistant, meaning they almost never get antibiotics, and they are not treated with growth hormones. Yak is a species of bovine that can be cross-bred with American cows, but they have more similarities to the American bison than to cattle. In Tibet, yaks are a central part of the culture. They are extremely agile animals (more like goats than cows), and are often used as pack animals. In addition to meat, they provide milk, fiber, and hide products.[173]

Yams [*Vegetable*] Yams are high in carbohydrates, fiber, Vitamin C, and B-complex Vitamins (B6 (pyridoxine), B1 (thiamine), B2 (riboflavin), B9 (folic acid), B5 (pantothenic acid), and B3 (niacin)). They also possess small amounts of Vitamin A and beta-carotene but good amounts of minerals copper, potassium, manganese, iron, phosphorus, magnesium, and calcium. This plant is a perennial vine cultivated for its large, edible, underground tuber, which can grow up to 120 pounds in weight. Yam is similar in appearance to sweet potato but not at all related to it. Yams are larger in size, features thick, rough, dark brown to pink skin, depending up on cultivar type, whereas sweet potatoes are relatively smaller in size and possess very thin peel. See also Potatoes – A Staple Worldwide under Food for Thought, under "P" and also Root Vegetables under Food for Thought, under "R."

Yeast Extract [*Fungus*] Yeast is a source of protein, iron, and selenium, and a very good source of B-complex Vitamins (B1 (thiamine), B2 (riboflavin), B3 (niacin), B6 (pyridoxine), and B9 (folic acid)), and minerals magnesium and potassium. Yeast extract is made by extracting the cell contents (removing the cell walls). It is used as a food additive, flavoring, or as a nutrient for bacterial culture media.

Yellow Turnip. See "Rutabaga."

Yerba Mate [*Herb*] Yerba mate is a herb used for tea that contains Vitamins C, A, E, B-complex Vitamins (B3 (niacin), B1, B2 (riboflavin), and B5 (pantothenic acid)), and minerals potassium, magnesium, phosphorus, calcium, and iron. An evergreen member of the holly family, it contains several antioxidants, including beta-carotene. It grows wild in Argentina, Chile, Peru, and Brazil, but is most abundant in Paraguay where it is cultivated. The plant is classified according to herbal medicine as aromatic, stimulant, bitter, astringent, and diuretic. The tea is known to combat fatigue and stimulates the mind. See "Herbs" for general information. See also Herbaceous Cooking under Healthy You, under "H."

Yogurt [*Dairy*] Yogurt is high in protein and fat. Yogurt is a good source of Vitamin D and B-complex Vitamins (B12 (cobalamin), B2 (riboflavin), B5 (pantothenic acid)), along with minerals calcium, potassium, zinc, iron, and magnesium. Yogurt contains healthy bacteria lactobacillus and bifidobacteria that help boost the immune system. Look for "contains active yogurt cultures" on the label. For those who find milk difficult to digest on its own, they may find yogurt a good milk substitute. Through the fermentation process, yogurt gains enzymes that pre-digest the casein proteins that can be hard for many to digest. Probiotics have been promoted as the new trend in yogurt. Probiotics, such as lactobacillus and acidophilus, are considered "good" bacteria that we generally want in large numbers in digestive tract and small intestine because they can be beneficial to your health and boost your immune system. Prebiotic supplements contain the nutrients these bacteria need to grow and thrive. According to *HealthCastle.com*, probiotics may improve the bio-availability (absorption) of nutrients such as B-complex Vitamins and minerals. This potential benefit is important to individuals who have taken antibiotics, as antibiotics destroy both "good" and "bad" bacteria.[174] In addition yogurt may help prevent colds. Researchers in Sweden gave 262 people a supplement with lactobacillus (healthy bacteria) and found they were 2.5 times less likely to catch a cold than the group who took the placebo![175] See also Menopause – Can Food Help the Transition? under Food and You or Your Environment, under "M."

Yolk [*Egg*] The center of the egg – the yolk – is high in fat and protein. Yolks are an excellent source of Vitamins A, D, E, K, and B-complex Vitamins (B12 (cobalamin), B5 (pantothenic acid), B2 (riboflavin), B9 (folic acid) and choline), and minerals phosphorus, selenium, iron, and zinc. All poultry produce eggs with varying but high nutrient content in their yolks, including chickens, ducks, geese, quail, emus, etc. See also The Egg under Food for Thought, under "E" and also How Can We Hold onto Yesterday's Memories? under Food and You or Your Environment, under "Y."

Youngberries [*Fruit*] These berries are rich in Vitamin A, C, and B1 (thiamine), the mineral calcium, and cellulose. They belong to the blackberry family. They ripen two weeks earlier than blackberries and are purple-black in color. See also "Berries" for general information.

Yuca [*Vegetable*] See "Cassava."

FOOD FOR THOUGHT

Miracle of Yeast

What Is Yeast? Yeast is a microscopic type of fungi that contains only a single cell and reproduces by budding. Some yeast may form long chains similar to those formed by molds. There about 1,500 species of yeast currently known.

> **All yeast are fungi
> but not all fungi are yeast.**

Before the mid-nineteenth century bakers and brewers knew very little about the nature of the organisms that helped make their products rise and taste delicious.

The experiments of French microbiologist Louis Pasteur (1822–1895) showed that fermentation could only take place in the presence of living yeast cells. He also deduced that anaerobic conditions (meaning no oxygen) were necessary for proper fermentation of wine and beer (in the presence of oxygen, yeast converts alcohol to acetic acid, a.k.a. vinegar).

Brewer's yeast is added to liquids derived from grains and fruits to brew beer and wine. Yeast that occurs naturally on the skins of grapes also plays a vital role in fermentation, converting the sugars of grapes into alcohol for wine production.

Baker's yeast is different than brewer's yeast. This yeast, used in dough, breaks down some of the starch and sugar present in the mixture, producing carbon dioxide. The carbon dioxide bubbles through the dough, forming many air holes and causing the bread to rise. Since oxygen is present, no alcohol is produced when the bread is rising.

In recent times, ethanol-tolerant yeast was used in the production of alternative energy sources. Yeast is placed in huge vats of corn or other organic material. When fermentation takes place, the yeast converts the organic material into ethanol fuel.

Yeast is a phylum of the Fungi family (meaning a subdivision of a group of organisms that have the same body plan). Fungi live in dark or light places as they digest simple organic foods like paper, cardboard, glues, and starch. They are helpful when they digest logs, twigs and leaves, produce antibiotics, or help make cheeses. They are problematic when they grow in and on houses and people and damage them. Some of the main fungi important to food are noted below.

- *Penicillium* is the mold that many know as a producer of penicillin, which has saved countless lives around the world.
- *Saccharomyces* is the genus name for common yeast used for leavened and baked bread, beers, wines and whiskeys. People all over the earth celebrate this good yeasts on a daily basis.
- *Saccharomyces boulardii*, or S. boulardii, is found in all of our probiotic liquids. S. boulardii is considered an immune system booster because it stimulates your body's production of antibodies, helps reduce antibiotic side effects associated diarrhea, controls candida, has shown promise in controlling Clostridium difficile (C.difficile), one of the most common causes of infectious diarrhea in the world.
- *Aspergillus* is a less familiar name, but this genus of mold is responsible for allergy and pulmonary conditions in both humans and animals. Aflatoxins, produced by some species of *Aspergillus*, are dangerous carcinogenic biochemicals released into contaminated batches of corn, peanuts and other nut and grain products.
- *Candida albicans* is yeast found in humans that may cause irritating infections of the mouth, gastrointestinal tract, and other mucosal areas of the body if they are out of balanced with good bacteria. Candidiasis is the medical term for a yeast infection.[176]

Just like bacteria, there are good and bad yeast and it is important to try to maintain more of the good kind in your body for optimal health. Eating fermented foods in moderation can boost the good yeast but too much sugary and refined food will feed the bad kind, causing bloating, fatigue, and brain fog! Remember to enjoy bread, beer, and wine in moderation (I do!) but don't overindulge too often or your body may start complaining loudly.

FOOD AND YOU OR YOUR ENVIRONMENT

How Can We Hold onto Yesterday's Memories?

My mother died a few years ago of dementia or Alzheimer's so I know how emotionally difficult this disease can be to families as they watch their loved one slip away day by day. My mother was a highly intelligent and kind woman who could devour a book in one day. She loved the classics as much as an Agatha Christie detective story but her disease robbed her of her intellect, joy, and even her personality.

Alzheimer's disease is the most common cause of dementia in people aged 65 and older. According to the Alzheimer's Association, up to 5.3 million Americans are suffering from this disease and every 70 seconds a new person is diagnosed. Some memory loss with age is normal but Alzheimer's and other forms of dementia cause a severe and often rapid mental decline. Studies are linking dementia to long-term inflammation in the body so foods that possess anti-inflammatory properties may delay age-related cognitive disorders or slow down the brain-wasting destruction.

> Forgetting where you put your pen is just forgetfulness; forgetting what a pen is for may be an early sign of a problem.

Given how precious our memories are and how important cognitive health is for a happy and long life, below are some of the top foods to help protect and preserve your brain and memory power.

1. **Almonds:** Almonds and other nuts contain Vitamin E in good quantities. According to the Alzheimer's Association, scientists believe that Vitamin E may delay the process and prevent Alzheimer's progression. A Dutch study assessed the brain health and diets of 5,395 people over the age of 54 who had no signs of dementia. Over the course of 10 years, 465 participants developed dementia, 365 of whom were diagnosed with Alzheimer's disease. After adjusting for other risk factors, such as a genetic predisposition to Alzheimer's, age, education, alcohol intake, smoking habits, body mass index, and supplement use, researchers found that people with the highest consumption of Vitamin E from food were 25% less likely to develop dementia than those who ate the least amount of Vitamin E.[177] Other high quality nuts include pumpkin, sesame, and sunflower. Aim for a handful of raw, unprocessed almonds for maximum benefit.

2. **Apples:** Apples contain quercetin (found in the skin) that has been found to protect the brain from damage associated with Alzheimer's disease according to a study conducted by Cornell University.[178] Other foods that contain quercetin include onions, lovage, and some berries like cherries, raspberries, and cranberries also contain small amounts. Apples also contain Vitamin C, which works to balance neurotransmitters associated with memory.

3. **Asparagus:** Asparagus contains high amounts of Vitamin B9 (folic acid) which has properties that lower homocysteine levels. Homocysteine is an amino acid or protein building block that we produce in our body but when in excess it is linked with cognitive impairment. Conversion of homocysteine requires Vitamins B9, B12 (cobalamin), and B6 (pyridoxine), which neutralize homocysteine's toxicity by transforming it into useful substances. A Korean study in 2008 found that individuals who were deficient in Vitamin B9 were 3.5 times more likely to develop dementia. One cup of asparagus spears will fulfill nearly 66% of your daily folic acid needs.[179]

4. **Coconut Oil:** Made up of medium chain fatty acids, it is known as MCT oil. With ingestion, the liver converts MCT oil to ketones. Since Alzheimer's patients' brains have difficulty metabolizing glucose, the brain's main source of energy, ketones act as an alternative source.[180] Caprylic acid is the active ingredient of a prescription-only "medical food" designed to treat Alzheimer's disease. Caprylic acid is also a medium chain triglyceride produced through coconut oil processing. A study presented at the Sixth Annual World Molecular Imaging Congress on September 2013 concluded that a 45-day regimen of the "medical food" prescription was effective in improving brain function in some Alzheimer's patients.[181]

5. **Coffee/Tea:** Regular consumption of green tea may enhance memory and mental alertness and slow brain aging. White and oolong teas are particularly brain healthy. Coffee also has brain-protecting properties, although the maximum you should drink is 2-4 cups daily, otherwise it can affect your sleep and cause the jitters. Caffeine has been suggested to have a protective effect against dementia. This new study comes from the University of Kuopio, Finland, and the Karolinska Institute in Stockholm, Sweden. Results showed that moderate coffee drinkers had a 65% lower risk for dementia and Alzheimer's disease later in life than the other groups.

6. **Free-Range Eggs:** Eggs are full of choline and omega-3 fatty acids (especially free-range organic ones). Humans can produce the mineral choline in small amounts only so they must also consume some in the diet to maintain good health. Choline is a key building block for memory because acetylcholine, the main brain chemical for memory, is made from choline. A deficiency in this chemical is probably the single most common cause for declining memory. In addition, rResearch shows that the omega-3 fatty acids that are present in high quality eggs help

reduce inflammation and prevent Alzheimer's disease. Eaten in moderation they are a great source of other vital vitamins and minerals as well as being a complete protein source.

7. **Turmeric:** A buildup of plaque in the brain is believed to contribute to death of brain cells, causing Alzheimer's disease. Studies have shown that curcumin, an active component in turmeric, is an effective substance that removes plaque. Turmeric is also a top anti-inflammatory food.

Your brain is a powerhouse of performance and directs almost all of your body functions. Its preferred fuel is glucose and complex carbohydrates like fruit, vegetables, and whole grains will supply the perfect energy. Your brain is over 60% fat too, so healthy fats like olive oil, avocados, nuts, and fish can also improve memory. Remember for brain health it is not just what you eat, but what you don't that helps too, so avoid too many additives, artificial sweeteners, and excess meat with saturated fat and antibiotic and hormone residues. Avoid refined sugar as there is also evidence to suggest that diets high in simple carbs can greatly increase the risk for cognitive impairment in older adults

In addition, certain supplements have been researched for their memory-boosting benefits. Vitamin B9 (folic acid), Vitamin B12 (cobalamin), Vitamin D, magnesium, fish oil, evening primrose oil, lecithin, and PS (phosphatidylserine) are believed to preserve and improve brain health. Studies of ginkgo biloba and coenzyme Q10 have yielded some results, and may also be helpful in the prevention or delay of Alzheimer's and dementia symptoms. Remember to always check with your doctor or health care provider if you want to add supplements to your loved one's medication for memory loss or are considering it yourself for early signs. The good news is that medical technology is now available that can enable the earlier detection of cognitive loss associated with dementia which would offer earlier intervention and aim for extended quality of life.

Other than food, other ways to avoid mental decline and Alzheimer's include keeping mentally active with games like Sudoku and bridge, reducing excessive stress, keeping active physically and socially, and getting quality sleep. Our memories are precious and an integral part of who we are so let's keep our brains healthy for as long as we can to protect the incredible treasure chest of our lives' recollections and adventures.

HEALTHY YOU

Young at Heart-Health – Benefits of Play

We can all get caught up in the seriousness of life. Bills, responsibilities, and caring for loved ones but what about just letting go and having some fun! I don't mean being reckless and going on a drinking binge either, just good old fashioned fun and play.

As adults, the goal of play is to forget about work and commitments and enjoy time without the need to accomplish anything except enjoying yourself. This could include a long walk along the beach, sharing jokes with a co-worker, dressing up for Halloween, or going on a last minute adventure with a friend or spouse. By giving yourself permission to play with the care-free attitude of childhood, you can reap the health benefits of lowered stress, improved brain function, and better relationships.

George Bernard Shaw said, "We don't stop playing because we grow old; we grow old because we stop playing." Being playful and young at heart will boost your energy and even improve your resistance to disease, so give it a try.

"Give a man a fish and you feed him for a day.
Teach a man how to fish and you feed him for a lifetime."

Lao-Tzu

(Zhou Dynasty, Chinese philosopher and poet)

Zucchini, Zucchini, Everywhere

When a friend's family moved to a more rural area, her father decided that he would take up small-scale farming. He had never had a backyard garden before so he bought packs of seeds and planted them all in a small plot.

One of the seed packs contained zucchini and he planted every seed diligently. Zucchini can be a prolific producer and a whole pack ended up overtaking the garden. To the amazement of the whole family, zucchini kept growing and growing. The family ended up giving away huge amounts of this delicious vegetable to every neighbor or new friend they met.

They were lovingly referred to as the Zucchini family for several years afterwards. They learned their lesson quickly though and planted accordingly the next year!

REAL "Z" FOODS

Zest [*Fruit*] Zest refers to the peel of citrus fruits like oranges and
lemons. It is very high in fiber, Vitamins C, and A, and has good
amounts of B-complex Vitamins (B6 (pyridoxine), B1 (thiamine), B5 (pantothenic acid), B2 (riboflavin), B9 (folic acid),

B3 (niacin)) along with minerals copper, calcium, iron, and some magnesium. Make sure to wash your fruit before zesting it.

Zucchini [*Vegetable*] Zucchini (or courgettes) and marrow are summer squashes belonging to the cucurbit family. They contain good amounts of carbohydrates, fiber, Vitamins C, A, B6 (pyridoxine), and some fiber, Vitamin K, and other B-complex Vitamins (B2 (riboflavin), B9 (folic acid), and B1 (thiamine)). It has small amounts of minerals manganese, iron, and phosphorus, and contains good amounts of antioxidants including carotenes, lutein and zeaxanthin. See also "Squash" for general information.

Zyphome [*Vegetable Classification*] Zyphomes are a classification of root vegetable and include ginger, ginseng and arrowroot. See "R" for nutrients in common zyphomes.

FOOD FOR THOUGHT

Zone and Other Diet Fads – How to Stop the Yo-Yoing

Have you ever gone on a diet? There are many that you may have heard of, including Zone Diet, Atkins, Paleo Diet, South Beach, or, even the food fad, and unhealthy Grapefruit Diet.

People trying to lose weight quickly may be tempted to try a diet fad that claims you will lose weight rapidly. Unfortunately, diet fads that promise rapid weight loss often lack proper nutrition principles and may lead to short-term and long-term problems. Diets with a deficiency in Vitamin D cause Ricketts, a painful bone disease, Beriberi is a disease caused by a deficiency in Vitamin B1 (thiamine), Pellagra is caused by Vitamin B3 (niacin) deficiency, and we've all heard of the sailor's disease, Scurvy, caused by Vitamin C deficiency. Today, according to many reports, many people are also magnesium deficient because they aren't eating enough greens and this is affecting metabolism and body organs. Remember that getting all your nutrients is important so look for diets that offer you all the nutrients you need before you jump in!

The only healthy way to lose weight is through a balanced diet and exercise program. There is much debate about ideal portions of protein, carbohydrate, and fat. Some diets recommend eating a diet high in carbohydrates and low in protein and fat and others, like Atkins and Paleo, suggests carbohydrates (especially grains) are all but eliminated especially for weight loss. Historically, traditional diets were about (40% complex carbs, 20% proteins, 40% fat) and some experts recommend a balance of nutrients (40% complex carbs, 30% protein 30% fat) is best.

Arctic cultures have diets up to 80% fat (fat has twice the calories as protein and carbohydrates) and are usually not as overweight as the rest of us. Vegetarian, Vegan, or Macrobiotic-based diets eliminate meat and some dairy. Some groups talk about food as being acid-forming like sugar and meat, or alkaline-forming like vegetables and fruit and recommend striking a balance. *Fit for Life* authors Harvey and Marilyn Diamond recommend eating only fruit in morning, starch at lunch, and protein at night. You can even find diets based on your blood type, metabolic type, or many other body type characteristics as well.

Have your ever tried a diet only to find your weight yo-yoing down and back up again? The addictive pattern of over-eating is hard to break unless there is an internal emotional shift that allows you to give up bad habits permanently and replace them with better eating habits. As a child, I was pudgy but not overweight by today's standards. I was eating a lot of processed and sugary foods that left me feeling tired and foggy and constantly craving more. I now realize I was craving more because there were not enough nutrients in my diet!

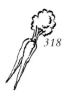

> Kick the yo-yoing pattern. Eat healthy, whole
> foods and move more. It may be a longer
> journey but it will be a healthier one too.

Special diet foods with artificial substitutes for fat and sugar should also be avoided. Ever notice how no packaged foods are ever low in fat, low in sugar, *and* low in sodium? That's because when they lower one of these ingredients, they increase the others to make it tasty so you'll buy it again.

In 1968, scientists at Procter and Gamble developed a special oil replacement called "olestra" that was supposed to be helpful in lowering cholesterol. The olestra molecules were so large and fatty that they could not be metabolized by enzymes and bacteria in the gut and were neither absorbed nor digested. But, it also caused severe abdominal cramping, loose stools, and inhibited the absorption of some vitamins and other nutrients like Vitamins A, D, E, and K! There were countless adverse reactions to this so-called "diet food" and finally in 2002, after decades of debate, the fat substitute was removed from products.

Weight loss can be very difficult for many and cause pain and emotional suffering. Trying to focus on buying whole foods, including high amounts and varieties of vegetables and fruits, high quality protein from wild-caught fish, free-range animals and eggs, dairy and legumes, quality fats high in omega-3 fatty acids, a blend of complex whole grains (and some gluten grains even for those who can tolerate gluten), plenty of high quality herbs and spices, quality water and teas will give you a framework to start the journey towards a new weight along with moderate amounts of exercise. The journey to a new weight should be enjoyed and every victory along with way celebrated! If you find any set-backs along way, or feel the need to indulge occasionally, forgive yourself immediately and start over the next day as the new you will be grateful for sticking to your goals. I have benefited greatly from coaching in my life for sports, work and personal goals. I highly recommend working with a qualified Nutritionist or coach to achieve your weight loss goals. Good Luck and good eating!

FOOD AND YOU OR YOUR ENVIRONMENT

Can We Reach Zero Tolerance Standards in Food Safety?

Over the past few years we've been hearing about more and more food safety scandals and food contamination issues. Whether it is the U.K. horsemeat scandal of 2013, the 2012 E. coli bacteria found in XL Foods that prompted a massive recall, or the 2008 Chinese milk scandal where milk and infant formulas were tragically mixed with melamine, affecting over 300,000 victims, it makes you wonder, "How safe is our food?"

In 2008 Maple Leaf Foods had to issue a major recall on meat because of a listeria outbreak at a processing plant that killed more than 20 people and made dozens sick, even though the government had increased the number of food inspectors by 700 and passed new legislation aimed at helping the Canadian Food Inspection Agency respond quickly to food safety issues.[182] The horsemeat scandal has prompted Nestle to suspend deliveries of all its products that included beef because "traces of horse DNA" were found in the meat and the levels found were above the 1% threshold the U.K.'s Food Safety Agency uses to indicate likely adulteration or gross negligence.[183]

In food safety policy, a "zero tolerance" standard generally means that if a potentially dangerous substance (whether microbiological, chemical, or other) is present in or on a product, that product will be considered adulterated (meaning mixed with impurities) and unfit for human consumption.[184] For the most part, food companies make a huge effort to combat bad bacteria, like E.coli, salmonella, botulism, listeria, and other toxins like mercury to make sure the food we eat is healthy and germ free. But it is impossible to have zero tolerance because it can sometimes take a while to detect an incident or negligence.

There are approximately 110,000 cases of E. coli in the United States each year. Children, the elderly, and those in developing countries are most at risk.[185] The U.S. Center for Disease Control estimates that food borne diseases result in 76 million instances of illness, 32,5000 hospitalizations, and 5,000 deaths each year. One-third are traced to salmonella, listeria, and toxoplasma, and another third are traced to a variety of specific bacteria or parasites. Many cause intestinal infections, including campylobacter, certain E. coli strains, viruses like hepatitis A, and parasites like cryptosporidium, blastocystis, and various amoebas, including giardia from contaminated waters.[186]

Overall, safety standards are good at most plants and some companies are starting to raise contract food workers' salaries and offer benefits to ensure they don't come to work when they are ill and can contaminate food.

How can we avoid getting sick from food? Louis Pasteur, the famous scientist known for his research into fermentation, pasteurization, microbes, and contagious disease stated, "The microbe (germ) is nothing. The terrain (milieu) is everything." What he implied was that we need to strengthen our systems so that germs have a minimal effect. His comments reinforce the importance of working to create a healthier body, or "terrain," so hostile to bad bacteria and organisms that it simply rejects them.

At home, you can protect yourself from germs by simply washing your hands regularly with plain old soap and water. Remember to wipe down and sterilize all surface areas when you handle raw meat and cook your meat thoroughly to ensure any harmful bacteria are killed. You can also protect yourself by boosting your immune system with specific foods and ensuring you eat plenty of healthy probiotic-rich foods to promote healthy gut flora. Our gut flora contains the fighting bacteria that will help kick butt on any invading pathogens and get rid of them before they do us harm.

> Healthy gut flora contains the fighting bacteria that will help kick butt on any invading pathogens.

The good news is that most companies are working really hard to ensure that food is safe and pathogens are kept to acceptable low amounts. An exciting new technology that incorporates probiotics in cleaning products is showing great promise as a superior way to keep harmful bacteria at bay in medical, manufacturing, and home applications. The research is impressive and the products are out-performing regular cleaners. The benefit also includes better health for the people (or animals) living in these facilities as they are not exposed to toxic chemicals and the cleaners are doing a better job of keeping harmful bacteria away because they contain live "good" bacteria cultures. I think we will see more of these products being used successfully in our food processing plants as well to ensure zero tolerance is maintained.

HEALTHY YOU

Zero Calories

I love food and love to eat but resting our systems occasionally with short-term fasting has been shown to boost our health and cleanse our over-worked livers. Research indicates that the benefits of Intermittent Fasting (IF) include:

- decreased cardiovascular disease risk,
- decreased cancer risk,

- lower diabetes risk (at least in animals, data on humans were less clear),
- improved cognitive function,
- protection against some effects of Alzheimer's and Parkinson's diseases, and
- weight benefits.

A fast eliminates most food, but not water, and can often include high-nutrient vegetable juices. Fasting should only be done for a short period (1-3 days) with frequent fluid intake and should be stopped immediately if there are any side effects.187

Not everyone should fast. Children, diabetics, pregnant and lactating women, or those with serious health issues should avoid fasting and it is always a good idea to talk to your doctor or health-care provider before you try a fast.

Giving our systems a rest is a good idea in principal and has been a practice among many health focused societies over thousands of years.

What *your* Body Needs *and* Why

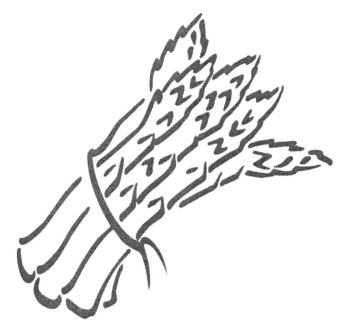

We have listed nutrients in the foods from A-Z and you may be wondering what they do in your body. We all need water, fiber, carbohydrates, protein, fats, and vitamins and minerals for optimal health, but what do they do for us?

In this section, we will go over in detail the three macronutrients – carbohydrates, fats, and protein – as well as vitamins and minerals along with the health-boosting antioxidants that support our immune systems and fight disease and infection. We will also touch on the role of other key dietary needs like – water and fiber – that are important to a well-functioning body. Feel free to refer back to this section to see what each food component does for the body at any time. Don't feel you have to remember all the information and feel free to skip sections or read only the parts that are of interest to you.

But before we get into the specifics of the various nutrients and food components, let's talk briefly about diet in general.

WHAT'S IN A DIET?

Now, when I say diet, I'm not talking about reduced calorie intake, I'm talking about following a specific eating pattern. There are a number of choices and all can have implications for you.

A *carnivore* is a person that eats other animals (or fish). Carnivore refers mostly to an exclusive diet of meat whereas omnivore refers to a person that eats both meat and plants. Most humans eat both meat and plants and are called omnivores.

A *vegetarian* is a person who does not eat meat and relies mainly on plant food for their diet. There are, however, several types of vegetarian diets.

- Flexitarian: describes someone who is mostly vegetarian but will eat meat occasionally.
- Pollo-Vegetarian: will eat chicken and fish but not red meat.

- Pescatarian: is a diet that excludes meat and fowl, but will eat fish and seafood.
- Lacto-ovo Vegetarian: is a diet free of meat, fowl, and fish, but includes dairy and eggs. This is the most common kind of vegetarian.
- Lacto-Vegetarian: is a vegetarian diet that includes dairy but not eggs.
- Vegan: is a vegetarian diet that excludes all meat, fish, fowl, dairy, eggs, and honey. This is the strictest form of vegetarianism.

There are many reasons why people choose a specific diet. For some people it is due to their upbringing, while others cite health issues or religious reasons. Other diets exist, including the Macrobiotic diet with an emphasis on balancing yin and yang foods, or even a raw food diet, which I personally do not recommend for extended periods of time. Cultures with the longest life-spans focus on diets with small amounts of high quality protein and fat, and large amounts of complex carbohydrates; mostly from vegetables and fruit.

THE LIFE-SUSTAINING DRINK – WATER

After oxygen, water is the most important thing that our bodies need for survival. The body could survive for a while without food, but it would only last a few days without water.

Lack of water can eventually lead to fatigue, or even more serious issues if dehydration occurs over extended periods. Most experts recommend drinking six to eight glasses of filtered water daily and/or eating water-rich foods like leafy greens and fruit to stay properly hydrated. Don't wait until you are thirsty to drink and remember caffeine, sugar, and alcohol are dehydrating so compensate by drinking extra water when you indulge.

WHAT IS FIBER?

Fiber comes from plant foods like fruits, vegetables, grains, nuts, and legumes. It is a type of carbohydrate that the body can't digest. Unlike starches and sugars (other kinds of carbohydrates), fiber contributes no calories or food energy. Instead of being broken down and absorbed into the bloodstream, fiber passes through the entire digestive system and takes up more space than food, making you feel fuller after you eat it. There are two types of fiber: soluble and insoluble.

In your stomach, soluble fiber dissolves, making other food components like fats and sugars less available for absorption. This is good news because this action helps to reduce cholesterol and causes other components like sugar to be absorbed more slowly, keeping blood sugar levels steadier. Foods that contain soluble fiber include legumes, barley, oat bran, chia seeds, flax seeds, psyllium husk, fruits, and vegetables.

Insoluble fiber doesn't dissolve in your stomach and aids in preventing constipation and other digestive disorders like diverticulosis and irritable bowel syndrome. The best food sources of insoluble fiber include whole grains, corn, oat bran, nuts, flax seed, and the skins and peels of fruits and vegetables.

Most foods contain a mixture of soluble and insoluble fiber. The inside of apples, for example, provide soluble fiber and the skins contain mostly insoluble fiber.[1] Many adults don't get enough fiber in their diet. Depending on how many calories are consumed, women need about 25 grams of fiber per day, and men need 38 grams per day, according to the Institute of Medicine.

WHAT ARE CARBOHYDRATES?

In the body carbohydrates provide energy or assist in the transport of energy. Foods typically high in carbs are breads, pasta, grains, vegetables, and some fruit.

Carbohydrates provide fuel for the central nervous system, muscular system (which uses the glycogen present in the muscle cells and the glucose in the bloodstream) and supply much needed dietary soluble and insoluble fiber. Carbohydrates are the body's preferred source of energy, followed by fat then protein.

When too many carbohydrates are consumed – that is, more carbohydrates than the body needs to function – they are turned into fat (glycogen) and stored in the liver and muscles and, in smaller amounts, in the other organs and tissues of the body. In order to keep a healthy weight and body mass, your body needs to exert exercise, to expend the additional carbs.

When carbohydrates are insufficient in the diet (as during a fast or on a weight-loss diet), stored fat (or glycogen) is broken down into glucose to make up the deficit. Some amino acids, instead of being used to make proteins, are broken down and used as carbohydrates to supply energy. The formation of glucose from amino acids is called gluconeogenesis. This phenomenon enables one to maintain normal blood sugar levels during a fast.

The average 1,800-calorie-a-day diet should contain between 210 and 290 grams of carbohydrates each day, which is equal to 45-65% of your daily calories. Since they are the main fuel for our body and brain, carbohydrates should make up about half of our daily calories. It is important to choose complex carbohydrates from whole foods, instead of simple carbohydrates like refined sugar.

> Yes, you need carbohydrates! In fact, half of 1,800 daily caloric intake should be of complex carbohydrates.

WHAT ARE FATS?

Fat is one of the three macronutrients (along with protein and carbohydrates) that supply calories to the body. Fat is essential for the proper functioning of the body.

Our bodies can make carbohydrates but not fat or protein. The body stores excess carbs and protein as fat. Fat serves as the storage substance for the body's extra calories and is also an important energy source. When the body has used up available calories from carbohydrates, which occurs after the first 20 minutes of exercise, it begins to depend on the calories from fat.

Fats provide essential fatty acids, which are not made by the body and *must* be obtained from food. They are important for controlling inflammation, blood clotting, and brain development. Healthy skin and hair are maintained by fat. Fat helps the body absorb and transport fat-soluble Vitamins A, D, E, and K through the bloodstream. Remember it is important to get fat in your diet!

Fats can get confusing and experts even disagree on recommendations. There are "good" fats and "bad" fats. Good fats help the body function properly and bad fats cause problems in the body when there are too many eaten or they collect in our arteries. The average 1,800-calorie diet should have between 40 and 65 grams of fat per day (20-35% of calories). The type of fat you eat is very important for proper health.

What Is Cholesterol?

Burgers, bacon, fries. Yes, they can be delicious but they are also high in cholesterol. Cholesterol is a waxy substance produced by the liver and found in certain foods.

We need cholesterol to make Vitamin D and some hormones, such as stress and sex hormones, build cell walls, and create bile salts that help us digest fat. Our liver produces about 1,000 milligrams of cholesterol a day or about 80% of the body's needs and the rest must be obtained through diet.

Lipids are fats that are found throughout the body. Cholesterol is a type of lipid and is found in foods from animal sources. This means that eggs, meats, and whole-fat dairy products (including milk, cheese, and ice cream) have cholesterol and vegetables and fruits have little or none. Because cholesterol can't travel alone through the bloodstream, it combines with certain proteins that pick up and transport it to different parts of the body. When this happens, the cholesterol and protein form a lipoprotein together.

The two most important types of lipoproteins are *high-density lipoproteins* (or HDL) and *low-density lipoproteins* (or LDL). You've probably heard people call LDL cholesterol "bad cholesterol" and HDL cholesterol "good cholesterol" because of their very different effects on the body. Most cholesterol is LDL cholesterol, and this is the kind that's most likely to clog the blood vessels, keeping blood from flowing through the body the way it should. On the other hand, HDL cholesterol removes cholesterol from the blood vessels and carries it back to the liver, where it can be processed and sent out of the body. It is the hero of the fats!

However, LDL also has some redeeming factors. It acts as a Band-Aid in the arteries when free radical damage creates micro tears in the arteries. High levels of LDL in our bodies are due to inflammation. Reduce the inflammation, and the LDL will be reduced. Finally, LDL is the preferred cholesterol of the brain so don't be afraid to have a little in your body!

The Omega Fat Family

What Are They and Why Do We Need Them?

Omega-3 and omega-6 are types of essential fatty acids – meaning we cannot make them on our own and have to obtain them from our diet. In modern diets, there are few sources of omega-3 fatty acids, mainly the fat of cold-water fish such as salmon, sardines, herring, mackerel, black cod, and bluefish, and grass-fed livestock. There are also omega-9 fatty acids but they are described as "non-essential," because our bodies can make them from other things we eat. The main omega-9 is oleic acid, found in oils like olive, canola, peanut, and sunflower.

There are two critical omega-3 fatty acids that the body needs – eicosapentaenoic acid, called EPA, and docosahexaenoic, or DHA. Vegetarian sources, such as walnuts and flax seeds, contain a precursor omega-3 (alpha-linolenic acid called ALA) that the body can convert to EPA and DHA. EPA and DHA are the building blocks for hormones that control immune function, blood clotting, and cell growth as well as components of cell membranes.

Our current diet of processed foods and processed vegetable oils has too much of the omega-6 fats (found in vegetable oils) and not enough omega-3 which we need in about equal portions. In general, however, you can cut down on omega-6 levels by reducing consumption of processed and fast foods and polyunsaturated vegetable oils (corn, sunflower, safflower, soy, and cottonseed) and by eating more oily fish (or taking fish oil supplements), walnuts, flax seeds, and omega-3 fortified eggs, organic or free-range eggs. DHA is the predominant omega-3 fatty acid in the brain and the retina, so an adequate supply is essential for proper brain, eye, and nerve functions. Low levels of DHA are linked to Alzheimer's and dementia.

Alpha-Linolenic Acid (ALA) is in the omega-3 family because it can be converted into the other long-chain omega-3 fats, EPA and DHA. Sources include flax seeds (as well as flax oil and ground flax seed), linseed oil (the seeds themselves are a lower source), hemp seeds, chia, walnuts, some sea vegetables, and dark green leafy vegetables. Optimal balance of omega-3 to omega -6 in the diet is a 1:1 ratio, but in most developed countries there are far more omega-6 fatty acids in food and the diet.[2]

Types of Fat – Food Sources

Saturated Fats

Good in small amounts, saturated fats are solid at room temperature, which is why it is also known as "solid fat." They are found mostly in animal products, such as milk, cheese, and meat, and are calorie dense. Poultry and fish have less saturated fat than red meat. Saturated fat is also found in some tropical oils like coconut and palm). These fats provide the building blocks for cell membranes and a variety of hormones and hormone-like substances.

Unsaturated Fats

Like saturated fat, unsaturated fats have a lot of calories and are good in moderation and necessary in our diets. However, they are liquid at room temperature. Most (but not all) liquid vegetable oils are unsaturated. (The exceptions include coconut, palm, and cocoa butter oils.) There are two types of unsaturated fats.

- **Monounsaturated Fats:** Examples include olive, canola and peanut oil.
- **Polyunsaturated Fats:** Examples include safflower, sunflower, sesame, corn, and soy.

Unlike butter or coconut oil, polyunsaturated vegetable oils can't be easily extracted simply by pressing or separating naturally. Most are chemically removed, deodorized and altered using chemicals and energy intensive processes. These oils are believed by some experts to be highly unstable and to oxidize easily in the body (if they haven't already oxidized during processing or by light exposure while sitting on the grocery store shelf). Oxidized oils can cause inflammation in the body. The best vegetable oils to use are extra virgin cold pressed as they do not undergo high pressure heat extraction in the manufacturing process.

Trans-Fatty Acids

These fats form when vegetable oil hardens (a process called hydrogenation) and can raise LDL levels (bad cholesterol) in the body.

They can also lower HDL levels (good cholesterol). These are bad fats, and should be avoided completely. Trans-fatty acids are found in fried foods, commercially baked goods (donuts, cookies, and crackers), processed foods, and margarines.

> **Run! Run away very fast from Trans-Fatty Acids and Hydrogenated Fats.**

To identify trans fats use the ingredient list, not the food label or advertising on the front of the box and look for a lack of the terms hydrogenated/shortening/hydrolyzed. Canadian laws dictate that manufacturers can have up to 0.2 grams of trans-fatty acid per serving and still be labeled as trans-fat free on the packaging. In the U.S. they can still retain 0.5 grams per serving and make this claim.

Hydrogenated and Partially Hydrogenated Fats

Because hydrogenated oils contain high levels of trans-fatty acids, which are linked to heart disease, they are considered bad fats and should be consumed in limited amounts. These fats are oils that have become hardened (such as margarine). Partially hydrogenated means the oils are only partly hardened.

WHAT IS PROTEIN?

Proteins are compounds composed of carbon, hydrogen, oxygen, and nitrogen, which are arranged in strands of amino acids. There are 21 amino acids, 9 of which are "essential" (cannot be made by the human body) and must be obtained from food. All food contains some amount of amino acids.

A complete protein source is one that contains all the essential amino acids in useful portions. All animal protein is complete, while most plant-based protein sources are incomplete and must be combined properly with complementary foods to obtain all essential amino acids.

The amino acids of protein play an essential role in the cellular maintenance, growth, and functioning of the human body. Serving as the basic structural molecule of all the tissues in the body, protein makes up nearly 17% of total body weight. Proteins are vital to basic cellular and body functions, including cellular regeneration and repair, tissue maintenance and regulation, hormone and enzyme production, fluid balance, and the provision of energy.[3] It is the primary component of muscles, skin, nails, eyes, neurotransmitters (cell-to-cell communication in the brain in the form of melatonin and serotonin), and all internal organs especially the heart. Protein is responsible for growth and maintenance of all body tissues as well as transporting minerals. Protein is the last energy source to be used by the body after carbohydrates and fat.

Proteins are the basis of the following structures within the body:

- **Enzymes:** complex proteins that act as catalysts that stimulate biochemical reactions (digestion, detoxification, etc.). Their activity depends on the presence of adequate amounts of vitamins and minerals, particularly magnesium.
- **Hemoglobin:** our red blood cells (RBC) need iron to form the iron-bearing protein hemoglobin – that is the key component of the RBC. Hemoglobin carries the oxygen and nutrients to the tissues of the body. If iron is low, look at protein levels in the diet.
- **Hormones:** Some primary protein hormones are insulin (controls blood sugar), thyroid (controls metabolism), and cortisol (increases with stress).
- **Antibodies:** part of the immune system.

Sources of Protein

Animal proteins, such as eggs, cheese, milk, meat, and fish, are complete proteins that provide all the essential amino acids for the body. Plant proteins, such as legumes (e.g., dried beans, chickpeas, soybeans, lentils, etc.), grain, corn, nuts, vegetables, and some fruits, when combined properly (such as brown rice and beans) provide good but incomplete sources of protein for our diets on their own. Other sources include soy, quinoa, chia seeds, hemp, nuts and seeds, and chlorella. You need to get 10-35% of your calories from protein. This means approximately 50-145 grams of protein each day depending on your size. To figure out the minimum amount of protein you need, multiply 0.8 grams of protein by your weight in kilograms. (If you don't know your weight in kilograms, find it by dividing your weight in pounds by 2.2). A 75-gram serving of meat, chicken, or fish has about 18-22 grams of protein. A cup of milk, a 50-gram serving of cheese or 3/4 cup of beans has 10 grams. Vegetables, fruit, and grains also have protein which will easily get you to the daily recommendation. Many Americans actually consume too much protein rather than not enough. Researchers have shown that excess protein can cause mineral loss and increase the risk of developing kidney stones.

WHAT ARE VITAMINS AND MINERALS?

Vitamins and minerals are nutrients that the human body requires to function properly. Vitamins act mainly as *coenzymes* for the enzymes that are the catalysts for chemical reactions in our bodies. Minerals assist the body, like vitamins, in energy production and other chemical reactions.

The foods we ingest are the sources of these vitamins and minerals. Some examples of important vitamins and minerals our bodies need are Vitamins D and A, and minerals calcium iron, magnesium, and potassium.

The Role of Vitamins and Minerals in the Human Body

It's important to remember that there are six nutrients essential for energy, proper functioning of the organs, utilization of food, and cell growth. They are carbohydrates, proteins, fats, vitamins, minerals, and water. These nutrients are absorbed by the body through the digestive process that breaks down the nutrients into small fragments using enzymatic actions. These are then absorbed through the walls of the digestive tract and eventually enter the bloodstream to be used by the body.

Vitamins are essential to sustain life and we must get them from our natural foods or dietary supplements. The nutrition they provide helps us feel better, more energetic, and assists the body with normal functions. Vitamins and minerals are necessary for our growth, vitality, and well-being. On the following pages are the main vitamins and their primary functions.

Recommendations for each vitamin vary greatly with size, age, and level of health or activity so I won't give exact recommendations. They are often listed as Recommended Dietary Allowance (RDA), Tolerable Upper Intake Level (UL) or Daily Value (DV) numbers tailored to men, women, and specific age groups. If you eat the recommended amounts of fat, complex carbohydrates, and protein from a variety of whole food sources, you should be covering your vitamin and mineral requirements each day.

VITAMINS[4]

Vitamin A (Retinol)

- **Function:** Important for healthy bones, teeth, mucus membranes, and skin. Aids vision, especially in the dark. Carotenoids, which are other forms of Vitamin A, are powerful antioxidants. A study by the University of Arizona found that Vitamin A has a protective affect against many types of cancer. As an antioxidant, it protects cell membranes and fatty tissue, helps repair damage caused by air pollutants, and boosts the immune system. Vitamin A is fat-soluble and found in animal products but can be made by the body from its precursor, beta-carotene.

- **Sources:** Meat, eggs, oily fish, liver, fortified dairy (milk and cheese), and kidney. Carotenoids (beta-carotene) is found in carrots, sweet potatoes, apricots, cantaloupe, broccoli, spinach, pumpkin, and all other green and orange fruits and vegetables.
- **Deficiency in Diet Causes:** Poor night vision, eye problems, weakened immune system, infection.

B-Complex Vitamins

In nature, none of the B-complex Vitamins are found in isolation. There are many of them and they often work together synergistically, thus they are called B-complex Vitamins. The B-complex Vitamins are the catalytic spark plugs of our body.

> **The B-complex Vitamins are the catalytic spark plugs of our body.**

Vitamin B1 (Thiamine)

- **Function:** Protects the heart and the nervous system from the build-up of toxic substances and is needed to convert carbohydrates and fats into energy.
- **Sources:** Lean meats, particularly pork, fortified bread and cereals, whole grains, dried beans, potatoes, spinach, nuts, peas, and yeast.

- **Deficiency in Diet Causes:** Tiredness and fatigue, muscle weakness, nerve damage, confusion, enlarged heart.

Vitamin B2 (Riboflavin)

- **Function:** Vital for growth, the production of red blood cells, and releasing energy from food.
- **Sources:** Poultry, lean meat, eggs, milk, fish, yogurt, yeast, soybeans, legumes, almonds, leafy green vegetables, and fortified breads and cereals.
- **Deficiency in Diet Causes:** Skin disorders, dry and cracked lips, bloodshot eyes, sore throat. B2 deficiency is not common in the developed world.

Vitamin B3 (Niacin)

- **Function:** Maintains healthy skin and keeps the digestive system working well. Helps open up the capillaries and thus improve circulation and detoxification.
- **Sources:** Poultry, lean meat, peanuts, legumes, potatoes, milk, eggs, liver, heart, kidney, fortified breakfast cereals, broccoli, carrots, avocados, tomatoes, dates, sweet potatoes, whole grains, and mushrooms.
- **Deficiency in Diet Causes:** Skin disorders, fatigue, depression and diarrhea.

Vitamin B5 (Pantothenic Acid)

- **Function:** Needed for the metabolism and synthesis of all foods. One of the key nutrients needed to support our stress glands.
- **Sources:** Eggs, meat, liver, dried fruit, fish, whole grain cereals, dried beans. B5 is found in all foods in small quantities.
- **Deficiency in Diet Causes:** A deficiency in this case is extremely rare, however, symptoms may include tiredness and a loss of feeling in the toes.

Vitamin B6 (Pyridoxine)

- **Function:** Required for the formation of red blood cells and various neurotransmitters. Helps to maintain nerve function, a healthy immune system, and healthy antibodies.
- **Sources:** Lean meat, eggs, chicken, liver, fish, beans, nuts, whole grains and cereals, bananas, and avocados.
- **Deficiency in Diet Causes:** Skin disorders, mouth sores, confusion, depression, and anemia.

Vitamin B7 (Biotin)

- **Function:** Essential in the metabolism and synthesis of essential fatty acids, carbohydrates, and fats, and the release of energy from these foods. Keeps hair, skin, and nails healthy.
- **Sources:** Found in almost all types of food. High amounts are present in liver, butter, yeast extracts, eggs, dairy produce, and fortified cereals.
- **Deficiency in Diet Causes:** Rare but symptoms include hair loss or brittle hair, skin rashes, and fungal infection. Could lead to depression and muscular pain.

Vitamin B9 (Folic Acid)

- **Function:** Required for the production of red blood cells, DNA, and proteins in the body. Important for the growth and repair of cells and tissues and is especially important during pregnancy to prevent babies being born with spina bifida.
- **Sources:** Leafy green vegetables, citrus fruits, beans, wheat germ, fortified cereals, liver, pork, poultry, broccoli, yeast, asparagus.
- **Deficiency in Diet Causes:** Anemia, incorrect absorption of essential nutrients, and neural tube defects in babies.

Vitamin B12 (Cobalamin)

- **Function:** Required for the metabolism process and to maintain the nervous system, energy, and mental health.
- **Sources:** Eggs, shellfish, poultry, meat, dairy products, liver, and fortified cereals.
- **Deficiency in Diet Causes:** Tiredness and fatigue, tingling and numbness in the hands and feet, loss of memory, anemia, and confusion.

Other B-complex Vitamins include choline, inositol, paba, B13 or Orotic Acid, B15 or Pangamic Acid, and B17 or Laetrile.

Vitamin C (Ascorbic Acid)

- **Function:** Required daily for the formation of collagen, which helps to maintain skin, teeth, gums, tendons, and ligaments; aids in healing wounds quicker; strengthens the immune system and fights cancerous cells; required to form neurotransmitters, such as dopamine in the brain; assists in fighting cardiovascular disease by protecting the linings of arteries from oxidative damage; and helps to reduce any damage to the body from toxic substances and chemicals.
- **Sources:** Citrus fruits, melon, strawberries, blackcurrants, green peppers, tomatoes, broccoli, kiwi fruit, potatoes, dark green leafy vegetables, red peppers, squash, mango, papaya, cauliflower, pineapple, blueberries, raspberries, and cranberries.
- **Deficiency in Diet Causes:** Prone to infections, slower healing of wounds, dental and gum problems, fatigue, loss of appetite, dry skin, painful joints, anemia, and a slower metabolism.

Note: Vitamins C is the most widely used of all vitamin supplements. It became famous in the 1970s when Nobel Prize-winning scientist Linus Pauling advocated daily mega-doses of Vitamin C to prevent and ease the symptoms of the common cold. Many clinical studies show that Vitamin C is superior to over-the-counter medicines in reducing the symptoms, duration, and severity of colds.

Vitamin D

- **Function:** Needed to absorb calcium and strengthen bones and teeth and can prevent the onset of osteoporosis.
- **Sources:** Sunlight, dairy products, oily fish (and their oils), eggs, oysters, and fortified cereals.
- **Deficiency in Diet Causes:** Softening and weakening of the bones, insomnia, nervousness, and muscle weakness.

Note: Vitamin D is also known as the "sunshine" vitamin, as 15 minutes of exposure to the sunshine, three times a week will enable the body to manufacture all the Vitamin D that it needs.

Vitamin E (Tocopherol)

- **Function:** Important antioxidant that protects our cells and tissues from harmful substances and free radicals, prevents cardiovascular and heart disease, and may delay the ageing process. Vitamin E is a potent antioxidant by itself, but its effectiveness is magnified when taken with other antioxidants, especially Vitamin C, selenium, and beta-carotene.
- **Sources:** Vegetable oils, such as canola, palm, sunflower, olive and soybean, nuts, seeds, wheat germ, spinach, green leafy vegetables, asparagus, and cereals.
- **Deficiency in Diet Causes:** Not very common but may include some nerve damage.

Note: Past studies have demonstrated higher Vitamin E intake is associated with decreased incidence of heart disease in both men and women. In addition, Harvard Medical School reported that Vitamin E might play a role in helping people live longer, citing its role in strengthening the immune system.

> **Want to live longer? Get more Vitamin E into your diet to strengthen your immune system.**

Vitamin K

- **Function:** Essential for blood clotting, helps to maintain strong bones, and could prevent osteoporosis.
- **Sources:** Spinach, cauliflower, kale, green leafy vegetables, soybeans, spring onions, and pistachio nuts.
- **Deficiency in Diet Causes:** Deficiency is rare, as Vitamin K is manufactured in the body. Signs of deficiency include easy bruising and bleeding.

Vitamin P

Vitamin P, also called bioflavonoids, is water-soluble and enhances absorption of other vitamins, especially Vitamin C, stimulates bile production, lowers cholesterol, helps prevent cataracts, and has antibacterial properties. One bioflavonoid is rutin and can show sedative effects on the brain. Sources include peppers, grapes, buckwheat, and the white peel of citrus fruits.

Coenzyme Q10

Coenzyme Q10, also known as Vitamin Q to some nutritionists, is a nutrient every cell must have to produce energy and was first discovered in 1957. Antioxidant sources are found in all animal meats. Cholesterol drugs and statins interfere with absorption of Coenzyme Q10.

MINERALS

Minerals are just as crucial as vitamins in our system. For example, we need potassium to regulate the balance of water in our bodies. We need other important minerals, like magnesium, calcium, copper, zinc, selenium, each for specific reasons and functions in our bodies. There are two types of minerals – macro minerals and trace minerals – which the body needs to function well. Macro minerals are essential nutrients that the body needs in large amounts in order to work properly. Trace minerals, or micro minerals, are essential nutrients your body needs to work properly, but only in small amounts.

Macro Minerals[5]

Calcium

- **Function:** Important for healthy bones and teeth, helps muscles relax and contract, significant in nerve functioning, blood clotting, blood pressure regulation, and immune system health.
- **Sources:** Milk and milk products, canned fish with bones (salmon, sardines), fortified tofu and soy milk, greens (broccoli, mustard greens), and legumes.
- **Deficiency in Diet Causes:** Osteoporosis; impaired bone mineralization, which in children can cause rickets; osteomalacia (adult rickets) due to inadequate calcium in bones (often due to low magnesium and Vitamin D); tooth decay; brittle nails; and rheumatoid arthritis (autoimmune disease that causes tissue damage and chronic inflammation of the joints).

Inadequate calcium intake produces little or no obvious symptoms in the short term, because the body regulates blood calcium levels tightly by drawing calcium from bones. Excessive phosphorus or magnesium in the diet, or insufficient secretion of stomach acid (which happens in many people, especially the elderly) can also inhibit the uptake of calcium.

Vitamin D facilitates the absorption and utilization of calcium. If Vitamin D is lacking or not converted into its active form (perhaps due to problems in the liver or kidneys where this should take place), then calcium levels are impaired. Moderate exercise enhances calcium absorption while lack of exercise increases calcium loss, as does poor diet.

Chloride

- **Function:** Required for proper fluid balance, stomach acid.
- **Sources:** Table or sea salt (sodium chloride), soy sauce; salt substitutes, such as potassium chloride; seaweed (such as dulse and kelp); olives; rye; vegetables, like celery, lettuce, tomatoes; preserved meats.
- **Deficiency in Diet Causes:** Loss of appetite, muscle weakness, lethargy, and dehydration. Hypochloremia, chloride deficiency, is rare, because it is part of table salt, which is present in most foods. Hypochloremia can occur, however, for a variety of reasons that include excessive fluid loss due to prolonged diarrhea or vomiting or overuse of laxatives; burns; congestive heart failure; kidney disorders; and Addison's disease.

Magnesium

- **Function:** Needed for making protein, muscle contractions, nerve transmissions, and immune system health. Found in bones.
- **Sources:** Nuts and seeds; legumes; leafy, green vegetables; seafood; chocolate; artichokes; "hard" drinking water.
- **Deficiency in Diet Causes:** Over activation of nerve and muscle impulses leading to tremors, hyper-excitability or irritability or nervousness, muscle weakness, twitching, mental

confusion, disorientation; inhibition of Vitamin D metabolism causing calcium depletion, which is linked to low blood levels of potassium, increased risk of abnormal heart rhythms, headaches and migraines, depression, disturbed sleep, insomnia or sleepiness, and changes to the heart, resulting in increased heartbeat or abnormal heart rhythms (arrhythmia).

Note: Some studies showed that children with attention deficit hyperactivity disorder (ADHD) tended to have mild magnesium deficiency; those given magnesium supplements in addition to their ADHD medication displayed significantly decreased hyper-activity.

Although severe magnesium deficiency is rare, some doctors believe it is possibly one of the most under-diagnosed nutrient deficiencies in the developed world. Hypomagnesemia (low blood levels of magnesium) can be due to any of a variety of reasons, including a diet that is short of foods containing magnesium, a diet high in fats, protein, zinc, or Vitamin D foods, or a diet high in oxalic acid, such as chard, celery, cocoa, spinach, and tea, which inhibit magnesium absorption.

Phosphorus

- **Function:** Important for healthy bones and teeth; found in every cell of the body; part of the system that maintains acid-base balance.
- **Sources:** Meat, fish, poultry, eggs, milk.
- **Deficiency in Diet Causes:** Unusually low blood phosphate levels is called hypophosphatemia. Deficiency of phosphorus is extremely rare as it is present in most foods. It occurs mainly in near-starvation, anorexia, or severe alcoholism cases. Symptoms include poor bone formation and growth,

impaired bone mineralization that causes rickets in children, arthritic-like pain, increased susceptibility to infection, fatigue or muscle weakness, anemia, loss of appetite, and changes to weight.

Potassium[6]

- **Function:** Needed for proper fluid balance, nerve transmission, and muscle contraction. Potassium works with sodium and thus is needed in the proper ratio.
- **Sources:** Meats, milk, fresh fruits and vegetables, whole grains, legumes.
- **Deficiency in Diet Causes:** Hypokalemia is not common, as high potassium foods are widespread. It is mainly a result of severe malnutrition or mal-absorption cases. People with severe hypokalemia, for example due to diarrhea followed by dehydration, may need potassium administered intravenously together with other salts.

Sodium

- **Function:** Required for proper fluid balance, nerve transmission, and muscle contraction.
- **Sources:** Table salt, soy sauce, large amounts in processed foods, small amounts in milk, breads, vegetables, and unprocessed meats.
- **Deficiency in Diet Causes:** Sodium deficiency is extremely rare, but it can occur. Low concentration of sodium in the blood is known as hyponatremia, and can be dangerous. Symptoms of deficiency include dehydration, low blood sugar, heart palpitations, muscle cramps, weakness and lethargy, confusion, nausea and, seizures if left untreated.

Sulfur

- **Function:** Involved in cellular respiration, which in simple terms means it helps the cells use oxygen efficiently, resulting in improved cell activity and brain function. Sulfur helps the body rid itself of toxins. Found in keratin, it keeps hair, fingernails and skin strong and healthy. Produces collagen, which is present in the skin's connective tissues, helping to maintain the skin's elasticity, heal wounds better and faster. Sulfur also plays a very key role in the metabolism of several important B-complex Vitamins, including B1 (thiamine), B5 (pantothenic acid), and B7 (biotin). Sulfur is known as a detoxifier in
the body.
- **Sources:** Lean meats, poultry, fish, eggs and egg yolks, milk, legumes, garlic, cabbage, Brussels sprouts, onions, turnip, kale, lettuce, kelp, seaweed, and some nuts.
- **Deficiency in Diet Causes:** Skin problems or disorders, muscle pain, nerve disorders, circulatory trouble, arthritis, inflammation, damage resulting from free radicals, stress, infection, constipation, and wrinkles. However, most people get sufficient quantities of sulfur from their diets, so instances of deficiency are extremely rare.

Trace Minerals (Micro Minerals)

The body needs trace minerals in very small amounts. Note that *iron* is considered to be a trace mineral, although the amount needed is somewhat more than for other micro minerals.

> Don't let the term fool you. Iron is a
> trace mineral – you must have it
> but a little goes a long way.

Boron

- **Function:** Needed for healthy bones and cognitive function.
- **Sources:** Fruit, especially apples, vegetables, especially leafy greens, nuts, and grains.
- **Deficiency in Diet Causes:** A weakening of the bone structure; depressed brain functioning, especially cognition and mental alertness. Deficiency rare as very little is required on a daily base and it is found in many foods.

Chromium

- **Function:** Works closely with insulin to regulate blood sugar (glucose) levels and synthesis of cholesterol, fat, and protein.
- **Sources:** Brewer's yeast, egg yolks, molasses, and onions (raw). Also found in apples, bananas, oranges, grapes, vegetables, like alfalfa, broccoli, carrots, green beans, green peppers, mushrooms, potatoes, romaine lettuce, ripe tomatoes, spinach, dried beans, beer, cheese, liver, meat (beef, chicken, turkey), oysters, brown rice, wheat germ, whole grains (in the bran and germ).
- **Deficiency in Diet Causes:** Insulin resistance or glucose intolerance, which affects the ability of insulin to regulate blood sugar and leads to high blood sugar levels that may result in type 2 diabetes in older people; elevated blood insulin levels (hyperinsulinemia); high LDL cholesterol, low HDL cholesterol levels, and/or high triglyceride levels; and high blood pressure.

Copper

- **Function:** Part of many enzymes and needed for iron metabolism.

- **Sources:** Legumes, nuts and seeds, whole grains, organ meats, and drinking water.
- **Deficiency in Diet Causes:** Osteoporosis, and joint problems; retarded growth or abnormalities in bone development in infants and young children; anemia; loss of skin or hair color; impaired immune function; impaired nerve function; inelastic blood vessels; elevated LDL (bad) cholesterol and lower HDL (good) cholesterol levels; irregular heart beat; breathing difficulties; fatigue and weakness; skin sores and hypothyroidism.

Fluoride

- **Function:** Involved in formation of bones and teeth and helps prevent tooth decay.
- **Sources:** Drinking water (either fluoridated or naturally containing fluoride), fish, and most teas.
- **Deficiency in Diet Causes:** Poorly formed or weak teeth and increase in tooth decay; brittle or weak bones; and fractured hips in the elderly.

Note: Fluoride should not be swallowed as it may cause problems in the body, which has led to controversy over the addition of fluoride to water systems. Many countries have opted to remove it from municipal water with no change to dental health.

Iodine

- **Function:** Found in the thyroid hormone, which helps regulate growth, development, and metabolism.
- **Sources:** Seafood, foods grown in iodine-rich soil, iodized salt, bread, and dairy products.
- **Deficiency in Diet Causes:** Goiter (an enlarged thyroid gland) which may cause a choking feeling or difficulty with

breathing and swallowing; hypothyroidism (under-production of thyroid hormones) which can lead to hair loss, brittle nails, dry pale skin, anemia, fatigue or weakness, depression, irritability, poor memory, weight gain, muscle or joint pain, constipation, decreased libido, abnormal menstrual cycles; and impaired immune system.

Iron

- **Function:** Needed for energy metabolism and carrying oxygen in the blood (iron is part of hemoglobin, found in red blood cells, that carries oxygen in the body).
- **Sources:** Organ meats, red meats, fish, poultry, shellfish (especially clams), egg yolks, legumes, dried fruit, dark, leafy greens, iron-enriched breads and cereals, and fortified cereals. Animal sources are better absorbed than plant sources. Caffeine and dairy inhibit iron absorption and Vitamin C improves it.
- **Deficiency in Diet Causes:** Anemia, with symptoms that may include headaches, dizziness, irritability, pale skin, cold hands and feet, lack of energy, rapid heartbeat, low immune function, brittle nails, shortness of breath, lack of appetite, blood in stools, restless legs syndrome; increased intestinal inflammation or irritation; depression or apathy; insomnia or disturbed sleep; decrease in ability to concentrate; impaired mental skills that can affect memory and job performance; learning disabilities and short attention spans in children; irregular menstrual periods; and brittle hair and hair loss.

Manganese

- **Function:** Part of many enzymes.
- **Sources:** Dark green, leafy vegetables (broccoli, chard, collard greens, kale, mustard greens, romaine lettuce, spinach), avocados, pineapple, raspberries, nuts (almonds, peanuts, pecans,

walnuts), bananas, blueberries, figs, grapes, kiwifruit, strawberries, blackstrap molasses, maple syrup, black pepper, cinnamon, cloves, coriander seeds, garlic, peppermint, thyme, turmeric, egg yolks, beets, carrots, sweet potato, asparagus, celery, leeks, summer squash, seaweed, legumes (black beans, garbanzo beans (chickpeas), dried peas, green beans, pinto beans, lima beans, navy beans), soybeans and soybean products like tofu and tempeh, and whole grains (oats, brown rice, rye, whole wheat, quinoa, barley, spelt).

- **Deficiency in Diet Causes:** Nausea or dizziness, vomiting, skin rash, hearing loss, iron-deficiency anemia (due to manganese's role in iron utilization), high blood sugar levels (impaired glucose tolerance), blood cholesterol levels that are too low, impaired bone growth or skeletal abnormalities, especially in children, excessive bone loss, weak hair and nails, loss of hair color, and defective functioning of the reproductive system.

Molybdenum

- **Function:** Part of some enzymes needed for nitrogen metabolism, iron absorption, fat oxidation, and normal cell function.
- **Sources:** Legumes (beans, dried peas, lentils, garbanzo beans (chickpeas), pinto beans), brown rice, millet, cereal grains, whole grains, liver, nuts, and dark green, leafy vegetables.
- **Deficiency in Diet Causes:** Increased respiratory or heart rate, night blindness, mouth and gum disorders, sexual impotence in older males, and sulfite sensitivity.

Selenium

- **Function:** Works as an antioxidant; known to be very useful for patients who suffer with arthritis, osteoarthritis and rheumatoid arthritis.

- **Sources:** Brazil nuts (one of the most concentrated selenium food sources), organ meats (liver, kidney), mushrooms (button, shiitake, and reishi), fish (cod, flounder, halibut, herring, mackerel, salmon, smelts, red snapper, swordfish, and tuna), and shellfish (lobster, oyster, scallops, shellfish, and shrimp).
- **Deficiency in Diet Causes:** Weaker immune system leading to susceptibility to stress and illnesses; greater incidence of cancer, especially gynecological, gastrointestinal, esophageal, lung, and prostate cancer; rheumatoid arthritis; elevated blood pressure; risk of atherosclerosis leading to heart or coronary artery disease; impaired thyroid function leading to hypothyroidism symptomized by lethargy, fatigue, intolerance to cold, depression, constipation, weight gain, heavy menstruation, dry skin, and hair loss.

Zinc

- **Function:** Part of many enzymes needed for making protein and genetic material; functions in taste perception, wound healing, normal fetal development, production of sperm, normal growth and sexual maturation, immune system health.
- **Sources:** Meats, fish, poultry, leavened whole grains, vegetables, and pumpkin seeds.
- **Deficiency in Diet Causes:** Impaired sense of smell and taste, impaired immune function, susceptibility to pneumonia and other infections in malnourished children and the elderly, skin ulcers, slow wound healing, retarded growth in infants and children, delayed sexual maturation, impotence, reduced thyroid hormone output, lowered glucose tolerance with increased risk of diabetes, decreased metabolic rate, mental lethargy, depression, lack of appetite, unexplained weight loss, diarrhea, hair loss, skin rashes or skin lesions, eye lesions, and night blindness.

Other trace nutrients known to be essential in tiny amounts include cobalt, silicon, and vanadium.

- **Cobalt** works with copper to promote assimilation of iron.
- **Silicon** is needed for strong yet flexible bones and cartilage; skin, hair, nails, and connective tissue; helps prevent atherosclerosis; and protects against toxic aluminum. Sources include millet, corn, flax, and bone broth.
- **Vanadium** is needed for cell metabolism, formation of teeth and bones, plays a role in growth and reproduction, and controls cholesterol levels. Sources include buckwheat, olives, and grains. Deficiencies are linked to kidney disease.

Not all minerals are good for the body. For example, lead, cadmium, mercury, aluminum, and arsenic are considered safe in minute amounts but poison in large quantities. Minerals like calcium and magnesium and antioxidants protect against these toxic minerals and help the body eliminate them.[7]

BIOAVAILABILITY: WHAT DOES IT MEAN?

Some minerals are absorbed more readily into our bodies than others. For example, while some foods have a high calcium content, you might not actually be getting as much calcium from them as you think. Why? Because the body does not absorb calcium and other minerals the same way. The degree to which vitamins and minerals in food can be absorbed and used by the body is called "bioavailability."[8]

Bioavailability refers to the amount of a nutrient actually absorbed and used by your body. For calcium, this represents the amount of calcium incorporated into your bones. The amount of calcium you consume is much less important than the amount actually absorbed and used by your body.

Bioavailability – it's not just eating the
vitamins and minerals, your body
had to absorb them too!

The body absorbs more vitamins and minerals from dairy than it does from certain plant-based foods which contain substances that impair full mineral absorption. For example, rhubarb appears to be one of the best plant sources of calcium. However, though this vegetable contains more calcium than milk, you would have to eat more than 4 cups of rhubarb for your body to absorb as much calcium as it would get from a single cup of milk. This is important to remember as you strive to get more vitamins and minerals in your diet. Having an adequate supply of digestive enzymes also helps with proper absorption.

WHAT ARE ANTIOXIDANTS?

Antioxidants are a broad group of compounds that destroy single oxygen molecules (also called free radicals) or bad guys in the body. They protect against "oxidative" damage to your cells and keep your cells healthy. Essential to good health, antioxidants are found naturally in a wide variety of foods and plants, including many fruits and vegetables. The most commonly known antioxidants are Vitamin C, Vitamin E, and beta-carotene. Others include grape seed extract, Vitamin A, selenium, coenzyme Q10, resveratrol, quercetin, lycopene, etc. Antioxidants are grouped into two broad categories – flavonoids and non-flavonoids.

Flavonoids[9]

Flavonoids are a group of antioxidant compounds found primarily in plants. They are primarily known as pigments, producing yellow or red/blue pigmentation in flower petals. There have been over 4,000 identified and they can be sub-divided into seven groups, including anthocyanins (found in red- and blue-colored food such as berries, grapes, and red wine), flavanols like catechins (found in tea, cocoa, red grapes, and berries), flavonones (found in citrus fruits), flavonoids like quercetin (found in onions, scallions, kale, and broccoli), flavones (found in parsley, thyme, and hot peppers), and isoflavones like genistein (found in soy and legumes).

Non-flavonoids

Non-flavonoid antioxidants can be broken down into three categories – vitamins, minerals, and plant pigments including Vitamin C and E, selenium, beta-carotene, lutein (found in spinach, kiwi, Brussels sprouts, and dark green vegetables), and lycopene (found in tomatoes, pink grapefruit, and watermelon). Lycopene is believed to protect against prostate cancer and boost heart health.[10]

Many herbs and medicinal plants are good natural sources of antioxidants. A diet rich in Vitamins A, C, E, and beta-carotene may help reduce the risk of some cancers, heart disease, cataracts, and strokes. Many experts agree that these nutrients are best consumed as food.

WHAT ARE PHYTOCHEMICALS?

Phytochemicals are naturally occurring chemicals in plants that provide flavor, color, texture, and smell. Phytochemicals have potential health benefits, as they may boost enzyme production or activity, which may, in turn, block carcinogens, suppress malignant cells, or interfere with processes that can cause heart disease and stroke. Together the phytochemical compounds in fruits and vegetables help scavenge harmful oxygen derived free radicals from the body and protect us from cancers, diabetes, degenerative diseases, and infections.[11]

Phytochemical-rich foods include cruciferous vegetables (e.g., broccoli, Brussels sprouts, cauliflower, cabbage), umbelliferous vegetables (e.g., carrots, celery, parsley, parsnips), allium vegetables (e.g., garlic, onions, leeks), berries, citrus fruits, whole grains, and legumes (e.g., soybeans, beans, lentils, garbanzo beans, peanuts).

There are many other nutrition points to cover on what your body needs and why. We have covered many here that I hope are useful to you as a reference guide.

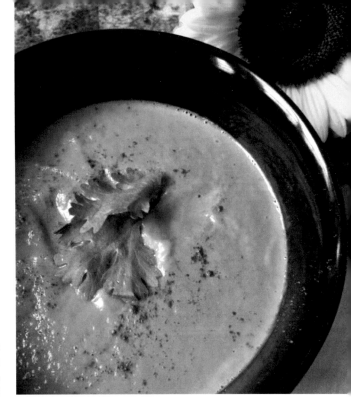

Incredible Spicy Butternut
Squash Soup (page 381)

Photo credit: MashnDashMeals
(www.facebook.com/mashndashmeals)

High Protein Cookie
Dough Balls (page 380)

Photo credit: MashnDashMeals
(www.facebook.com/mashndashmeals)

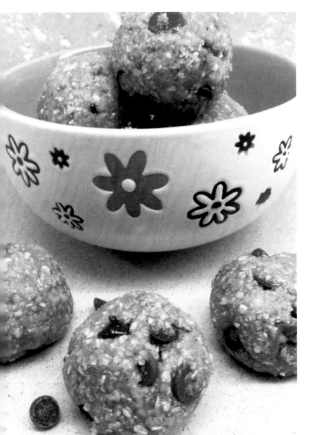

Cauliflower Lentil Indian Soup

Virtuous Brownies (page 415)

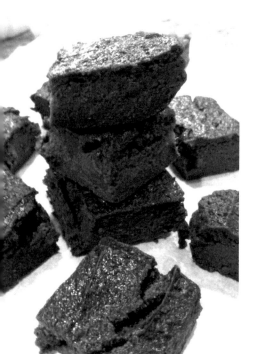

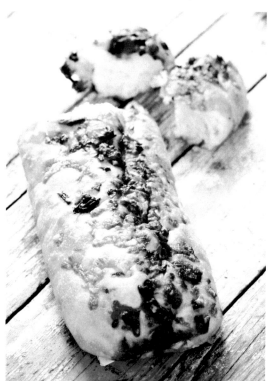

Fresh Loaf

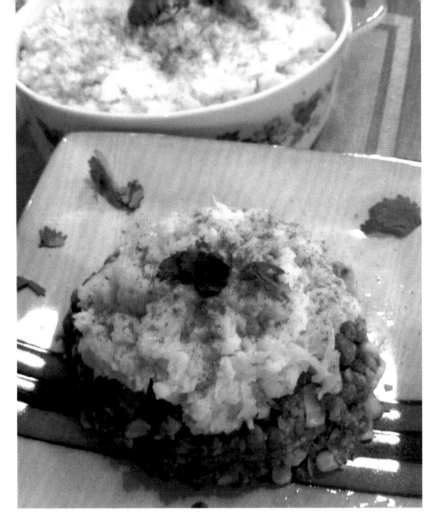

Lentil Shepherd's Pie with Cauliflower Topping (page 389)

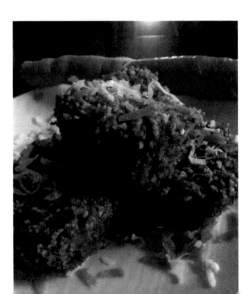

Dairy-free, Morning Glory
Muffins (page 369)

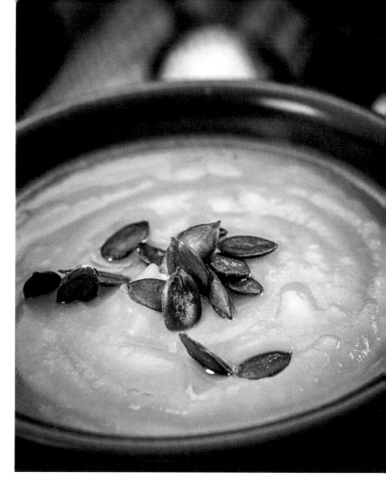

Pure Pleasure Pumpkin
Soup (page 400)

Photo credit: iStock

Salad

Photo credit: iStock

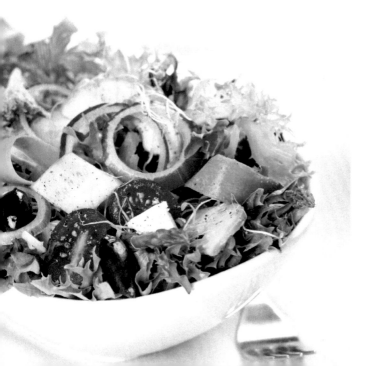

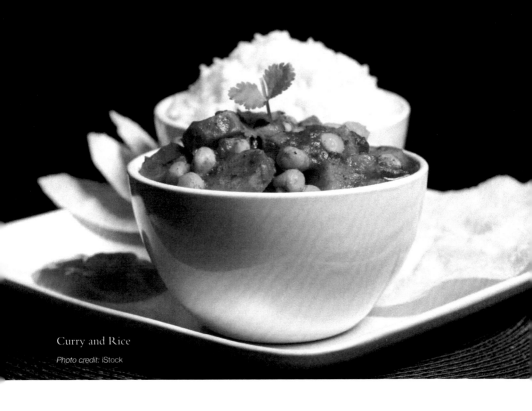

Curry and Rice

Photo credit: iStock

Frittata with Tomatoes

Photo credit: iStock

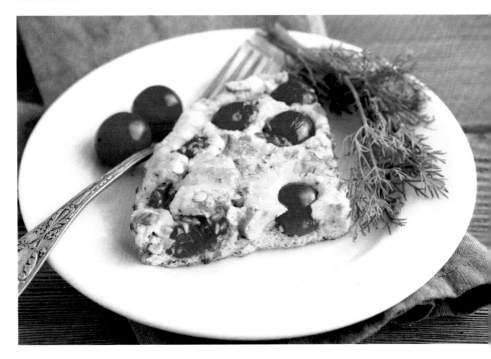

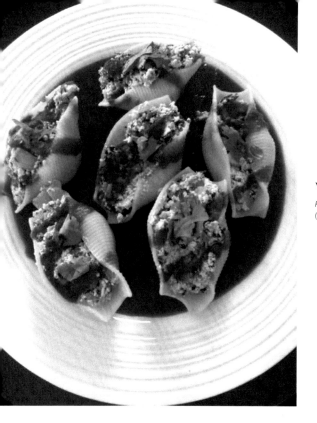

Vegan Stuffed Pasta Shells

Photo credit: MashnDashMeals
(www.facebook.com/mashndashmeals)

Summer Chickpea Salad with
Lime Vinaigrette and Basil

Photo credit: MashnDashMeals
(www.facebook.com/mashndashmeals)

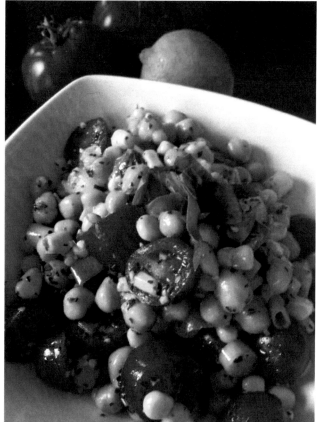

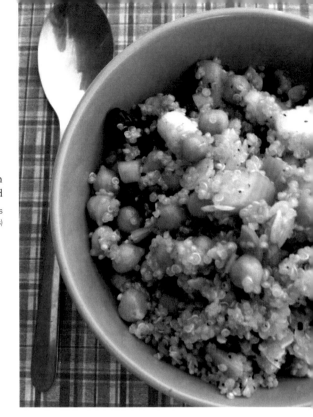

Quinoa and Apple Salad with Cranberry and Almond

Photo credit: MashnDashMeals
(www.facebook.com/mashndashmeals)

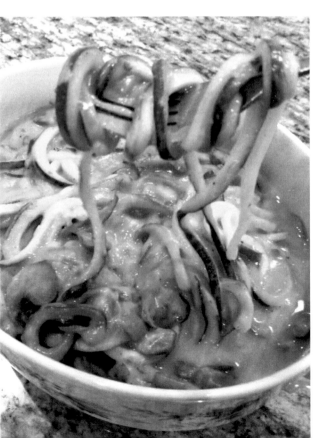

Zucchini Noodles with Rosemary Butternut Cream Sauce

Photo credit: MashnDashMeals
(www.facebook.com/mashndashmeals)

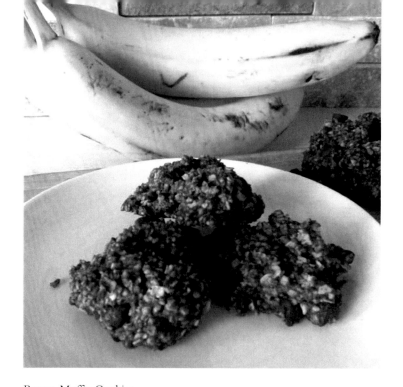

Banana Muffin Cookies

Photo credit: MashnDashMeals (www.facebook.com/mashndashmeals)

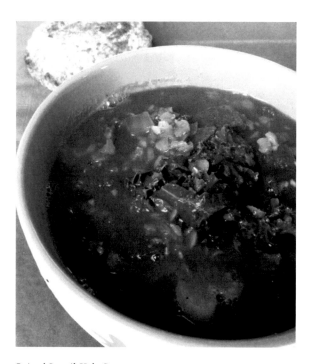

Spiced Lentil Kale Soup

Photo credit: MashnDashMeals (www.facebook.com/mashndashmeals)

Recipes *from* A to Z

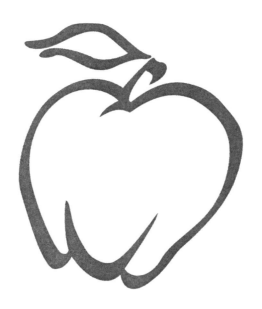

"A party without cake is just a meeting."
Julia Child
(1912-2004, American chef, author, and television personality)

Before we explore some tasty and nutritious recipes, I wanted to give you some simple guidelines for improving flavor and nutrients.

- In the recipes that follow, I won't note it, but wherever you can try to find organic varieties for eggs (or free range or farm fresh), beef, chicken, dairy, and vegetables, especially those that are more prone to pesticide residues like apples, blueberries, strawberries, lettuce, cucumbers, spinach, potatoes, bell peppers, and green beans.

- I also believe it is helpful to use high quality oils (see Oils Are Fats under Food for Thought, under "O") so I recommend using extra virgin olive oil for most recipes, and coconut oil or cultured butter for baking but feel free to substitute oils according to your taste.

- I do have many gluten-free flours listed or often use spelt, which isn't gluten-free but easy to use and a nice change from whole wheat. You can always revert to whole wheat or your flour of choice for most recipes if you prefer that taste instead.

- I use a lot of herbs and spices in these recipes because they are loaded with antioxidants. While fresh herbs are good, they are not always practical so I recommend investing in some high quality dried herbs. I also use sea salt infused with herbs and vegetables regularly (I like Herbamare by A. Vogel).

- You can always substitute refined sugar for sucanat, honey, maple syrup, or even xylitol or molasses, etc., according to your preferences to upgrade nutrients or reduce sugar content.

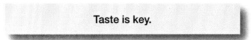

Taste is key.

For each recipe, I've provided a short introduction highlighting some of the health benefits in the particular dish and you can check the A-Z of Foods section for in-depth information on power ingredients as well.

I value flavor enormously too so I want you to love the food you eat and enjoy it! I tried to put an assortment of recipes for vegetarians, meat lovers, gluten-free diets, and those with a sweet tooth and focused on recipes that take less than an hour to prepare to accommodate busy work and life schedules! I hope you enjoy the healthy food and are able to incorporate some of these into your weekly meal plans!

I have a book full of other recipes but wanted to keep this a food information book and not a cook book, so keep visiting my website at *www.abc-soffood.com* for new recipes and health tips down the road.

Bon appetite!

"Tis an ill cook that cannot lick his own fingers."
William Shakespeare
(1564-1616, English poet, playwright, actor)

Anti-Inflammatory Chicken Curry

Meat Lovers/Gluten Free

The combination of spices and jalapeno pepper in this dish will help regulate cholesterol and improve blood flow. The vegetables offer antioxidants, vitamins, and minerals, and the broccoli, onions, and garlic will boost liver function. Finally the cashews supply extra magnesium and selenium for improved health, circulation, and metabolism.

Ingredients
1-3 garlic cloves, minced
1/2 cup chopped broccoli
1/2 cup snow peas
1 green onion, diced
1 red pepper, sliced
2 tablespoons chopped cashews (or almonds)
1/2 teaspoon peeled and minced fresh ginger root
1 small jalapeno pepper, minced
1 1/2 teaspoons curry powder
sea salt and pepper to taste
1 teaspoon extra virgin olive oil (or coconut oil)
2-4 ounces (60-120 g) chicken breast cut into bite-sized pieces

1/4 – 1/2 cup veggie stock, if needed for moisture
1/2 cup cooked brown rice (or quinoa)

Directions

Combine the garlic, broccoli, snow peas, green onion, red pepper, cashews, minced ginger, jalapeno pepper, curry powder and sea salt and pepper in a bowl and set aside.

Heat the oil in a small skillet over medium heat. Add the chicken and sauté until lightly browned.

Combine the veggies and chicken into a larger saucepan. Simmer covered for 10 minutes or until chicken is fully cooked, adding the vegetable stock if necessary.

Serve over rice (or quinoa).

Serves: 4

Asparagus and Mushroom Pasta

Vegetarian Delight/Gluten Free

Asparagus, the first green of spring, is loaded with folic acid (Vitamin B9), important for production of red blood cells and proteins in the body, including hormones. Mushrooms are rich in the mineral selenium, which boosts our immune system, and herbs like parsley, oregano, rosemary, and thyme are antioxidants that reduce inflammation in the body. The olive oil is full of heart-healthy monounsaturated fats that help lower LDL cholesterol in the body. Eating some gluten-free meals gives the digestive system a rest from wheat but this recipe can be made using regular noodles if desired.

Ingredients

1 bunch asparagus
2 cups shitake mushrooms
2 tablespoons extra virgin olive oil
1/2 cup green onions, sliced
1/2 cup leeks, chopped
1/4 teaspoon each oregano, rosemary and thyme to season
1/4 cup white wine

1/2 cup vegetable broth
4 tablespoons cultured butter
sea salt and ground pepper
1 8-ounce (240 g) package buckwheat or quinoa pasta
1 tablespoon chopped parsley
parmesan cheese, to taste

Directions

After washing thoroughly, cut off ends of asparagus and mushrooms and slice into small pieces.

In a large skillet heat oil over medium-high heat. Add mushrooms, then onions, leeks, and herbs and cook until softened. Finally, add asparagus for a few minutes.

Add wine and vegetable broth and simmer until the liquid has evaporated. Add butter and toss until melted and season with salt and pepper.

Meanwhile in a large pot of of boiling salted water, cook pasta of choice according to package directions. Drain. Toss with sauce and add parsley and fresh parmesan cheese.

Serves: 4

B

> *"The discovery of a new dish does more for the happiness of the human race than the discovery of a star."*
> Jean Anthelme Brillat-Savarin
> (1755-1826, French lawyer and politician,
> known as an epicure and gastronome)

Delicious Beef Burgundy

Meat Lovers

A classic in French cooking, using grass-fed or pasture-raised beef increases the heart-healthy omega-3s in this healthier version. This dish's herbs and spices work as antioxidants to reduce free radicals and the carrots are full of beta-carotene, important for eye health. Mushrooms are full of selenium, a potent antioxidant, and onions and garlic are excellent detoxifiers and good for liver and cell health. Red wine (in moderation) contains resveratrol, a powerful antioxidant that helps prevent coronary disease. Use less meat and more vegetables to reduce saturated fat intake.

Ingredients
2 tablespoons olive oil
1-2 pounds (1/2 to 1 kg) round steak (try to find grass-fed or
    pasture-raised for more omega-3s and flavor), cut into small pieces
3 tablespoons whole spelt or whole wheat flour (or any other
    gluten-free flour if preferred)
3 onions, sliced
2 cups beef broth or water
1 1/2 cups dry red wine

1 teaspoon sea salt
freshly ground black pepper
3-4 garlic cloves crushed
1/2 teaspoon each of rosemary and thyme
Dash of cinnamon
4-6 large diced carrots
2 1/2 cups sliced fresh wild mushrooms (shitake or oyster)
3-4 bay leaves
Rice or noodles

Directions

In a large stock pot over medium-high heat, heat the oil and add the beef pieces. Sprinkle the flour over the beef and add onions. Brown the onions and meat on all sides.

Pour in broth/water and red wine. Sprinkle in salt, black pepper, garlic, and herbs and spices. Add in diced carrots and mushrooms.

Bring to a boil and add bay leaves. Cover, and reduce heat. Simmer for 1 1/2 hours or until beef is tender, stirring occasionally.

Liquid should just cover everything. If necessary, add some more wine to cover. Cook until everything is tender.

Serve over rice or noodles.

Serves: 4

Banana Bars

Sweet Tooth/Gluten Free

Bananas provide a powerhouse of nutrition in these tasty bars. High in potassium, bananas are good for regulating blood pressure, proper fluid balance, nerve transmission, and muscle contraction. Walnuts contain high amounts of omega-3s, important for heart and brain health, as well as magnesium. The recipe contains gluten-free coconut flour which is higher in protein and fiber than grain flours and contains metabolism-boosting medium-chained fatty acids. Ground flax increases omega-3 fatty acid intake.

Ingredients

2 large or 3 small very ripe bananas
1 1/2 cups coconut flour
1/3 cup coconut oil, or cultured butter, melted
1/3 cup raw honey or real maple syrup
4 free-range eggs
1 1/2 tablespoon ginger
2 teaspoons cinnamon
2 teaspoons ground flax
2 tablespoons cocoa
1 teaspoon ground cardamom
1 teaspoon baking soda
2 teaspoons apple cider vinegar
1/2 cup walnuts, chopped

Directions

Preheat the oven to 350°F. Grease a 9 x 9 glass baking dish with coconut oil or line it with parchment paper.

In a food processor, blend together everything except the baking soda, vinegar and walnuts until combined. Add the baking soda, vinegar and chopped walnuts, blend quickly and pour into the prepared dish.

Bake for about 30-40 minutes until a toothpick comes out clean.

Serves: 6-8

C

"One cannot think well, love well, and sleep well,
if one has not dined well."
Virginia Woolf
(1882-1941, English writer)

Hearty Homemade Chicken Soup

Meat Lovers

A classic for curing colds and of moms everywhere, this version is loaded with iron and nutrient-dense vegetables, like spinach and kale along with antioxidant-rich herbs, and immune-boosting garlic and onions. Simmering chicken bones brings added flavor and nutrients into the broth and is delicious.

Ingredients
1 (2-3 pound/1-1.5 kg) free-range whole left over chicken, cooked
3 stalks celery with leaves, chopped
2 cups carrots, chopped
1 cup frozen peas
1/2 cup frozen kernel corn
2 onions, chopped
1/2 bunch spinach, chopped finely
1-2 large leaves kale, chopped into small pieces
3 cans low-sodium, chicken broth
1/4 teaspoon fresh garlic, crushed
1/4 teaspoon each dried thyme, basil, parsley, dill, and poultry seasoning
freshly ground pepper

Directions

Bone last night's left over chicken and place chicken carcass and bones in a large pot and cover with water. Place leaves of celery in pot and bring to boil, then reduce heat and simmer about 40-60 minutes. You can leave the bones in the pot overnight for more flavor before making soup if desired.

When cool enough to handle, strain the cooking liquid, discard celery tops, any bones, and place cooking liquid in a large pot. Place celery, carrots, onion, spinach, and kale in pot with chicken broth. Add garlic and other seasonings. Let simmer.

Cut up meat (deboned earlier) into bite-size pieces and add to pot.

Cook until vegetables are tender and flavors are well blended, stirring often (up to 90 minutes or longer). Tastes even better the next day.

Serves: 6

Curried Chickpeas with Carrots and Peas

Vegetarian Delight

Fiber- and protein-rich chickpeas form the nutritional base of this dish, along with antioxidant-dense spices, immune-boosting onion and garlic, and circulation-enhancing cayenne and turmeric. The peas and carrots provide vital vitamins and minerals.

Ingredients

2 tablespoons organic butter
1 onion, finely chopped
2 cloves of garlic, minced
1/2 teaspoon ground ginger (or 1 tablespoon minced)
1/2 teaspoon cumin
1/2 teaspoon coriander
1/2 teaspoon turmeric
1/2 teaspoon cayenne pepper
1 19-ounce (540 ml) can of chickpeas
1-2 large organic carrots, diced
1/2 cup frozen peas
1 cup fresh parsley, chopped

Directions

Heat butter, onion, garlic, and ginger until onion has softened.

Add seasonings and stir for 2 minutes until soft.

Add liquid from can of chickpeas and boil vigorously until liquid has reduced to 1/3 of original.

Add chickpeas and warm. Add cut carrots and frozen peas and simmer for 20-25 minutes.

Garnish with parsley and serve over rice.

Serves: 4

*"As long as you have food in your mouth, you have
solved all questions for the time being."*
Franz Kafka
(1883-1924, German-language writer)

Dairy-free, Morning Glory Muffins

Sweet Tooth/Gluten Free

These are the perfect breakfast muffins when served with some almond butter and a bowl of fruit or as an afternoon power snack on their own. They contain fiber-rich oats, while protein and magnesium are found in the nuts. The carrots are a good source of beta-carotene, cinnamon regulates blood sugar levels, and the natural sweeteners will satisfy any sweet tooth.

Ingredients
1 cup garbanzo and fava, almond, or coconut flour
1/2 cup oats
2 teaspoons baking powder
2 teaspoons cinnamon
1/2 teaspoon sea salt
1/4 teaspoon nutmeg
2 free-range eggs
1 cup unsweetened applesauce
1/4 cup maple syrup

2 teaspoons pure vanilla extract
1/2 cup melted coconut oil
2 cups carrots, shredded
1/2 cup unsweetened shredded coconut
1/2 cup organic raisins
1/3 cup raw pecans, chopped
1/3 cup raw almonds, chopped

Directions

Preheat oven to 350°F. Grease a muffin tin with coconut oil or line with paper muffin cups.

In a large bowl combine flour, oats, baking powder, cinnamon, sea salt, and nutmeg. In a separate bowl, combine eggs, applesauce, maple syrup, and vanilla. Stir coconut oil into the wet mixture.

Add the dry mixture to the wet and combine, but do not over mix. Fold in the carrots, coconut, raisins, pecans, and almonds. Scoop muffin mix into muffin tins. They do not rise a lot, so you can fill the batter up to the top.

Bake for 30-35 minutes.

Serves: 12 muffins

Delightful Berry Crumble

Sweet Tooth/Gluten Free

This dessert contains fiber-rich oats, vitamin- and antioxidant-dense apples and berries, and blood-sugar regulating cinnamon, along with omega-3-rich flax. Cloves are a powerhouse of nutrients and act to boost digestion and reduce body inflammation. Coconut oil is easy to digest and boosts metabolism.

Ingredients

4 organic apples

1 cup mixed frozen berries (blueberries, strawberries, raspberries, and blackberries)

3/4 unsweetened apple sauce

1 cup old-fashioned oats

4 tablespoons amaranth, coconut, or almond flour

4 tablespoons light brown sugar

1 teaspoon cinnamon

1 teaspoon ground flax or ground chia

1/2 teaspoon ground cloves

1/2 teaspoon cardamom or ginger

1 tablespoon coconut oil

1 tablespoon cultured unsalted butter, cut in small pieces

Directions

Preheat oven to 350°F and grease 12 x 18 baking dish with coconut oil.

Quarter apples, remove cores, and cut into thin slices. Place apples and berries in baking dish and coat evenly with applesauce.

In bowl mix together oats, flour, sugar, cinnamon, flax, cloves, and cardamom or ginger. Work coconut oil and butter into dry ingredients, mixing with fingers. Sprinkle oat mixture over apples and berries.

Bake 30-35 minutes, until topping is golden.

Serve with organic ice cream. Yum!

Serves: 4-6

*"If more of us valued food and cheer and song above
hoarded gold, it would be a merrier world."*
J.R.R Tolkien
(1892-1973, English writer, philologist, and university professor)

Energy Smoothie

Sweet Tooth

Rich in calcium, goat's milk is easier to digest than cow's milk for many people. The bananas provide potassium for blood pressure regulation and power berries for high antioxidants, along with probiotic kefir to boost your immune system. Spirulina is a powerhouse of protein and nutrients and great for detoxing the blood and supporting the liver and immune system. It also contains ground flax that is high in omega-3s and other iron-rich greens for a nutrient packed morning drink.

Ingredients
1 cup goat's milk or yogurt
2 tablespoons plain kefir
1 banana, fresh or frozen
1/2 to 1 cup frozen berries (blueberries, raspberries, strawberries, and
    blackberries)
1 tablespoon ground flax seeds
1 scoop spirulina powder or handful of chopped greens (kale, spinach,
    swiss chard, barley grass, etc.)
1 tablespoon raw honey or maple syrup, if desired to sweeten

Directions

Blend all ingredients in a food processor or blender until smooth and drink immediately.

Serves: 1

Easy Cauliflower Soup

Vegetarian Delight

The main ingredient, cauliflower, contains liver-supporting compounds, along with detoxifying onion and leek. Anti-inflammatory spices like turmeric and cayenne to support circulation and lower cholesterol. The cauliflower and celery are rich in fiber.

Ingredients
1 large cauliflower, washed
1 leek, washed and sliced
2 tablespoons butter or olive oil
1 onion, chopped
1-2 stalk celery, chopped
1 teaspoon salt
1/2 teaspoon pepper
1/2 teaspoon turmeric
1/2 teaspoon cayenne
4 cups vegetable stock
grated cheese, to taste

Directions
Slice the cauliflower finely into small pieces.

Chop leek and cook for 1-2 minutes in butter or oil until softened.

Add the cauliflower, onion and celery. Stir in sea salt, pepper, turmeric, and cayenne.

Cover with vegetable stock and cook for 5-10 minutes until the cauliflower is tender. Remove from the heat.

Puree with a good blender. Add additional filtered water (1-2 cups) to desired consistency.

Serve warm soup with grated Parmesan, cheddar, or gruyere on top. Enjoy.

Serves: 4

Fish on the Grill – Succulent Salmon

Meat Lovers

Great on the grill, salmon provides a good source of protein and omega-3 fatty acids. Digestion-boosting raw apple cider vinegar, power herbs for antioxidants, and probiotic soy sauce complete the nutritional impact of this dish.

Ingredients
1 large wild-caught salmon fillet
2 tablespoons lemon juice
2 tablespoons raw apple cider vinegar
1 teaspoon maple syrup
1 1/2 teaspoons dried parsley
1/2 teaspoon dried rosemary
1 teaspoon garlic powder
1 teaspoon soy sauce
sea salt and pepper

Directions

Place fish, skin side down, on grill pan. Combine the lemon juice, vinegar, maple syrup, parsley, rosemary, garlic powder, and soy sauce. Pour over fish. Sprinkle with salt and pepper.

Marinate fish in sauce for 1-2 hours in fridge.

Place pan on grill. Cover grill and cook over medium heat for 15-20 minutes or until fish flakes easily with a fork.

Serves: 4

French Fries Bistro Style with Parsley and Garlic

Vegetarian Delight

Adding healthy oils and baking is a far healthier option than store-bought frozen fries! Organic potatoes are high in fiber, Vitamin C, and B-complex Vitamins. The skin contains many nutrients so leave it on! Garlic is a great immune boost and the parsley adds flavor and antioxidants. Easy to make and a winner every time in my household!

Ingredients

4 medium organic potatoes (about 13/4 pounds/720 g), unpeeled
2 tablespoons coconut oil, extra virgin olive oil, or peanut oil
1/4 cup fresh parsley, chopped
2 garlic cloves, minced
coarse sea salt

Directions

Position rack in center of oven and preheat to 425°F.

Cut potatoes lengthwise into 1/3-inch thick slices, and then cut again lengthwise into 1/3-inch wide strips. Combine potatoes, oil, and garlic in large bowl; toss to coat well.

Place potatoes on large baking sheet; spread in single layer. Sprinkle with sea salt.

Bake about 40 minutes, turning and rearranging potatoes frequently, until potatoes are deep golden brown. Top with parsley before serving.

Serves: 4

G

> "Fill your bowl to the brim and it will spill. Keep
> sharpening your knife and it will blunt. Chase after
> money and security and your heart will never unclench.
> Care about other people's approval and you will be their
> prisoner. Do your work, and then step back.
> The only path to serenity."
>
> Lao Tzu
> (604-531 BC, Chinese philosopher, poet, and founder of Taoism)

Greek Salad with Avocado and Mixed Greens

Vegetarian Delight

This salad is a powerhouse of fiber and nutrients. Tomatoes contain lycopene, which is great for heart health, and peppers, which are loaded with antioxidants. Onions and radicchio are great for the liver and avocados are a great source of monounsaturated oils for heart health. Mixed greens are loaded with minerals and magnesium and sprouts are a powerhouse of nutrients and enzymes needed for healthy digestion!

Ingredients
Vinaigrette
1 teaspoon Dijon mustard
1/2 cup raw apple cider vinegar
1 tablespoon sucanat or maple syrup
2/3 cup extra virgin olive oil
1/3 cup flax oil

dried herbs, including any of basil, parsley, marjoram, tarragon, lovage,
   dill, and fennel
salt and pepper to taste

Salad
1 large cucumber
2-3 medium tomatoes
1/2 red pepper
1/2 green pepper
1/2 yellow pepper
1/2 medium red onion
mixed greens, three to four handfuls
1/2 cup radicchio pieces
1 large avocado peeled, pitted, and cubed
sprouts (radish, alfalfa, mung bean, etc.), large handful
1 cup black olives
2 cups feta cheese

Directions
Vinaigrette
Mix all together in a small jar and shake. Set aside.

Salad

Cut the cucumber lengthways and then slice it; place it in a mixing bowl.

Cut the tomatoes into wedges and add to the mixing bowl.

Clean the peppers and cut into chunks; mix with the cucumber and
tomatoes.

Slice the red onion and add to the mixed vegetables. Add mixed greens,
radicchio and avocado.

Top with sprouts of your choice!

Toss in dressing as desired and mix well until all ingredients are covered.

Top with black olives and crumbled feta cheese.

Serves: 3-4

Grape and Fruit Salad

Sweet Tooth

Antioxidant-rich berries load this salad with Vitamin C, fiber, and potassium. Grapes are packed with resveratrol, a powerful antioxidant that helps prevent coronary disease. The almonds and pecans add protein and minerals, while the yogurt adds calcium and probiotics to boost the immune system and celery adds fiber to this delicious dessert.

Ingredients
1 red apple, cored and chopped
1 granny smith apple, cored and chopped
1 cup red grapes
1 nectarine, pitted and sliced
1 green melon, seeds removed and balled or peeled and cut into cubes
3/4 cup blueberries
3/4 cup strawberries, sliced
1/2 cup blackberries
2 stalks of celery, sliced finely
1/2 cup dried cranberries
1/2 cup almonds, chopped
1/2 cup pecans, chopped
1 small tub of buffalo or plain organic yogurt

Directions

In a large bowl, combine fruit, celery, and nuts.

Mix in yogurt.

Chill until ready to serve.

Serves: 2-4

"Knowledge is knowing that a tomato is a fruit;
wisdom is not putting it in a fruit salad."
Miles Kington
(1941-2008, British journalist, musician, and broadcaster)

Healthy and Tasty Hamburger Patties

Meat Lovers

Since many of us love burgers, I have included a healthier upgrade that is delicious and easy to prepare. Using grass-fed hamburger meat is a great choice for boosting mega-3 heart-healthy fatty acids and the herbs help to neutralize any carcinogens from the BBQ. You can even make these gluten free by using gluten-free breadcrumbs (Mary's can be found in most stores).

Ingredients
1 pound (480 g) lean ground beef (grass fed, free range, or organic)
1/2 cup spelt breadcrumbs
1 free-range egg
2 tablespoons lemon juice
2 tablespoons fresh basil, chopped
1 tablespoon fresh thyme, chopped
1 tablespoon fresh rosemary, chopped
1 tablespoon chives, chopped
1/2 teaspoon salt
1/4 teaspoon black pepper

Directions

Preheat grill to medium-high heat.

In a large mixing bowl, combine all ingredients until well mixed.

Split mixture into eight equal portions. Shape into rectangular patties about 5-6 inches long.

Place patties on lightly oiled grill and cook for 8-10 minutes on each side.

Remove from heat and serve on buns or between Portobello mushroom caps.

Serves: 6-8

High Protein Cookie Dough Balls

Sweet Tooth

From www.facebook.com/mashndashmeals
Delicious magnesium-dense dark chocolate makes for a tasty and protein-rich treat. This easy recipe also contains fiber-rich oats, high protein flours, and nut butter.

Ingredients
1 1/2 cup rolled oats
2 tablespoons coconut oil
3 tablespoons nut butter (can be, sugar-free peanut or almond butter)
1/4 cup pure maple syrup
1 teaspoon pure vanilla extract
3/4 cup almond meal
4 tablespoons dark chocolate chips

Directions

In a food processor, blend the oats to a fine powder (flour).

In a large bowl, combine the coconut oil, nut butter, maple syrup, and vanilla. Beat with a hand mixer until smooth. Add the almond meal, and oat flour and beat again until combined. Fold in chocolate chips.

Roll the dough into small balls and place on cookie sheet.

Freeze the bites for 5-10 minutes or until firm.
Serves: 4

"Ice-Cream is exquisite. What a pity it isn't illegal."
Voltaire
(1694-1778, French Enlightenment writer, historian, and philosopher)

Incredible Spicy Butternut Squash Soup

Vegetarian Delight

Warm and delicious soup always feels good and this one is good for you too. Squash, celery, and potatoes supply the fiber and minerals, while the jalapeno peppers and onions provide circulation-boosting compounds. And the carrots provide lots of antioxidants too! Yum.

Ingredients
2 tablespoons butter
1 small onion, chopped
1 stalk celery, chopped
1 medium carrot, chopped
2 medium potatoes, peeled and cubed
1 medium butternut squash, peeled, seeded, and cubed
1 sweet potato, peeled and cubed
1 32-ounce (980 ml) container vegetable stock
1 jalapeno pepper, chopped finely (for heat)
dash of hot sauce to taste
salt and pepper to taste

Directions

Melt the butter in a large pot, and cook the onion, celery, carrot, potatoes, squash, and sweet potato 5 minutes, or until lightly browned. Pour in enough of the stock to cover vegetables. Add chopped jalapeno pepper and hot sauce. Bring to a boil. Reduce heat to low, cover pot, and simmer 40 minutes, or until all vegetables are tender. Transfer the soup to a blender, and blend until smooth. Return to pot, and mix in any remaining stock to attain desired consistency. Season with salt and pepper.

Serves: 4

Irresistible Power Oatmeal

Gluten Free

Oats contain high amounts of soluble fiber that can help reduce cholesterol and keep blood sugar levels steadier. Quinoa is a high-protein grain that gives this oatmeal added crunch, while the kefir adds probiotics and calcium. The ground flax adds heart- and brain-healthy omega-3s and the pumpkin seeds provide additional omega-3s as well as zinc, which is important for our immune system and protein generation. This recipe is loaded with fiber and steel cut oats are minimally processed.

Ingredients

4 cups filtered water
1/2 teaspoon sea salt
1 cup steel cut oats (I like Bob's Redmill)
1/2 cup quinoa
handful of organic raisins
2 large handfuls minimally processed pumpkin seeds
2 tablespoons ground flax
1 cup plain organic kefir
handful of berries
1 tablespoon maple, agave syrup, or raw honey

Directions

Bring 4 cups of filtered water to a boil with sea salt. Add steel cut oats and quinoa and reduce heat for about 10-15 minutes, until liquid is absorbed.

Turn off the heat and add raisins, pumpkin seeds, and flax. Stir in kefir. Let sit for 5-10 minutes and top with berries and maple syrup, or natural sweetener of choice.

Serves: 4

*"After a good dinner one can forgive anybody,
even one's own relations."*
Oscar Wilde
(1854-1900, Irish writer and poet)

Jamaican Goat Curry

Meat Lovers

Try this dish for a taste of the islands. It contains high amounts of lean protein, heart- and circulation-boosting ginger, garlic, curry, and habanero, and lycopene-rich tomatoes. The herbs are high in antioxidants and the potatoes and carrots contain Vitamin cup for the immune system. The olive oil helps to reduce cholesterol. Coconut milk is rich in a type of saturated fat called "lauric acid" that can help boost HDL in the body, which may lessen chances of heart disease.

Ingredients
3 pounds (1.5 kg) goat (or any lean game like venison)
sea salt
1/4 cup extra virgin olive oil
6-8 tablespoons curry powder
2 tablespoons allspice
2 onions, chopped
1-2 habanero or hot peppers, seeded and chopped
2-inch piece of ginger, peeled and minced
4-5 cloves garlic, peeled and chopped
2 15-ounce (480 ml) cans coconut milk

1 15-ounce (480 ml) can of tomato sauce or crushed tomatoes
1-2 carrots, peeled and sliced
3 cups water
1 tablespoon dried thyme
5 Yukon gold potatoes, peeled and cut into 1-inch chunks

Directions

Cut the meat into large chunks. If you have bones, you can use them, too. Salt everything lightly and set aside to come to room temperature for about 30 minutes.

Heat the olive oil in a large pot over medium-high heat. Mix in 2 tablespoons of the curry powder and allspice and heat briefly. Place the meat in the curried oil in batches, browning on all sides and set aside in a bowl.

Add the onions and habanero to the pot and sauté, stirring from time to time, until the onions start to brown. Sprinkle some salt over them as they cook. Add the ginger and garlic, mix well and sauté for another 1-2 minutes.

Put the meat (and bones, if using) into the pot, along with any juices left in the bowl. Mix well. Pour in the coconut milk, tomatoes, carrots and 5 tablespoons of the curry powder. Stir to combine. Add water along with thyme and potatoes. Bring to a simmer and cook until the meat is falling-apart tender, which will take at least 2 hours. Longer if you have a mature goat.

Note: This recipe works well in a slow cooker to save time.

Serve with Jamaican rice and peas, or coconut rice with kidney beans.

Serves: 6

Juicing in the Morning!

Sweet Tooth

Juicing makes nutrients easier to absorb or more "bioavailable." All these recipes contain high amounts of Vitamin C to help keep immune systems strong along with vitamin- and mineral-rich vegetables. Juicing raw vegetables provides vital enzymes needed to properly digest food. Combine this drink with small amounts of healthy protein for a great start to super charge your day!

To make the following recipes you do need a home juicer. All recipes are for one serving.

Ingredients

Apple Breeze
2 apples, seeded
2 stalks celery
1/4 lemon

Lemon Veggie Delight!
4 carrots
2 stalks celery
4 kale leaves (can also try bok choy or spinach)
1 lemon

Detoxifying Sweet Beets
1-2 medium-sized fresh beets
2 stalks celery
1-2 carrots
2 kale leaves
Optional: you can add more carrots, beet greens, or a wedge of lemon

Directions
Place all in blender and puree until liquefied.

Serves: 1

Kamut Grain Pancakes

Gluten Free

The whole grains in this recipe are packed with fiber and B-complex Vitamins. Buckwheat is loaded with flavonoids, particularly rutin, that protect against disease and help to lower cholesterol. Incorporated are ground flax for added omega-3s, antioxidant-rich berries, cinnamon to regulate blood sugar, and kefir to boost healthy gut flora.

Ingredients
1 cup kamut flour
1/2 cup buckwheat flour
2 tablespoons ground flax (salba)
1 teaspoon baking soda
1 teaspoon kefir
1/4 teaspoon salt
1 1/2 cups cow or goat milk (or water)
3 tablespoons olive oil
1/2 teaspoonful cinnamon
1-2 teaspoons agave nectar or maple syrup (optional)
fresh or frozen fruit (e.g., blueberries, raspberries, strawberries)
    (optional)

Directions

Preheat a non-stick griddle or large skillet. In a large bowl, whisk the flours, baking soda, kefir, and salt.

In a 2-cup measure, combine the milk or water, oil, cinnamon, and agave nectar or maple syrup. Pour into the flour mixture, and whisk just until combined. Don't beat or over mix.

Drop by spoonful (2 per cake) onto the griddle or skillet. Add fruit to the pancakes. Cook until the tops are bubbly and edges are brown. Turn and cook until light brown.

Serves: **4**

Kale and Lentil Soup

Vegetarian Delight

Delicious and sustaining, this soup contains fiber- and protein-rich lentils and black beans, along with magnesium- and iron-dense kale. It is packed with liver-supporting onion, garlic, and leeks and Vitamin C-rich potatoes. Meat lovers can add small amounts sliced hot Italian sausage to add spice and additional protein.

Ingredients

2 tablespoons unsalted cultured butter
1 large sweet onion, chopped
1-2 leeks, stems trimmed and chopped
4 stalks celery, chopped
4 medium red potatoes, chopped
1 carrot, chopped
3 cloves garlic
1/4 teaspoon ground allspice
1/4 teaspoon cumin seeds
1/4 teaspoon cayenne pepper
1/8 teaspoon ground cloves
1 dash pepper

1 quart (950 ml) vegetable broth
1 cup dry red lentils
1 15-ounce (480 ml) can black beans
2 cups water
1 1/2 cups kale, roughly chopped
1/4 cup fresh cilantro, chopped

Directions

Melt the butter in a large saucepan over medium heat. Stir in the onion, leeks, and celery. Cook until tender. Mix in the potatoes, carrot, and garlic. Continue to cook and stir for about 5 minutes, until the potatoes are well coated with butter. Season the mixture with allspice, cumin, cayenne pepper, cloves, and pepper.

Pour in the vegetable broth, and mix in the lentils and beans. Add water, increasing the amount as necessary to cover all ingredients. Bring to a boil, reduce heat, and stir in the kale. Cook, stirring occasionally, 35-45 minutes, until the lentils are tender.

Mix in the cilantro. Continue cooking about 5 minutes, or to desired thickness.

Serve with hearty sourdough rye bread or top it with melted cheese.

Serves: 4

*"The only time to eat diet food is while you're waiting
for the steak to cook."*
Julia Child
(1912-2004, American chef, author, and television personality)

Lentil Shepherd's Pie with Cauliflower Topping

Vegetarian Delight

From www.facebook.com/mashndashmeals
The lentils and chickpeas in this dish provide a big hit of fiber and vegetable protein, along with liver-supporting onions, garlic, and cauliflower. It has antioxidant-boosting mushrooms, carrots, and herbs and Omega-3-rich flax. Enjoy!!

Ingredients
1 head of cauliflower, broken into florets
1 tablespoon ground flax seed
3 tablespoons of water
1 medium onion, diced
1 teaspoon olive oil
2 cloves garlic, minced
2 large carrots, chopped
1/2 cup mushrooms, chopped

2 cups lentils, cooked
1 cup chickpeas, mashed
1/2 cup frozen corn
1 tablespoon rosemary, chopped
1 tablespoon fresh sage, chopped
1 tablespoon fresh thyme, chopped
salt and pepper to taste
1/8 cup almond milk

Directions

Preheat oven to 400°F. Lightly grease casserole dish.

Place cauliflower in large pot and cover with water. Cook until cauliflower is soft and can be mashed.

Meanwhile in small bowl mix flax seed and 3 tablespoons of water and set aside.

In large skillet fry onions with 1 teaspoon olive oil for about 3 minutes. Add garlic, carrots, mushrooms, lentils, chickpeas, corn, rosemary, sage, and thyme. Cook for another 5 minutes.

Add in flax mixture.

Place mixture in the bottom of casserole dish.

Mash cauliflower and add almond milk. Place on top of vegetable and lentil mixture.

Bake for 30 minutes.

Serves: 4-6

Lime Coconut Tilapia

Meat Lovers

Having very low levels of mercury, tilapia is an excellent freshwater fish for eating – it's delicious too. In this dish, tilapia contributes a big hit of omega-3 fatty acids and protein. Immune-boosting Vitamin C comes from the limes, liver-supporting elements are found in the garlic, and the spinach supplies iron and magnesium. Easy and quick to make!

Ingredients
juice and zest of 3 limes (save 1 tablespoon for dressing)
4 cloves garlic, minced
1/4 teaspoon sea salt
1/4 teaspoon pepper
3 tablespoons coconut oil, melted
4 tilapia fillets
8 cups fresh spinach

Directions
Heat cast iron skillet over medium high heat.

In small bowl combine lime juice, zest, garlic, salt, pepper and 1 tablespoon of coconut oil. Coat tilapia fillets with marinade mixture on both sides.

Melt 1 tablespoon of coconut oil in the skillet and place fillets, two at a time, in pan and cook 4-5 minutes on each side.

In a large bowl toss spinach with remaining tablespoon of coconut oil and 1 tablespoon reserved lime juice.

Serve the fish over the spinach.

Serves: 4

*"The only real stumbling block is fear of failure.
In cooking you've got to have a what-the-hell attitude."*
Julia Child
(1912-2004, American chef, author, and television personality)

Mixed Vegetable Stew

Vegetarian Delight

This hearty and flavorful veggie stew is full of fiber, vitamins, minerals, and protein-rich legumes. The spices and herbs are packed with anti-inflammatory antioxidants and the onions and garlic support cells and the immune system.

Ingredients
1 tablespoon extra virgin olive oil
1 onion, chopped
2 stalks celery, chopped
2 red bell peppers, chopped
2 garlic cloves, minced
3 cups vegetable broth
3 cups well-scrubbed or peeled yams or sweet potatoes, cubed
1 medium eggplant, cut into cubes
2 cups diced tomatoes (canned or fresh)
2 cups cooked chickpeas
1 cup cooked black beans
1 tablespoon lemon juice

2 teaspoons grated ginger
2 teaspoons each ground cumin, curry powder, ground coriander,
    chili powder, turmeric, salt, pepper
handful fresh cilantro, chopped
brown rice or whole grain bread

Directions

Sauté the onions, celery, peppers and garlic in olive oil until veggies soften.

Add the rest of the ingredients, except cilantro, and bring to a boil. Reduce to a simmer and cook, covered, for 20-30 minutes.

Add cilantro and simmer for 5 more minutes.

Serve over brown rich or with whole grain bread.

Serves: 4-6

Marvelous Meatloaf

Meat Lovers/Gluten Free

Born out of the Depression, this "All-American" meal has been upgraded to a healthy but still delicious choice with grass-fed beef, rich in omega-3 fatty acids and CLA. Additionally, the herbs provide powerful antioxidants, the onions and garlic support liver health, and the tomatoes are loaded with lycopene, a heart-boosting antioxidant. The spices rev up circulation and support heart health, while reducing inflammation.

Ingredients

1 28-ounce (796 ml) can tomato sauce
1/4 cup packed sucanat, molasses, or light brown sugar
1/2 teaspoon mustard
1/2 teaspoon chili powder
1/4 teaspoon ground cloves
1 garlic clove, minced
1 1/2 tablespoons Worcestershire sauce
3/4 teaspoon dried oregano
3/4 teaspoon crushed red pepper flakes
1 dash hot pepper sauce
3/4 pound (360 g) lean ground beef (free range or grass fed)

1/4 pound (120 g) lean ground turkey (or additional 1/4 pound
    (120 g) lean ground beef)
1 large free-range egg, lightly beaten
1 cup dried gluten-free bread crumbs
1/2 teaspoon salt
1/4 teaspoon ground black pepper
1 tablespoon instant chopped onion

Directions

Preheat the oven to 350°F.

In a small bowl, combine the tomato sauce, sugar, mustard, chili powder, cloves, garlic, and Worcestershire sauce. Mix well. Set aside half the tomato mixture and place the other half in a large bowl.

Add all the remaining ingredients to the bowl. Mix well with your hands. Shape the mixture into a loaf, either rounded or rectangular, and place in a baking pan. (If desired, place loaf on a metal rack; I use a round, perforated rack that allows the fat to drip through to the bottom of the pan and keeps the fat away from the loaf during baking).

Make an indentation in the center of the loaf and pour the reserved tomato mixture into this indentation.

Bake for 45 minutes, or until the loaf is nicely browned.

Serves: 4-6

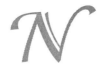

"You can't just eat good food. You've got to talk about it too. And you've got to talk about it to somebody who understands that kind of food."
Kurt Vonnegut
(1922-2007, American writer)

Noodles (Soba) with Vegetables

Vegetarian Delight

Loaded with power vegetables, this tasty dish provides fiber- and protein-rich legumes and liver-supporting onions, garlic, and scallions. The ginger aids digestion and reduces body inflammation, while the carrots are full of antioxidant beta-carotene. And the mushrooms, full of selenium, boost the immune system.

Ingredients
4 scallions, chopped, separating the green stems from the white bulbs
2 teaspoons chopped cilantro
2 large garlic cloves, minced
4 teaspoons ginger, grated
1 tablespoon rice vinegar
1 1/2 tablespoon soy sauce
2 tablespoons raw honey
1 1/2 teaspoons red-pepper flakes

1 cup bok choy, chopped
1 cup cooked red lentils
1 large carrot, grated
1 teaspoon dark sesame, peanut, or extra virgin olive oil
1 1/2 teaspoons coconut oil
1 1/2 cups shitake mushrooms, sliced
6 ounces (180 g) soba noodles

Directions

Combine 2 cups of water with scallion whites, cilantro, garlic, and ginger in large cast iron skillet. Stir in rice vinegar, soy sauce, raw honey, red-pepper flakes, and simmer 10 minutes.

During last 2 minutes of cooking, add chopped bok choy, red lentils, grated carrot, and dark sesame, peanut, or extra virgin olive oil. Remove from heat and cover.

Heat coconut oil in medium skillet over medium-high heat. Add sliced shitake mushroom caps and cook until golden brown.

Prepare soba noodles according to package directions. Divide noodles, sauce, mushrooms, sliced scallion greens among four bowls.

Serves: 4

Noontime Lentil, Wild Rice and Quinoa Salad

Vegetarian Delight

A great cold salad to bring to work, it's packed with fiber-rich wild rice, quinoa, and lentils. The protein hit comes from the almonds and legumes and the antioxidants from the spices and cranberries. Lasts for days in the fridge for prolonged enjoyment!

Ingredients

Salad
1/2 cup wild rice, cook
2/3 cup green or brown lentils, cooked
1/2 cup quinoa, cooked
1/2 cup dried cranberries
1/4 cup red onion, finely chopped
1/3 cup slivered almonds, roasted (or pumpkin seeds)

Vinaigrette
1/4 cup raw apple cider vinegar
1 teaspoon Dijon mustard
1/2 teaspoon raw honey
1/2 teaspoon salt
1/2 teaspoon ground coriander
1/4 teaspoon each turmeric, paprika, nutmeg and cardamom
Pinch of cayenne, cinnamon and ground cloves
1/4 cup flax or extra virgin olive oil

Directions

Combine all salad ingredients.

Mix dressing and add to salad.

Serves: 4

Spicy Okra Stew

Vegetarian Delight

Okra has a unique flavor that is a nice change from the usual vegetables! In this dish, the vegetables provide a good source of fiber, vitamins, and minerals, while spices like turmeric, cayenne, garlic, and chili powder are heart healthy. And it's loaded with antioxidants and nutrients.

Ingredients
1 1/2 pounds (720 g) okra
1 medium yellow or red onion
1 cup celery, sliced
1 cup carrots, sliced
1 green pepper, seeded and diced
1 red pepper, seeded and diced
3 medium tomatoes (canned tomatoes work just fine in this recipe)
3 cloves garlic, minced
1 tablespoon extra virgin olive oil or avocado oil

1 1/2 teaspoons chili powder
2 teaspoons cumin seeds
1 teaspoon turmeric
1/4 teaspoon cayenne (optional)
1/2 teaspoon sea salt, plus more to taste
1 tablespoon lemon juice
1 teaspoon raw brown sugar or sucanat

Directions

Trim off the stem ends from the okra and cut the pods into 1/4- to 1/2-inch slices. Set aside.

Peel and thinly slice onion and set aside. Slice celery and carrots and dice peppers and set aside.

Chop the tomatoes and mince the garlic and set them both aside.

Heat oil in a large cast iron frying pan or sauté pan over high heat. Add onion and cook, stirring frequently, until onions start to brown.

Add garlic and cook, stirring, about 30 seconds. Add chili powder, cumin seeds, turmeric, and cayenne, if using, and cook, stirring, another 30 seconds.

Add okra, stir to coat with onion-spice mixture. Add tomatoes, any juices they've released, salt, and 1/2 cup water. Add peppers, celery and carrots. Stir to combine and cover.

Reduce heat to maintain a steady simmer and cook until okra is tender and flavors are blended, 10-15 minutes.

Stir in lemon juice and add more salt to taste, if you like. Top with raw sugar or sucanat if desired. Serve hot or warm.

Serves: 4-6

Pure Pleasure Pumpkin Soup

Vegetarian Delight

Pumpkin, rich in fiber, Vitamins A and C, and beta-carotene, combine with heart- and circulation-promoting spices and liver-supporting onions and garlic for a warm soup during cold fall nights.

Ingredients

6 cups of homemade pumpkin puree (or the equivalent in canned
   pumpkin puree)
4 tablespoons unsalted butter
2 medium yellow onions, chopped
2 teaspoons garlic, minced
1/8 to 1/4 teaspoon crushed red pepper flakes
2 teaspoons curry powder
1/2 teaspoon ground coriander

Pinch ground cayenne pepper (optional)

5 cups of vegetable broth (or chicken broth if you don't desire a vegetarian dish)

1/2 cup sucanat, sugar, or maple syrup

2 cups of milk

1/2 cup cream or yogurt

pumpkin seeds, toasted, for garnish

Directions

To make your own pumpkin purée, cut a sugar pumpkin in half, scoop out the seeds, and place face down on a baking pan. Bake at 350°F until soft, about 45–60 minutes. Cool and scoop out the flesh. (Puree or mash for other recipes calling for puree). Freeze whatever you don't use for future use.

Melt butter in a 4-quart saucepan over medium-high heat. Add onions and garlic and cook, stirring often, until softened, about 4 minutes. Add spices and stir for a minute more.

Add pumpkin puree and 5 cups of broth; blend well. Bring to a boil, reduce heat, and simmer for 10–15 minutes.

Transfer soup, in batches, to a blender or food processor. Cover tightly and blend until smooth. Return soup to saucepan.

With the soup on low heat, add brown sugar and mix. Slowly add milk while stirring to incorporate. Add cream or yogurt. Adjust seasonings to taste. If a little too spicy, add more cream to cool it down. You might want to add a teaspoon of salt.

Serve in individual bowls. Sprinkle the top of each with toasted pumpkin seeds.

Serves: 4-6

Q

> *"Tomatoes and oregano make it Italian; wine and tarragon make it French; sour cream makes it Russian; lemon and cinnamon make it Greek; soy sauce makes it Chinese; garlic makes it good."*
> Alice May Brock
> (1941– , American restaurateur, painter, designer, and subject of Arlo Guthrie song, Alice's Restaurant)

Quinoa Spaghetti Squash

Vegetarian Delight

Have your spaghetti and get some fiber and nutrition too! This recipe contains fiber-rich spaghetti squash and quinoa, along with protein, and high levels of nutrients and iron from the greens of spinach and kale. Liver-supporting shallots and antioxidant-rich basil and cardamom add to this delicious powerhouse of flavor.

Ingredients
1 spaghetti squash
1 tablespoon agave nectar or maple syrup
2 tablespoons extra virgin olive oil, divided
2 tablespoons raw honey
3/4 cup quinoa
1 shallot, minced

3 tablespoons lemon juice
1 teaspoon ground cardamom
1/3 cup basil, chopped
1 pear, diced
2 cups baby spinach or kale
salt and pepper, to taste
parmesan to taste

Directions

Preheat oven to 425°F.

Cut squash in half and seed it. Mix the maple syrup and 1 tablespoon of the olive oil. Rub generously onto the flesh of the squash. Roast cut side down, for about 20 minutes. Turn the squash cut side up and cook another 15–20 minutes, until it a fork pierces it easily. The cooking time will depend on the size of the squash you use.

While squash is cooking, prepare the quinoa. Bring 1 1/2 cups water to a boil and add the quinoa. Cover and simmer for about 10 minutes, until the liquid is absorbed. Remove and transfer to a mixing bowl.

Add the shallot, lemon juice, cardamom, remaining olive oil, and honey, and stir. Allow to cool down and then add the basil, pear, and greens to combine. Remove the squash boats and let them sit about 5 minutes to cool down.

Fill each cavern with desired amount of quinoa mix. Sprinkle with fresh ground pepper and parmesan and serve.

Serves: 4

Rainbow Chard Omelet

Vegetarian Delight

Omega-3-rich eggs provide the protein in this recipe. But you also get liver-supporting onions, iron-rich swiss chard, calcium-rich goat's milk and cheese, and circulation-boosting paprika. And it's delicious and easy to prepare to boot.

Ingredients
2 tablespoons olive oil or safflower oil
1/4 cup onions, chopped
3 medium free-range eggs
2 tablespoons goat milk or cow milk
dash of lemon juice
1/2 teaspoon salt
1/2 teaspoon paprika
black pepper to taste
3/4 cup rainbow chard, chopped
1/4 organic goat cheese
parsley for garnish (optional)

Directions

Heat a medium size pan and add the olive oil, turning your burner to the medium setting. Add the onions and stir until soft and slightly browned.

During this time, prepare your egg mixture by first whisking the eggs in a bowl, and adding the milk, lemon juice, and spices.

Cook chard for 1 minute in pan then remove with onions.

Now pour in egg mixture. Cook for 2-3 minutes until the bottom begins to set, using a spatula to lift the edges so that the uncooked mixture can flow to the bottom of the pan. Turn the burner to a low setting; add back the onions and chard, spreading it evenly over the egg mixture. Let cook for another 30 seconds to 1 minute.

Sprinkle the top with goat cheese, let it melt, and with a spatula fold the omelet in half and slide it onto a plate.

Serves: 3

Raw Root Veggie Slaw

Vegetarian Delight

Rich in fiber and antioxidants, this root vegetable slaw can be topped with pumpkin seeds for additional protein. With heart healthy olive oil and metabolism-boosting raw apple cider vinegar, this is a great lunch to take to work. It stores for a week or more in the fridge!

Ingredients

2 carrots, peeled
1 beet, peeled
2 kohlrabi bulbs, peeled
1 parsnip, peeled
1 bulb celeriac, peeled
1/2 red cabbage, sliced
1 spring onion, white parts only, chopped finely
1 bunch parsley, chopped finely
2 tablespoons lemon juice and zest of half a lemon

1/2 cup extra virgin olive oil
3-5 tablespoons raw apple cider vinegar
1 teaspoon raw honey
pinch of sea salt
freshly ground black pepper
pumpkin seeds, for garnish

Directions

Grate root vegetables coarsely into a large bowl (carrots, beet, kohlrabi, parsnip, and celeriac). Add cabbage, onion, and parsley.

In a small bowl, mix lemon juice and zest with olive oil, apple cider vinegar, honey, salt and pepper. Pour over root slaw.

Top with a handful of pumpkin seeds for added crunch and protein and serve!

Serves: 4-6

"Fat gives things flavor."
Julia Child
(1912-2004, American chef, author, and television personality)

Super Spanish Rice

Vegetarian Delight

Using brown rice ups the fiber and B-complex vitamins in this classic Tex-Mex dish. But you also get liver-supporting onions and leeks, vitamin-rich vegetables, and an antioxidant boost from the spices and herbs.

Ingredients
1 cup brown basmati rice, organic, rinsed
2 cups vegetable stock
1 teaspoon butter
1/2 cup onions, diced
1/2 cup leeks, diced
1/2 teaspoon black pepper
1 teaspoon tamarind sauce
1 teaspoon paprika
1 teaspoon chili powder
1 teaspoon cumin
1/2 cup corn, frozen
1/2 cup frozen peas
1 cup tomatoes, diced
1/2 cup carrots, diced

Directions

Combine the rice and 2 cups stock; cook in rice cooker until tender.

In a sauté pan, heat butter. Add leeks, onions, pepper, tamarind sauce, and allow to brown. Add remaining spices, corn, peas, tomatoes, and carrots, and simmer 1-2 minutes.

Stir in vegetable mixture into cooked rice.

Serve as a side dish.

Serves: 4

Sweet Potato, Squash and Pumpkin Casserole

Vegetarian Delight/Gluten Free

This dish does contain some sugar and milk but those ingredients give great flavor to this delicious side dish. But there is also lots of nutrition with the beta-carotene-dense sweet potatoes, butternut squash, and pumpkin, omega-3-rich eggs, and cinnamon to regulate blood sugar. And pecans add protein, magnesium, and crunch.

Ingredients
3 cups sweet potato, sliced thin
1 cup butternut squash, sliced thin
1 cup pumpkin, sliced thin (or canned pumpkin puree)
1/2 cup raw sugar or sucanat
2 free-range eggs, beaten
1/2 teaspoon sea salt
4 tablespoons butter, softened
1/2 cup milk
1/2 teaspoon vanilla extract
1/2 cup raw honey
1/3 cup garbanzo and fava flour (I like Bob's Red Mill)
3 tablespoons butter, softened
1/2 cup chopped pecans

Directions

Preheat oven to 325°F. Prepare a 9 x 13 baking dish.

Put sweet potatoes, butternut squash, and pumpkin in a medium saucepan, with enough water to cover everything. Cook over medium high heat until tender; drain and mash.

In a large bowl, mix together the mashed vegetables, sugar, eggs, salt, butter, milk, and vanilla extract. Mix until smooth. Transfer to prepared baking dish.

In medium bowl, mix the honey and flour. Cut in the 4 tablespoon butter until the mixture is coarse. Stir in the pecans. Sprinkle the mixture over the sweet potato mixture.

Bake in the preheated oven 30 minutes, or until the topping is lightly browned.

Serves: 4

T

"All sorrows are less with bread."
Miguel de Cervantes Saavedra
(1547-1616, Spanish novelist, poet, and playwright)

Terrific Tabbouleh

Vegetarian Delight

A mid-eastern staple, this recipe gets fiber from bulgur, antioxidants from a variety of herbs, and protein and more fiber from chickpeas and black beans. Liver-supporting compounds come from the onions and garlic, while the tomatoes and olive oil provide heart healthy elements. Finally vegetables like cucumber, carrots, and peppers supply a powerhouse of vitamins and enzymes.

Ingredients
1 cup fine bulgur or cracked wheat
4 green onions, chopped
4 tomatoes, seeded and chopped
2 carrots, grated
1 bunch fresh parsley, finely chopped
1 bunch fresh mint, finely chopped
1 red, yellow, orange or green pepper, chopped
1/2 English cucumber
1 19-ounce (540 ml) can chickpeas
1 19-ounce (540 ml) can black beans
2 cups feta cheese, crumbled

Vinaigrette
2/3 cup extra virgin olive oil
1/2 cup fresh lemon juice (we add lemon zest too)
2 teaspoons garlic, minced
salt and freshly ground pepper

Directions

Soak bulgur or cracked wheat in hot water for 20 minutes. Drain well, pressing out excess water.

Add remaining salad ingredients to grains in a large bowl.

Combine dressing ingredients in a jar with a tight-fitting lid and shake to blend. Pour over salad and toss until well mixed. Stores up to 1 week.
Serves: 4-6

Tantalizing Slow Cooker Turkey

Meat Lovers

This recipe contains lean protein, vitamin- and fiber-rich root vegetables, liver-supporting onions and garlic, probiotic-rich soy sauce, and antioxi-dant-rich, anti-inflammatory herbs. It is easy to prepare and tastes delicious. As an added bonus, turkey contains high amounts of tryptophan that helps make the happy hormone serotonin! Enjoy.

Ingredients
1 bone-in turkey breast (3 pounds/1.5 kg)
2 tablespoons butter, softened
1 tablespoon soy sauce
1 tablespoon fresh parsley, finely chopped
1/2 teaspoon dried basil
1/2 teaspoon dried sage
1/2 teaspoon dried thyme
1/2 teaspoon dried rosemary
1/4 teaspoon ground black pepper
2-4 large cloves garlic, minced

1 large carrot, peeled and sliced
2 large potatoes, cut into chunks
1 small turnip, peeled and cut into cubes
1 large onion, chopped
2 stalks celery, chopped

Directions

Place turkey breast into a slow cooker. Combine butter, soy sauce, parsley, basil, sage, thyme, rosemary, black pepper, and garlic in a small bowl until smooth. Brush herb mixture over the turkey breast. Cover with vegetables and put lid on slow cooker.

Cook 4-6 hours on high or 8-10 hours on low, until turkey is tender.

Serves: 4

U

> *"He who distinguishes the true savor of his food
> can never be a glutton; he who does not
> cannot be otherwise."*
> Henry David Thoreau
> (1817-1862, American author, poet, philosopher, naturalist)

Unbelievable Lemon Shrimp

Meat Lovers

Shrimp supply lean protein and omega-3 fatty acids that support heart and brain health. This dish also supplies Vitamin C from the lemon, liver-supporting garlic and antioxidant-rich herbs. It is easy to prepare and delicious.

Ingredients
3 tablespoons unsalted, cultured butter, divided
1 1/2 pounds (720 g) peeled and deveined jumbo shrimp
1 teaspoon sea salt
2 teaspoons garlic, minced
2 tablespoons fresh lemon juice
2 tablespoons chopped parsley fresh (or 1 tablespoon dried)
1 tablespoon chopped dill-fresh (or 1/2 tablespoon dried)
1/4 teaspoon freshly ground pepper

Directions

Melt 1 tablespoon butter in a large, non-stick skillet over medium-high heat. Add half the shrimp to pan and sprinkle with half the salt. Sauté 2 minutes or until almost done. Transfer shrimp to a plate.

Melt another tablespoon of butter, add the remaining shrimp and salt to pan, and; sauté until almost done. Transfer to plate.

Melt remaining tablespoon of butter in pan. Add garlic and cook 30 seconds, stirring constantly. Stir in shrimp, lemon juice, parsley, dill, and pepper; cook 1 minute or until shrimp are done.

Serve over rice or noodles.

Serves: 4

*"Cookery means ... English thoroughness, French art,
and Arabian hospitality; it means the knowledge of all
fruits and herbs and balms and spices;
it means carefulness, inventiveness, and watchfulness."*
John Ruskin
(1819-1900, English art critic)

Virtuous Brownies

Sweet Tooth/Gluten Free

These grain-free brownies are delicious and nutritious. They contain high protein, gluten-free flours and ground nuts along with omega-3-rich eggs and flax, and a hit of beta-carotene from sweet potato. So packed with nutrients, they're almost too good to be true.

Ingredients
2 1/4 cups ground walnuts (or ground almonds or a combination)
1/2 cup hemp flour (or garbanzo and fava flour)
1/4 cup ground chia seeds (or flax meal)
1/2 cup unsweetened cocoa powder
1 teaspoon baking soda
2 teaspoons baking powder (gluten free)
1/8 teaspoon sea salt
1 cup agave nectar (or maple syrup or mixture of half of each)
1/4 cup pureed sweet potato
3 free-range eggs
1/4 cup unsweetened applesauce

Directions

Bake 1-2 sweet potatoes until soft. Remove the skin and puree in blender or food processor until smooth. Set aside 1/4 cup. Keep remainder in fridge for a week or freeze for later use.

Preheat oven to 350°F and grease and line with parchment an 8-inch square pan.

In a large bowl mix ground nuts, flour, chia seeds, cocoa powder, baking soda and powder, and salt until blended.

Add agave and sweet potato puree and mix until blended.

Beat in the eggs one at a time. Add the applesauce and mix until blended.

Pour into prepared pan and bake at for 25-30 minutes, or until a toothpick inserted in the center comes out clean.

Serves: 4-6

"First we eat, then we do everything else."
M.F.K. Fisher
(1908-1992, American food writer)

Warm Mushroom Salad

Vegetarian Delight

This salad is packed full of fiber, power greens, antioxidants, and protein. The mushrooms add the antioxidant–rich, immune-boosting mineral selenium and the dressing has olive oil for heart health along with liver-supporting garlic. Served warm, this is a delicious and impressive dish for entertaining.

Ingredients
1 1/2 to 2 cups mixed mushrooms and portobellos
1-2 red peppers
1 cup green beans
1 cup asparagus, ends trimmed and chopped
3/4 cup olive oil, divided
6 teaspoons balsamic vinegar (regular)
1/2 cup slivered almonds
1 teaspoon Dijon mustard
1 garlic cloves, minced
freshly ground pepper
1 large package mixed greens
soft goat's cheese (chèvre)
1 pint (950 ml) cherry tomatoes

Directions

Chop mushrooms, red pepper, green beans, and asparagus. Sauté them in 1/4 cup olive oil in cast iron pan until just slightly firm. Remove vegetables and add balsamic vinegar.

Heat slivered almonds for 2-3 minutes until lightly browned. Remove.

Mix remaining olive oil (1/2 cup), Dijon mustard, garlic, and pepper in a small bowl. Heat in pan for 1 minute to warm.

Add warm vegetables to mixed greens and top with crumbled cheese. Mix in warmed dressing and serve immediately topped with lightly roasted slivered almonds and cherry tomatoes.

Serves: 4-6

Winter Roasted Vegetables

Vegetarian Delight

This recipe includes liver-supporting Brussel sprouts, beta-carotene-rich sweet potatoes and squash, antioxidant-boosting herbs, and heart- and circulation-supporting cayenne! It can be prepared with just one vegetable if preferred or a combination of two or three together for maximum nutrient impact. The olive oil will add flavor and support heart health and the coconut will boost metabolism.

Ingredients

2 cups of Brussels sprouts, stemmed, trimmed, and halved

4-5 sweet potatoes, cut in large chunks

1 small butternut squash or pumpkin, peeled, seeded, and cut into large
    chunks

1/4 cup each of extra virgin olive oil and coconut oil (less if you
    choose to prepare fewer vegetables)

3/4 tablespoon cayenne

1 tablespoon dried rosemary, or 2 fresh sprigs chopped

1 tablespoon dried thyme (or 2 tablespoons fresh, chopped)

pinch of sea salt

freshly ground black pepper to taste

Directions

Preheat oven to 375°F.

Put vegetables and oil in a large baking dish. Coat with cayenne and other
herbs and mix.

Cook for 20-30 minutes, turning once or twice to coat oil and cayenne
evenly.

Serve as a tasty side dish.

Serves: 4

*"What is patriotism but the love of the food
one ate as a child?"*
Lin Yutang
(1895-1976, Chinese writer, translator, linguist and inventor)

Xceptional Chili

Meat Lovers

Legumes make this dish rich in fiber, protein, and nutrients, along with a powerhouse of circulation-boosting herbs and spices, iron-dense molasses, heart-supporting tomatoes, and antioxidant-rich peppers. There is even a substitute to make this a delight for vegetarians too. It is even more delicious the next day.

Ingredients
2 tablespoons olive oil
1 large onion, diced
1 large stalk celery, diced
1 medium red bell pepper, diced
1 medium green bell pepper, diced
1 pound (480 g) free-range, ground turkey (substitute tempeh for vegetarians)
6 to 8 cloves garlic, minced

2 to 3 Serrano or jalapeno peppers, seeded and minced

2 teaspoons good quality chili powder

1 teaspoon fresh, toasted cumin seeds, ground

1 1/2 teaspoons dried winter savory

1/2 to 1 teaspoon salt

1 to 2 teaspoons organic tamari soy sauce (or Bragg's Aminos gluten-free soy sauce)

1 15-ounce (480 ml) can dark red kidney,

1 15-ounce (480 ml) can pinto beans

1 15-ounce (480 ml) can black beans (or start with 1 pound (480 g), dried and soak overnight)

1 28-ounce (796 ml) can tomatoes, chopped

1 to 2 tablespoons molasses

few dashes Angostura bitters

1 ounce (30 g) bittersweet chocolate

1/4 cup each fresh chopped parsley and cilantro

Directions

Heat the oil in a large skillet and sauté the onion for a minute. Add the celery and bell peppers and sauté 2 or 3 minutes.

Add the ground turkey (or tempeh) and stir for 5 minutes. Add the garlic, chili peppers, chili powder, cumin, savory, and 1/2 teaspoon salt. Sprinkle with the tamari or Bragg's Aminos; stir for a few minutes. Add the beans, tomatoes, molasses, and bitters, stir well and cook over medium heat, just simmering for 15 minutes.

Taste for seasoning; add more chili powder, cumin, salt, tamari, or molasses if necessary. Add the chocolate and fresh herbs, stir well, and cook for 5 minutes more.

Serve hot with grated cheese if desired.

Serves: 4-6

Xtra Delicious Carrot Muffins

Sweet Tooth

Using whole grains provides a good source of B-complex Vitamins to these tasty morsels. Cinnamon helps to regulate blood sugar, while eggs provide a source of omega-3s and protein. The vegetables supply loads of vitamins and fiber, with carrots specifically bringing beta-carotene and zucchini providing Vitamin K to the mix.

Ingredients

1 1/2 cups sprouted flour (can use regular)
1 cup whole spelt flour
1 cup sucanat (or raw honey)
2 teaspoons baking powder
2 teaspoons baking soda
2 teaspoons cinnamon
1/2 teaspoon nutmeg
4 free-range eggs
1 cup extra virgin olive oil or melted butter
3 cups carrots, grated
1/2 cup zucchini, grated
1 cup walnuts (or other nuts), chopped
1/2 cup raisins

Directions

Preheat oven to 350°F. Lightly grease or line muffin tray.

Mix together all dry ingredients. (If using honey, combine with the egg mixture.)

Beat eggs and add oil or butter.

Combine dry ingredients with egg mixture. Fold in carrots, zucchini, raisins, and nuts.

Pour into prepared muffin tray. Bake for 20-25 minutes or until set.

Enjoy!

Serves: 6

y

*"Find ecstasy in life;
the mere sense of living is joy enough."*
Emily Dickinson
(1830-1886, American poet)

Yummy Red Cabbage Stir Fry

Meat Lovers

Quick and easy to prepare, the vegetables in this dish provide antioxidants, vitamins, and minerals, as well as liver-supporting compounds. The garlic and onions boost cell development and the immune system, while the circulation system gets help from the ginger and cayenne.

Ingredients
2 tablespoons Asian sesame or peanut oil, divided
1 medium-size red onion, cut lengthwise into 1/3-inch-thick slices
8 ounces (240 g) skinless, boneless chicken, cut into bite-sized pieces
1 tablespoon fresh ginger, peeled and minced
3 garlic cloves, minced
2 cups red cabbage, sliced
2 cups mixed broccoli and cauliflower, chopped
1 cup snow peas
3 tablespoons hoisin or soy sauce
3/4 cup chopped fresh cilantro
Chinese hot sauce to taste

Directions

Heat 1 tablespoon oil in large non-stick skillet over medium-high heat. Add onion and sauté until soft.

Season chicken with salt and pepper. Add remaining 1 tablespoon oil to skillet. Add chicken, ginger, and garlic. Stir-fry 1 minute.

Add cabbage, broccoli, cauliflower, and snow peas and stir fry until chicken is cooked through and cabbage is wilted but still slightly crunchy, 2-3 minutes.

Stir in hoisin sauce. Season to taste with salt and pepper. Mix in cilantro.

Transfer stir-fry to serving bowl. Serve with rice or soba noodles.

Serves: 4

Yellow Potato Salad

Vegetarian Delight

A healthy option for your summer BBQ gatherings, Yukon gold potatoes add potassium and vitamin C, as well as a rich color. Fiber is provided by liver-supporting shallots, the olive oil promotes heart health and a variety of herbs supply a variety of antioxidants. It also has raw apple cider vinegar to boost metabolism and stores well for about a week.

Ingredients

2 pounds (1 kg) of Yukon golden potatoes
3 tablespoons shallots, chopped
1/2 tablespoon Dijon mustard
1 tablespoon grainy mustard
1 tablespoon raw apple cider vinegar, or to taste
1/2 teaspoon black pepper
1/2 teaspoon sea salt
3 tablespoons extra virgin olive oil
2 tablespoons fresh parsley, chopped
1 tablespoon fresh dill, chopped

Directions

Cook potatoes with salted water (about 1/2 teaspoon) until tender. Drain.

Whisk together shallots, mustards, vinegar, pepper, and salt in a large bowl. Add oil, whisking until blended.

When potatoes are cool, cut into bite-sized chunks and add to vinaigrette along with parsley and dill. Toss to combine.

Serve warm or at room temperature.

Serves: 4

Zucchini Spaghetti with Spinach Pesto Sauce

Vegetarian/Gluten Free

The spaghetti contains fiber and vitamins in this dish – in the form of zucchini. Garlic provides liver-supporting compounds, the spinach is full of iron that boosts red blood cell production, and mushrooms aid the immune system. Cashews supply the protein and magnesium.

Ingredients
1 packed cup baby spinach
1 small bunch basil
1/4 cup cashews
1 garlic clove
1 cup extra virgin olive oil
salt and freshly ground pepper, to taste
4 medium zucchini
2-3 roasted red peppers, sliced
1 cup shitake or oyster mushrooms, sliced
freshly grated parmesan
freshly ground pepper
handful chopped cashews

Directions

Add spinach, basil, cashews, garlic, olive oil, and salt and pepper to blender. Pulse until smooth, adding more olive oil, if needed, to make a smooth pesto. Taste and adjust for seasoning.

Using a spiralizer or vegetable turning slicer, turn zucchini into long spaghetti strands. Add zucchini strands to large pot of salted, boiling water and blanch for 15-30 seconds. Drain well.

Sauté roasted red peppers and mushrooms in olive oil until soft.

Toss zucchini spaghetti with pesto. Add roasted red peppers and mushrooms. Top with cashews, freshly ground pepper and parmesan to taste. Enjoy.

Serves: 4

Zucchini Chocolate Chip Cookies

Sweet Tooth

Just because they're cookies doesn't mean they can't also pack in some nutrients. These treats get a super hit of omega-3 fatty acids from eggs, hemp, flax, and walnuts. Besides the blood-sugar-regulating cinnamon and the whole grains full of B-complex Vitamins, the fiber and Vitamin K in zucchini can't be beat. And the dark chocolate adds sweet delight! They can be made without nuts to pack in kids' lunches.

Ingredients

1 free-range egg, beaten
1/2 cup butter, softened
1/2 cup brown sugar
1/3 cup raw honey
1 tablespoon vanilla extract
1 cup whole wheat flour
1 cup whole spelt flour (or 2 cups spelt flour and no wheat flour)
1 tablespoon ground flax seed
1 tablespoon hemp protein
1/2 teaspoon baking soda

1/4 teaspoon salt
1/4 teaspoon cinnamon
1/4 teaspoon nutmeg
1/2 cup walnuts, chopped
1 cup zucchini, finely shredded
12 ounces (360 g) dark chocolate chips (Fair-trade chocolate preferred)

Directions

Preheat oven to 350°F and lightly grease a cookie sheet (or use parchment).

Combine egg, butter, sugar, honey, and vanilla extract in large bowl.

Combine flours, flax seed, hemp, baking soda, salt, cinnamon, nutmeg, and walnuts in a separate bowl.

Slowly blend dry mixture into the wet mixture.

Stir zucchini and chocolate chips into other ingredients.

Drop by spoonful onto prepared baking sheet and flatten with back of spoon.

Bake at 350°F for 12-15 minutes, until golden brown.

Serves: 6-8

Conclusion

"The journey of a thousand miles begins with a single step."

Lao-Tzu

(Zhou Dynasty, Chinese philosopher and poet)

We have covered a lot of information together about food and our food system. You may be wondering about what healthy eating and living advice will look like in 10, 20 or 50 years as the global population continues to grow.

Recently some authors have written books about the future of food and one author even speculates that meat could actually be grown out of a petrie dish in years to come and different fast-growing varieties of fish will become more popular, like the cobia which grows much quicker than salmon.

What new foods will be popular? African cuisine and grains like teff or new ideas from Asian or South American cuisine? Will Western countries ever actually eat insects? According to research published by Dennis Oonincx and colleagues from the University of Wageningen, Netherlands, beetle larvae (called mealworms) farms produce more edible protein than traditional farms for chicken, pork, beef or milk, for the same amount of land used.[1] Still, I admit that I am not ready to make bug pie part of my weekly menu.

The real food issues are about quality and sustainability. I wonder if more people will move back to local food systems with more organic food available at a lower price and less processed food. Will restaurants serve more "locally sourced" ingredients? Will we start eating more high-nutrient super greens that we now consider "weeds" or incorporate more existing draught and flood resistant plants into our diet? Norway has been building a heritage seed bank in their frozen tundra to save seeds and preserve biodiversity. Will farmers start to diversify the crops they are growing to meet demand for more quality and variety of foods and incorporate more grown-in-the-wild perennial plants? Will more people compost, grow vegetables or herbs, or have more of a permaculture landscape on their land?

Some speculate that in years to come agriculture and the environment will be seen as one and the same. A new direction instead of agribusiness would be agri-environment where governments pay farmers to keep their soil healthy and offer multiple ways for farmers to make a healthy income other than their crops. I am sure farmers would welcome this scenario as multiple revenue streams are always a good idea in business. Ensuring farmers are paid well and respected for their work is the best way to ensure that we will have healthier food and people in the future. Farmers are the doctors of the land and caretakers of many plants so are a vital link to a cleaner brighter future. I'd like to see governments pay farmers who are taking the extra time to create healthier food and soil. If it costs tax payers a lot less than environmental clean-up, it may be a good investment on many fronts.

While some of our medical advances have extended the human life-span, we have not yet extended the human health-span given the drastic increases in chronic disease and discomfort.[2] As we recognize the importance of quality food and respect and compensate our farmers who grow it for us, chronic disease may be reduced and human ingenuity and productivity may find new and exciting directions for growing quality food for the growing planet and supporting maximum health and diversity. Personally I am looking forward to what the next few decades will bring!

"Hence we conceive of the individual animal as
a small world, existing for its own sake, by its
own means. Every creature has its own reasons to be.
All its parts have a direct effect on one another, a
relationship to one another, thereby consistently
renewing the circle of life."

Johann Wolfgang von Goethe
(1749-1832, German writer and statesman)

Endnotes

A to Z of Foods

1. Rowan Jacobsen, "The Importance of Bees to Our Food Supply" (March/April 2009) at *www.eatingwell.com*.
2. Amy Growell, "Eat Wild Amaranth" at *www.edibleaustin.com*.
3. John Chapman is remembered as Johnny Appleseed as he wandered around the U.S. in the first half of the 1800s planting apple seeds and transplanting saplings to establish apple orchards.
4. "Cloned Apples: Inside Science – Discoveries and Breakthroughs" at *www.ivanhoe.com*.
5. "New Secrets to Outsmarting Allergies," *Health Magazine*, April 2014.
6. For more types of berries, see *www.buzzle.com*.
7. Jessica Bernard, "The Nutritional Contents of Beef Bone Marrow" (October 25, 2012) at *www.livestrong.com*.
8. "The Difference Between Grass-Fed Beef and Grain-Fed Beef" at *www.marksdailyapple.com*.
9. Vandana Shiva, *Staying Alive: Women, Ecology, and Devleopment* (Vancouver BC: South End Press, 2010).
10. Dr. Mercola, "The Latest Weapon in the War on Cancer: Honey Bees" (November 24, 2012) at *www.mercola.com*.
11. Newcastle University, "Could Spiders be the Key to Saving our Bees?" (June 3, 2014) at *www.sciencedaily.com*.
12. McLaughlin, "Herbs Attract Pollinating Insects" at *www.vegetablegardner.com*.
13. "Counting Chickens," *The Economist*, July 27, 2011.
14. Diana Herrington, "10 Benefits of Carrots: The Crunchy Power Food" (2011) at *care2.com*.
15. See "Chlorella" on *www.WebMD.com*.
16. "What's New and Beneficial about Cremini Mushrooms" at *www.whfoods.com*.
17. Michael Pollan, *The Omnivore's Dilemna: A Natural History of Four Meals* (New York: The Penguin Press, 2006).
18. "Pesticide, Herbicide Use in U.S. Agriculture, 1960-2008" (June 2014) at *cornandsoybeandigest.com*.
19. "Rate of Cancer Highest in North America," *International Journal of Cancer*, 2002, Volume 97, pp. 72-81.
20. Lisa Garber, "6 Super-foods that Fight Cancer and Prevent Cancer" (September 11, 2012) at Natural Society.com.

[21] Christian Nordqvist, "What Is Vitamin D? What Are the Benefits of Vitamin D?" (September 2014) at *www.medicalnewstoday.com*.

[22] Read more at: *www.all4naturalhealth.com/dandelion-facts.html#ixzz2x1RWzioI*.

[23] Brett and Kate McKay, "Surviving in the Wild: 19 Common Edible Plants" (October 6, 2010) at *www.artofmanlyskills.com*.

[24] Dr. Mercola, "42 Flowers You Can Eat" (April 18, 2012) at *www.mercola.com* under Health Articles tab.

[25] Michael Moss, *Salt, Sugar, Fat: How the Food Giants Hooked Us* (Toronto, ON: McClelland and Stewart, 2014).

[26] "Do Gut Bacteria Rule Our Minds?" (August 2014) at *www.sciencedaily.com*.

[27] "The Truth About Overeating" (March 1996) at *www.medicalweightlossrx.com*.

[28] "Eggs and Heart Disease" at *www.hsph.harvard.edu/nutritionsource/eggs/*.

[29] Sharron Farlouis, "Interesting Facts about Elderberries" (June 24, 2012) at *www.helium.com*.

[30] "History of Egg Production: From Ancient Times" at *www.incredibleegg.org/egg-facts/basic-egg-facts/history-of-egg-production/from-ancient-times*.

[31] Wikepedia: "Chicken."

[32] Egg Nutrition Center, "Fun Facts About Eggs" (April 2014) at *www.wherefoodcomes-from.com*.

[33] David Wolfe, Jeff Beem-Miller, Allison Chatrchyan, and Lauren Chambliss, "Climate Change Facts: Farm Energy, Carbon, and Greenhouse Gases" (November 2011) Cornell Climate Change.

[34] Tom Philpott, "Why the Government Should Pay Farmers to Plant Cover Crops" (January 12, 2013) at *www.motherjones.com*.

[35] "Changing Global Diets Is Vital to Reducing Climate Change" (August 31, 2014) at *www. Science daily.com*.

[36] H Adlercreutz, "Phytoestrogens: Epidemiology and a Possible Role in Cancer Protection" *Environmental Health Perspectives*, Vol. 103, Supp. 7 (October 1995), pp. 103-112.

[37] Marion Nestle, Food Politics: How the Food Industry Influences Nutrition and Health (Oakland, CA: University of California Press, 2013).

[38] Wayne Roberts, *The No-Nonsense Guild to World Food*, 2nd ed. (Toronto, ON: Between the Lines, 2013).

[39] Barbara Kingsolver, *Animal, Vegetable, Miracle: A Year of Food Life* (New York: Harper-Collins, 2007).

[40] Vandana Shiva, *Manifestos on the Future of Food and Seed* (Cambridge, MA: South End Press, 2010))

[41] Annie Bond, "Why It Matters to Buy Heirloom Plants and Seeds" (November 28, 1999) at *www.care2.com*.

[42] "Garlic Facts Remedies and Health Benefits of Garlic" (March 9, 2008) at *www.dia-bled-world.com*.

[43] See articles by Connie Jeske Crane (Fall 2013) on *www.edibletoronto.com*.

[44] "Benefits of Grapefruit Seed Extract" at *www.globalhealingcentre.com*.

45 Jeffrey M. Smith, *Seeds of Deception: Exposing Industry and Government Lies About the Safety of the Genetically Engineered Foods You're Eating* (Portland, ME: Yes! Books, 2003).

46 Thomas Pawlick, *The End of Food: How the Food Industry Is Destroying Our Food Supply - and What You Can Do About It* (Vancouver, BC: Greystone Books Ltd., 2006).

47 Annie Bond, "Why It Matters to Buy Heirloom Plants and Seeds" (November 28, 1999) at *www.care2.com.*.

48 Dallas and Melissa Hartwig, *It Starts with Food: Discover the Whole30® and Change Your Life in Unexpected Ways* (Las Vegas: Victoria Belt Publishing, 2014).

49 University of Greenwich, "Drugs for Diabetes? Scientists Test the Power of Plants" (January 16, 2013) at *www.sciencedaily.com*.

50 Francina Marie Parks at *Knoji.com*.

51 "Many Apples a Day Keep the Blues at Bay" at *www.sciencedaily.com*.

52 University of Toronto, Rotman School of Management, "Like Some Happiness with That? Fast Food Cues Hurt Ability to Savor Experience" (June 2, 2014), at *www.dailyscience.com*.

53 Kimberley Cairns, "Foods that Make You Feel Happy" (April 17, 2014) at *eHow.com*.

54 Ibid.

55 Edward Clements, "Ten Delicious Body Building Foods that Increase Serotonin levels" (December 14, 2012) at *www.musclehealthfitness.com*.

56 "Serotonin" at *webmd.com*, Depression Health Center.

57 Centre for Disease Control and Prevention at *www.cdc.gov/Heart Disease/facts.html*.

58 Shereen Jegtiv, "Best Foods for Heart Health" (May 23, 2014) at *about.com*.

59 "Chemical Cuisine" at *www.cspinet.org*.

60 US Food and Drug Administration at *www.fda.gov*.

61 Andy Bellatti, "Opening Pandora's Lunchbox: Processed Foods Are even Scarier than You Thought" (February 26, 2013) at *www.grist.com*.

62 "Child Diet Linked to IQ" (February 8, 2011) at *www.nhs.uk.*

63 Michelle Green, "How to Boost Your Intelligence" at *eHow.com*.

64 "Juniper Berries Health Benefit" at *www.diethealthclub.com*.

65 Wayne Roberts, *The No-Nonsense Guide to World Food*, 2nd ed. (Toronto: Between the Lines Press, 2013) at page 68.

66 "Fast Fact About Deforestation" at *www.facingthefuture.org*.

67 Patel Raj, *Stuffed and Starved: Markets, Power and the Hidden Battle for the World's Food Systems* (Toronto: HarperCollins, 2010) at page 289.

68 Rick Smith and Bruce Lourie, *Slow Death by Rubber Duck: How the Toxic Chemistry of Everyday Life Affects Our Health* (Toronto: Random House of Canada.Ltd., 2009).

69 Ibid.

70 Shelley Frost, "The Importance of Eating Meals Together as a Family" (January 26, 2014) at *www.livestrong.com*.

71 Calia Roberts, "Difference in Pickling and Fermentation" at *eHow.com*.

72 J. Scott Smith, a food science professor, discovered rosemary's strength as part of a long-term project at Kansas State University.

[73] University of Arkansas, Food Safety Consortium, "To Block the Carcinogens, Add a Touch of Rosemary When Grilling Meats" (May 24, 2008) at *www.dailyscience.com*.

[74] Jo Jordan, "How to Use Food-Combining Techniques for Better Digestion" at *www.puristat.com*.

[75] Read more about lemons at *www.care2.com/greenliving/16-health-benefits-of-lemons*.

[76] Ken Robbins, *Food for Thought: The Stories Behind the Things We Eat* (New York: Roaring Brook Press (Macmillan), 2009).

[77] Jethro Kloss, *Back to Eden: The Classic Guide to Herbal Medicine, Natural Foods, and Home Remedies Since 1939* (Detroit: Lotus Press, 2004).

[78] Genevieve Jackson, "Cleansing Remedies Using Lemon and Water" (August 16, 2013) at *www.livestrong.com*.

[79] Diana Herrington, "16 Health Benefits of Lemons" (July 2012) at *www.care2.com*.

[80] Barbara Kingsolver, *Animal, Vegetable, Miracle: A Year of Food Life* (New York: Harper-Collins, 2007).

[81] Lierre Keith, *The Vegetarian Myth: Food, Justice and Sustainability* (Oakland, CA: PM Press, 2009) at pages 42-44.

[82] Joel Salatin, Folks, *This Ain't Right: A Farmer's Advice for Happier Hens, Healthier People, and a Better World* (New York: Center Street Books, 2011).

[83] Aimee Shea, "Vitamins and Minerals in Maca Root" (July 2011) at *www.livestrong.com*.

[84] Bess O'Connor, "Move Over Acai Berries: The next Wave of Superfoods Is Here" (December 2014) at *www.mindbodygreen.com*.

[85] International Potato Center, "Oca, Ulluco & Mashua" at *www. Cipotato.org*.

[86] American Society for Horticultural Science, "Anticancer Compound Found in Common Plant: American Mayapple" (September 2009) at *www.sciencedaily.com*.

[87] "Why Whole Milk Is the Healthiest Choice" (August 2009) at *www.care2.com*.

[88] Aurora Geib, "Top 10 Herbs and Spices for Strengthening your Immune System" (April 9, 2012) *www.naturalnews.com*.

[89] Emily Steiner, "How Reishi Combats Aging" in *Life Extension Magazine*, February 2013, pp. 82-90.

[90] Paul Stamets, *Mycelium Running: How Mushrooms Can Help Save the World* (Berkeley: Ten Speed Press, 2005).

[91] Paul Stamets, "Unusual & Interesting Facts About Mushrooms" (December 15, 2009) at *www.fungi.com* on Articles by Paul Stamets; and and Ken Robbins, *Food for Thought: The Stories Behind the Things We Eat* (New York: Roaring Brook Press (Macmillan), 2009).

[92] James F. Balch, Mark Stengler, and Robin Young Balch, *Prescription for Natural Cures: A Self-Care Guide for Treating Problems with Natural Remedies Including Diet, Nutrition, Supplements, and Other Holistic Methods* (Hoboken, NJ: John Wiley & Sons Inc, 2011).

[93] Cindy Ell, "Natural Herbal Remedies & Their Many Benefits" (May 18, 2011) at *www.livestrong.com*.

[94] Dr. Weil, "Balanced Living – Herbal Remedies" at *www.drweil.com*.

[95] Cathy Wong, "Top 15 Conditions for which People Seek Complementary/Alternative Therapies" (August 11, 2006) at *about.com*.

96 Diana Beresford-Kroeger, *The Global Forest: Forty Ways Trees Can Save Us* (New York: Penguin Books Ltd, 2010).

97 Ibid.

98 Mike Adams, "Heal Yourself in 15 Days by Correcting Your Nature Deficiency" (February 2010) at *www.naturalnews.com.*

99 Learn more at *www.naturalnews.com/028203_nature_deficiency_self_healing.html#ixzz2J695yuaZ.*

100 See *www.ecotherapyheals.com.*

101 Beth Lapin, "The Healing Power of Nature" at *www.innertapestry.org.*

102 Kathryn Rubin, "Healthy Eating: 7 Food Wonders of the Ancient World" (July 13, 2011) at *www.jpost.com.*

103 Shubhra Krishan, "8 Great Benefits of Onions" (November 30, 2012) at *www.care2.com.*

104 Mary G. Enig and Sally Fallon, *Nourishing Traditions: The Cookbook that Challenges Politically Correct Nutrition and the Diet Dictocrats,* 2nd ed. (Washington: New Trends Publishing, Inc., 2001).

105 Mary Enig, PhD, and Sally Fallon, "The Skinny on Fats" (January 1, 2000) at *www.westonprice.org.*

106 Sally Fallon and Mary Enig, PhD, *Nourishing Traditions,* supra, note 104.

107 Kendra Cherry, "Benefits of Positive Thinking" at *about.com.*

108 Jan Suszkiw, "Phytochemical Profilers Investigate Potato Benefits" from research of Duroy A. Navarre and Charles R. Brownare at the USDA-ARS Vegetable and Forage Crops Research Laboratory in Agricultural Research magazine (September 2007).

109 Asker Jeukendrup and Micheal Gleeson, "Dehydration and Its Effects on Performance" at *www.humankinetics.com.*

110 See *www.painkillerabuse.us.*

111 "What's New and Beneficial about Quinoa" at *www.whfoods.com.*

112 Danilo Alfaro, "Quinoa" at *about.com.*

113 Gray Graham, Deborah Kesten, Larry Scherwitz, *Pottenger's Prophecy: How Food Resets Genes for Wellness or Illness* (Amherst, Mass: White River Press, 2011), at page 61.

114 See *www.cdc.gov/pdf/factsaboutobesityin.*

115 Dr Paul Haider, "The Health Benefits of Silence" (October 16, 2012) at *www.paulhaider.com.*

116 From a study in the American Journal of Clinical Nutrition.

117 "What Is Raw Sugar" at *www.wisegeek.com.*

118 See *www.healwithfood.org/health-benefits/red-oak-leaf-lettuce.php#ixzz3GYCM3qFg.*

119 Jagg Xaxx, "The History of Root Cellars" at *eHow.com.*

120 "Keeping the Harvest Fresh" (July 7 2009) at *www.vegetablegardener.com.*

121 "Facts about Root Vegetables" at *www.goodhousekeeping.com.*

122 National Institute of Allergy and Infectious Diseases, "Understanding Autoimmune Disease" at *www.rightdiagnosis.com.*

123 Jaclyn Law, "Autoimmune Disease: The Body Against Itself" at *www.besthealthmag.com.*

124 Brindusa Vanta, "Vitamin D Deficiency in Autoimmune Disease" at *www.livestrong.com.*

125 Bidita Debnath, "Relationship Between Diet and Disease Activity" at *www.medindia.net*.

126 See more at *www.naturaltherapypages.com.au/article/drinking_water_to_manage_inflammation#ixzz35OcZUkEd*.

127 Roxanne Webber, "7 Shocking Food Waste Statistics" (June 2, 2011) at *www.chow.com/food-news*.

128 Jennifer Burdett, "Facts About Spice" at *www.eHow.com*.

129 "Super Food Series: Ocean Vegetables" (April 2009) at *www.wellandgooodblogspot*.

130 "The Nutrition of Edible Seaweed" at *fitday.com*.

131 Vinent Laruen, "Top 10 Superfoods: Goji Berries, Cinnamon, Turmeric and More" at *www.canadianliving.com*.

132 Adrian, "Health Benefits of Shiitake Mushrooms" (April 1, 2008) at *www.elements4health.com*.

133 Carolyn Green, "Sorghum Grain Nutrition" at *www.eHow.com*.

134 Jamie Ashcraft, "Explore the Health Benefits You Can Enjoy by Eating Spelt Today" at *www.histakes-spelt.ca*.

135 See FAQs at *www.australianspirulina.com.au*.

136 See *www.steviauniversity.com*.

137 Anxiety Statistics from *www.anxietycentre.com*.

138 Keri Glassman, "13 Foods that Fight Stress" at *www.prevention.com*.

139 See *Annesremedies.com*.

140 Michelle Schoffro Cook, "Insomnia Relief Never Tasted So Good" (August 22, 2014) at *www.care2.com*.

141 Andrew Weil, MD, "Tea and Health" at *www.inpursuitoftea.com*.

142 Preston Sullivan, "Sustainable Soil Management" (2004) at *www.attra.ncat.org*.

143 "Topsoil" under definition at *www.eHow.com*.

144 Jacqueline Jeanty, "What Are Three Ways to Preserve Topsoil" at *www.eHow.com*.

145 Kara Robinson, "10 Surprizing Health Benefits of Sex" at *www.webmd.com*.

146 Mike Adams, "Camu Camu: The Natural Vitamin C Powerhouse for Peak Mental Function and Nervous System Protection" (December 4, 2007) at *www.naturalnews.com*.

147 Kathryn Rubin, "Healthy Eating: 7 Food Wonders of the Ancient World" (July 13, 2011) at *www.jpost.com*.

148 Ibid.

149 "The Pre-Columbian Experience" at *www.allchocolate.com*.

150 Dr Jolie Bookspan, "Traveller's Stomach, Tips for Travelers" at *www.worldstogethertravel.com*.

151 "Rooftop Gardens" at *www.trentu.ca*.

152 Blair Kamin, "Ten Years of Green Roofs in Chicago" (April 20, 2010) at *www.chicagotribune.com*.

153 Cal Orey, *The Healing Powers of Vinegar: A Complete Guide to Nature's Most Remarkable Remedy* (New York: Kensington, 2012).

154 "Vitamins and Dietary Supplements" under Market Research, Consumer Health at *www.euromonitor.com*.

155 Carolyn Dean, M.D., N.D., *The Magnesium Miracle*, Revised and Updated Edition (Random House: Ballantine Books, 2014).

156 Adria Vasil, *Ecoholic Body: The Ultimate Earth-Friendly Guide to Living Healthy and Looking Good* (Toronto: Vintage Canada, a division of Random House, 2012).

157 Andy Bellatti, "Opening Pandora's Lunchbox: Processed Foods Are even Scarier than You Thought" at *www.grist.com*.

158 Adria Vasil, *supra*, note 156.

159 "Whole Grains A to Z" at *www.wholegrainscouncil.org*.

160 Ashley Adams, "Whey" at *about.com*.

161 Traci Joy, "The Health Benefits of Button Mushrooms" (2013) at *www.livestrong.com*.

162 Robert Glennon, *Unquenchable: America's Water Crisis and What To Do About It* (Washington, D.C.: Island Press, 2014).

163 University of Maryland Center for Celiac Research and Celiac (July 9, 2010) at *www.umm.edu/celiac*.

164 William Davis, M.D., *Wheat Belly* (London: HarperCollins, 2014).

165 Wayne Roberts, *No Nonsense Guide to World Food*, 2nd ed. (Toronto: Between the Lines Press, 2013).

166 Ibid.

167 Tom Philpott, "What Do Biofuels Have to Do With the Price of Tortillas in Guatemala" (January 9, 2013) at *www.motherjonuaryes.com*.

168 University of Illinois College of Agricultural, Consumer and Environmental Sciences, "Lower Nitrogren Losses with Perennial Biofuel Crops" (January 10, 2013) at *www.sciencedaily.com*.

169 Y. Zheng, et al., "Ensilage and Bioconversion of Grape Pomace into Fuel Ethanol" *Journal of Agricultural and Food Chemistry* 60(44):11128-11134.

170 Sandia National Laboratories, "Engineering Alternative Fuel with Cyanobacteria" (January 9, 2013) at *www.dailyscience.com*.

171 Adria Vasil, *supra*, note 156.

172 "Other Uses" at *www.pfaf.org*.

173 "All Natural Yak" at *www.penfoodnews.ca*.

174 "Nutrients in Yogurt" at *www.livestrong.com*.

175 Selene Yeager and the editors of Prevention magazine, *The Doctors Book of Food Remedies* (Emmaus, PA: Rodale Books, 2008).

176 G.J. Tortora, B.R. Funke, and C.L. Case, *Microbiology: An Introduction*, 10th ed. (Pearson Education, 2010).

177 Jill Provost, "Can Eating Almonds Improve Your Memory?" (July 2010) at *www.ivillage.com*.

178 Sussan S. Lang, "An Apple a Day Could Help Protect Against Brain-Cell Damage that Triggers Alzheimer's, Parkinsonis," (November 17, 2004) Cornell Studies.

179 "9 Brain Foods that Prevent Dementia and Alzheimer's Disease" at

theconsciouslife.com.

[180] Anjus Chiedozie, "Coconut Oil and Alzheimers Disease" at *www.eHow.com.*

[181] Clay McNight, "Coconut Oil and Alzheimers Disease" at *www.livestrong.com.*

[182] Allison Cross, "Canadians Kept in the Dark for Two Weeks Over Tainted Meat Scandal" (October 1, 2012) *National Post.*

[183] "Food Giant Nestle Recalls Products After Horse Meat Discovery" (February 19, 2013) at *www.cnn.com.*

[184] "Food Safety" at *www.wikipedia.com.*

[185] Angela Harris, "Spinach Recalled in 39 States Due to E. Coli Scare" (February 15, 2013) at *www.digitaljournal.com.*

[186] Elson M. Haas, MD, with Buck Levin, PhD, RD, *Staying Healthy with Nutrition: The Complete Guide to Diet and Nutritional Medicine*, revised edition (Berkeley: Ten Speed Press, 2006).

[187] Dr Andrew Weil, "Intermittent Fasting: A Healthy Choice" at *Huffingtonpost.com.*

What your Body Needs and Why

[1] Monica Reinagel, M.S, L.D/N., "What Is the Difference between Soluble and Insoluble Fiber" (May 6, 2010) at *www.nutritiondiva.com.*

[2] Andrew Weil, MD "Balancing Omega-3 and Omega-6" at *www.drweil.com.*

[3] "Protein" at *Encyclopedia.com.*

[4] "Vitamins – A General Guide to A, B, C, D, E and K" (2001) at *www.helpwithcooking.com.*

[5] Sarah Marshall, MD, and Rhonda O'Brien, "Minerals, Their Function and Sources" (February 4, 2011) at *www.emedicinehealth.com.*

[6] "Mineral Deficiency Symptoms, Benefits and Food Sources" at *www.healthsupplementsnutritionalguide.com.*

[7] Sally Fallon, *Nourishing Traditions: The Cookbook that Challenges Politically Correct Nutrition and the Diet Dictocrats* (Washington, D.C.: New Trends Publishing Inc., 2001).

[8] See *dairygoodness.ca.*

[9] *The Gale Encyclopedia of Alternative Medicine (The Gale Group Inc., 2005).*

[10] "Antioxidants 101: What Are Flavonoids, Non-flavonoids" at *fitday.com.*

[11] *The Gale Encyclopedia of Alternative Medicine: Nutrition* (The Gale Group, 2004).

Conclusion

1 "From Farm to Table Mealworms May be the Next Best Food" (December 19, 2012) at *www.sciencedaily.com.*

2 John Robbins, *Healthy at 100: The Scientifically Proven Secrets of the World's Healthiest and Longest-Lived Peoples* (New York: Random House Publishing Group, 2007).

Bibliography

Books and Articles

"9 Brain Foods that Prevent Dementia and Alzheimer's Disease" at *www.theconsciouslife.com*

"All Natural Yak" at *www.penfoodnews.ca*

"Benefits of Grapefruit Seed Extract" at *www.globalhealingcentre.com*

"Changing Global Diets Is Vital to Reducing Climate Change" (August 31, 2014) at *www. Science daily.com*

"Chemical Cuisine" at *www.cspinet.org*

"Child Diet Linked to IQ" (February 8, 2011) at *www.nhs.uk*

"Chlorella" on *www.WebMD.com*

"Cloned Apples: Inside Science – Discoveries and Breakthroughs" at *www.ivanhoe.com*

"Counting Chickens," *The Economist*, July 27, 2011

"Do Gut Bacteria Rule Our Minds?" (August 2014) at *www.sciencedaily.com*

"Eggs and Heart Disease" at *www.hsph.harvard.edu/nutritionsource/eggs/*

"Facts about Root Vegetables" at *www.goodhousekeeping.com*

"Fast Fact About Deforestation" at www.facingthefuture.*org*

"Food Giant Nestle Recalls Products After Horse Meat Discovery" (February 19, 2013) at *www.cnn.com*

"Food Safety" at *www.wikipedia.com*

"Garlic Facts Remedies and Health Benefits of Garlic" (March 9, 2008) at *www.diabled-world.com*

"History of Egg Production: From Ancient Times" at *www.incredibleegg.org/egg-facts/basic-egg-facts/history-of-egg-production/from-ancient-times*

"Juniper Berries Health Benefit" at *www.diethealthclub.com*

"Keeping the Harvest Fresh" (July 7 2009) at *www.vegetablegardener.com*

"Many Apples a Day Keep the Blues at Bay" at *www.sciencedaily.com*

"New Secrets to Outsmarting Allergies," *Health Magazine*, April 2014

"Nutrients in Yogurt" at *www.livestrong.com*

"Other Uses" at *www.pfaf.org*

"Pesticide, Herbicide Use in U.S. Agriculture, 1960-2008" (June 2014) at *cornandsoybeandigest.com*

"Rate of Cancer Highest in North America," *International Journal of Cancer,* 2002, Volume 97, pp. 72-81

"Rooftop Gardens" at *www.trentu.ca*

"Serotonin" at *webmd.com*, Depression Health Center

"Super Food Series: Ocean Vegetables" (April 2009) at *www.wellandgooodblogspot*

"The Difference Between Grass-Fed Beef and Grain-Fed Beef" at *www.marksdailyapple.com*

"The Nutrition of Edible Seaweed" at *fitday.com*

"The Pre-Columbian Experience" at *www.allchocolate.com*

"The Truth About Overeating" (March 1996) at *www.medicalweightlossrx.com*

"Topsoil" under definition at *www.ehow.com*

"Vitamins and Dietary Supplements" under Market Research, Consumer Health at *www.euromonitor.com*

"What Is Raw Sugar" at *www.wisegeek.com*

"What's New and Beneficial about Cremini Mushrooms" at *www.whfoods.com*

"What's New and Beneficial about Quinoa" at *www.whfoods.com*

"Whole Grains A to Z" at *www.wholegrainscouncil.org*

"Why Whole Milk Is the Healthiest Choice" (August 2009) at *www.care2.com*

Adams, Mike, "Camu Camu: The Natural Vitamin C Powerhouse for Peak Mental Function and Nervous System Protection" (December 4, 2007) at *www.naturalnews.com*

Adams, Mike, "Heal Yourself in 15 Days by Correcting Your Nature Deficiency" (February 2010) at *www.naturalnews.com*

Adlercreutz, H, "Phytoestrogens: Epidemiology and a Possible Role in Cancer Protection" *Environmental Health Perspectives,* Vol. 103, Supp. 7 (October 1995), pp. 103-112

Adrian, "Health Benefits of Shiitake Mushrooms" (April 1, 2008) at *www.elements4health.com*

Alfaro, Danilo, "Quinoa" at *about.com*

Allen, Will, *The Good Food Revolution* (New York: Penguin Group, 2012)

American Society for Horticultural Science, "Anticancer Compound Found in Common Plant: American Mayapple" (September 2009) at *www.sciencedaily.com*

Ashcraft, Jamie,"Explore the Health Benefits You Can Enjoy by Eating Spelt Today" at *www.histakes-spelt.ca*

Ashley Adams, "Whey" at *about.com*

Ashworth Suzanne, *Seed to Seed* (Decorah: Seed Savers Exchange Inc., 2002)

Balch, James F., Mark Stengler, and Robin Young Balch, *Prescription for Natural Cures: A Self-Care Guide for Treating Problems with Natural Remedies Including Diet, Nutrition, Supplements, and Other Holistic Methods* (Hoboken, NJ: John Wiley & Sons Inc, 2011)

Bateson-Koch, Carolee, *Allergies Disease in Disguise* (Summertown: Books Alive, 1994)

Beck, Alison, *The Canadian Edible Garden* (Edmonton: Lone Pine Publishing, 1971)

Bellatti, Andy, "Opening Pandora's Lunchbox: Processed Foods Are even Scarier than You Thought" (February 26, 2013) at *www.grist.com*

Bellatti, Andy, "Opening Pandora's Lunchbox: Processed Foods Are even Scarier than You Thought" at *www.grist.com*

Beresford-Kroeger, Diana, *The Global Forest: Forty Ways Trees Can Save Us* (New York: Penguin Books Ltd, 2010)

Bernard, Jessica, "The Nutritional Contents of Beef Bone Marrow" (October 25, 2012) at *www.livestrong.com*

Blythman, Joanna, *What to Eat* (London: HarperCollins, 2012)

Bond, Annie, "Why It Matters to Buy Heirloom Plants and Seeds" (November 28, 1999) at *www.care2.com*

Bond, Annie, "Why It Matters to Buy Heirloom Plants and Seeds" (November 28, 1999) at *www.care2.com*

Bookspan, Dr Jolie, "Traveller's Stomach, Tips for Travelers" at *www.worldstogethertravel.com*

Braly, James, MD and Hoggan, Ron MA, *Dangerous Grains* (New York: Penguin Putnam Inc., 2002)

Burdett, Jennifer, "Facts About Spice" at *www.ehow.com*

Cairns, Kimberley, "Foods that Make You Feel Happy" (April 17, 2014) at *ehow.com*

Campbell, Colin, PhD and Campbell, Thomas, MD, *The China Study* (Dallas: BenBella Books Inc., 2006)

Centre for Disease Control and Prevention at *www.cdc.gov/ Heart Disease/facts.html*

Cherry, Kendra, "Benefits of Positive Thinking" at *about.com*

Chiedozie, Anjus, "Coconut Oil and Alzheimers Disease" at *www.ehow.com*

Chopra, Deepak, *Grow Younger Live Longer* (New York: Harmony Books, 2001)

Clarke, Murray, ND, *Natural Baby-Healthy Baby* (Gold River: Authority Publishing, 2010)

Clements, Edward, "Ten Delicious Body Building Foods that Increase Serotonin levels" (December 14, 2012) at *www.musclehealthfitness.com*

Colbin, Annemarie, *Food and Healing* (New York: The Random House Publishing, 1986)

Cook, Michelle Schoffro, "Insomnia Relief Never Tasted So Good" (August 22, 2014) at *www.care2.com*

Crane, Connie Jeske, (Fall 2013) on *www.edibletoronto.com*

Cross, Allison, "Canadians Kept in the Dark for Two Weeks Over Tainted Meat Scandal" (October 1, 2012) *National Post*

Daniel, Kaayla, PhD, *The Whole Soy Story* (Washington: New Trends Publishing, 2005)

Davis, William, M.D., *Wheat Belly* (US: Rodale Inc, 2011)

Dean, Carolyn, MD, ND, *The Magnesium Miracle* (New York: Ballantine Books, 2003)

Debnath, Bidita, "Relationship Between Diet and Disease Activity" at *www.medindia.net*

Dr. Mercola, "42 Flowers You Can Eat" (April 18, 2012) at *www.mercola.com*

Dr. Mercola, "The Latest Weapon in the War on Cancer: Honey Bees" (November 24, 2012) at *www.mercola.com*

Egg Nutrition Center, "Fun Facts About Eggs" (April 2014) at *www.wherefoodcomesfrom.com*

Ell, Cindy, "Natural Herbal Remedies & Their Many Benefits" (May 18, 2011) at *www.livestrong.com*

Enig, Mary G. and Sally Fallon, *Nourishing Traditions: The Cookbook that Challenges Politically Correct Nutrition and the Diet Dictocrats*, 2nd ed. (Washington: NewTrends Publishing, Inc., 2001)

Enig, Mary, PhD, and Sally Fallon, "The Skinny on Fats" (January 1, 2000) at *www.westonprice.org*

Erasmus, Udo, *Fats that Heal Fats that Kill* (Summertown: Alive Books, 1986)

Farlouis, Sharron, "Interesting Facts about Elderberries" (June 24, 2012) at *www.helium.com*

Frost, Shelley, "The Importance of Eating Meals Together as a Family" (January 26, 2014) at *www.livestrong.com*

Garber, Lisa, "6 Super-foods that Fight Cancer and Prevent Cancer" (September 11, 2012) at *Natural Society.com*

Geib, Aurora, "Top 10 Herbs and Spices for Strengthening your Immune System" (April 9, 2012) *www.naturalnews.com*

Glassman, Keri, "13 Foods that Fight Stress" at *www.prevention.com*

Glennon, Robert, *Unquenchable* (Washington: Island Press, 2009)

Glennon, Robert, *Unquenchable: America's Water Crisis and What To Do About It* (Washington, D.C.: Island Press, 2014)

Gray, Graham, Deborah Kesten, Larry Scherwitz, *Pottenger's Prophecy: How Food Resets Genes for Wellness or Illness* (Amherst, Mass: White River Press, 2011)

Green, Carolyn, "Sorghum Grain Nutrition" at *www.ehow.com*

Green, Michelle, "How to Boost Your Intelligence" at *eHow.com*

Grott, David, *101 Foods that Could Save Your Life* (New York: Random House Inc., 2008)

Growell, Amy, "Eat Wild Amaranth" at *www.edibleaustin.com*

Haas, Elson M., MD, with Buck Levin, PhD, RD, *Staying Healthy with Nutrition: The Complete Guide to Diet and Nutritional Medicine*, revised edition (Berkeley: Ten Speed Press, 2006)

Haider, Dr Paul, "The Health Benefits of Silence" (October 16, 2012) at *www.paulhaider.com*

Harris, Angela, "Spinach Recalled in 39 States Due to E. Coli Scare" (February 15, 2013) at *www.digitaljournal.com*

Hartwig, Dallas and Melissa, *It Starts with Food: Discover the Whole30® and Change Your Life in Unexpected Ways,* (Las Vegas: Victoria Belt Publishing, 2012)

Hausman, Patricia and Hurley, Judith Benn, *The Healing Foods* (Pennsylvania: Rodale Press, 1989)

Herrington, Diana, "10 Benefits of Carrots: The Crunchy Power Food" (2011) at *care2.com*

Herrington, Diana, "16 Health Benefits of Lemons" (July 2012) at *www.care2.com*

Holford, Patrick, *New Optimum Nutrition for the Mind* (Laguna Beach: Basic Health Publications Inc., 2009)

International Potato Center, "Oca, Ulluco & Mashua" at *www. Cipotato.org*

Jackson, Genevieve, "Cleansing Remedies Using Lemon and Water" (August 16, 2013) at *www.livestrong.com*

Jacobsen, Rowan, "The Importance of Bees to Our Food Supply" (March/April 2009) at *www.eatingwell.com*

Jeanty, Jacqueline, "What Are Three Ways to Preserve Topsoil" at *www.ehow.com*

Jegtiv, Shereen, "Best Foods for Heart Health" (May 23, 2014) at *about.com*

Jeukendrup, Asker and Micheal Gleeson, "Dehydration and Its Effects on Performance" at *www.humankinetics.com*

Joachim, David and Schloss, Andrew, *The Science of Good Food* (Toronto: Robert Rose Inc., 2008)

Jordan, Jo, "How to Use Food-Combining Techniques for Better Digestion" at *www.puristat.com*

Joy, Traci, "The Health Benefits of Button Mushrooms" (2013) at *www.livestrong.com*

Junger, Alejandro, MD, *Clean Gut* (New York: Harper Collins, 2013)

Junger, Alejandro, MD, *Clean* (New York: Harper Collins, 2011)

Kamin, Blair, "Ten Years of Green Roofs in Chicago" (April 20, 2010) at *www.chicagotribune.com*

Keith, Lierre, *The Vegetarian Myth: Food, Justice and Sustainability* (Oakland, CA: PM Press, 2009)

Kendall-Reed, Penny ND and Reed, Stephen, MD, *Healing Arthritis* (Toronto: CCNM Press Inc., 2011)

Kingsolver, Barbara, *Animal, Vegetable, Miracle: A Year of Food Life* (New York: HarperCollins, 2007)

Kloss, Jethro, *Back to Eden: The Classic Guide to Herbal Medicine, Natural Foods, and Home Remedies Since 1939* (Detroit: Lotus Press, 2004)

Krishan, Shubhra, "8 Great Benefits of Onions" (November 30, 2012) at *www.care2.com*

Lang, Sussan S., "An Apple a Day Could Help Protect Against Brain-Cell Damage that Triggers Alzheimer's, Parkinsonis," (November 17, 2004) Cornell Studies

Lapin, Beth, "The Healing Power of Nature" at *www.innertapestry.org*

Laruen, Vinent, "Top 10 Superfoods: Goji Berries, Cinnamon, Turmeric and More" at *www.canadianliving.com*

Law, Jaclyn, "Autoimmune Disease: The Body Against Itself" at *www.besthealthmag.com*

Louv, Richard, *The Natural Principle* (New York: Workman Publishing, 2011)

Madison, Deborah, *Preserving Food Without Freezing or Canning* (Paris: Terre Vivante, 1992)

Manning, Richard, *Against the Grain* (New York: North Point Press, 2004)

Markham, Brett, *Mini Farming* (New York: Skyhorse Publishing, 2010)

Matsen, Jonn, ND, *Eating Alive* (Vancouver: Gordon Soules Book Publishers Ltd, 2012)

Mazo, Ellen, *The Immune Advantage* (London: Rodale Ltd., 2004)

McKay, Brett and Kate, "Surviving in the Wild: 19 Common Edible Plants" (October 6, 2010) at *www.artofmanlyskills.com*

McLaughlin, "Herbs Attract Pollinating Insects" at *www.vegetablegardner.com*

McNight, Clay, "Coconut Oil and Alzheimers Disease" at *www.livestrong.com*

Merrell, Woodson, MD, *The Source* (Toronto: Random House, 2008)

Miloradovich, Milo, *Growing and Using Herbs and Spices* (New York: Dover Publications Inc., 1980)

Moss, Michael, *Salt, Sugar, Fat: How the Food Giants Hooked Us* (Toronto, ON: McClelland and Stewart, 2014)

Murad, Howard, M.D, *The Water Secret* (Honoken: John Wiley & Sons, 2010)

Murray, Michael T, N.D, *Diabetes & Hypoglycemia* (Roseville: Prima Publishing, 1994)

Murray, Michael, N.D. & Joseph Pizzorno, N.D, *The Encyclopedia of Natural Medicine* (New York: Simon & Schuster, 2012)

Myss Caroline, *Anatomy of the Spirit* (New York: Crown Publishers, 1996)

Myss, Caroline, Ph.D, *Why People Don't Heal and How They Can* (New York: Crown Publishing Group, 1998)

National Institute of Allergy and Infectious Diseases, "Understanding Autoimmune Disease" at *www.rightdiagnosis.com*

Nestle, Marion, *Food Politics*: How the Food Industry Influences Nutrition and Health (Oakland, CA: University of California Press, 2013)

Newcastle University, "Could Spiders be the Key to Saving our Bees?" (June 3, 2014) at *www.sciencedaily.com*

Nordqvist, Christian, "What Is Vitamin D? What Are the Benefits of Vitamin D?" (September 2014) at *www.medicalnewstoday.com*

O'Connor, Bess, "Move Over Acai Berries: The next Wave of Superfoods Is Here" (December 2014) at *www.mindbodygreen.com*

Orey, Cal, *The Healing Powers of Vinegar: A Complete Guide to Nature's Most Remarkable Remedy* (New York: Kensington, 2012)

Parks, Francina Marie, at *Knoji.com*

Patel, Raj, *Stuffed and Starved: Markets, Power and the Hidden Battle for the World's Food Systems* (Toronto: HarperCollins, 2010)

Patel, Raj, *The Value of Nothing* (Toronto: Harper Collins Publishers Ltd, 2009)

Pawlick, Thomas, *The End of Food* (Vancouver: Greystone Books, 2006)

Pawlick, Thomas, *The End of Food: How the Food Industry Is Destroying Our Food Supply - and What You Can Do About It* (Vancouver, BC: Greystone Books Ltd., 2006)

Philpott, Tom, "What Do Biofuels Have to Do With the Price of Tortillas in Guatemala" (January 9, 2013) at *www.motherjonuaryes.com*

Philpott, Tom, "Why the Government Should Pay Farmers to Plant Cover Crops" (January 12, 2013) at *www.motherjones.com*

Plant, Jane, *Eating for Better Health* (Plymouth: Virgin Books, 2010)

Pollan, Michael, *In Defense of Food* (New York, Penguin Press, 2008)

Pollan, Michael, *Second Nature* (New York: Grove Press, 1991)

Pollan, Michael, *The Omnivore's Dilemma: A Natural History of Four Meals* (New York: The Penguin Press, 2006)

Provost, Jill, "Can Eating Almonds Improve Your Memory?" (July 2010) at *www.ivillage.com*

Robbins, John, *Healthy at 100* (New York: Random House, 2007)

Robbins, Ken, *Food for Thought: The Stories Behind the Things We Eat* (New York: Roaring Brook Press (Macmillan), 2009)

Roberts, Calia, "Difference in Pickling and Fermentation" at *ehow.com*

Roberts, Wayne, *No Nonsense Guide to World Food*, 2nd ed. (Toronto: Between the Lines Press, 2013)

Roberts, Wayne, *The No-Nonsense Guide to World Food,* 2nd ed. (Toronto: Between the Lines Press, 2013)

Robin, Marie-Monique, *The World According to Monsanto* (Paris: La Decouverte, 2008)

Robinson, Kara, "10 Surprizing Health Benefits of Sex" at *www.webmd.com*

Roth, Geneen, *Women, Food and God* (New York: Simon & Schuster Inc., 2010)

Rowland, David, *The Nutritional Bypass* (Parry Sound: Rowland Publications, 2012)

Rubin, Kathryn, "Healthy Eating: 7 Food Wonders of the Ancient World" (July 13, 2011) at *www.jpost.com*

Salatin, Joel, *Folks, This Ain't Right: A Farmer's Advice for Happier Hens, Healthier People, and a Better World* (New York: Center Street Books, 2011)

Sandia National Laboratories, "Engineering Alternative Fuel with Cyanobacteria" (January 9, 2013) at *www.dailyscience.com*

Schonwald, Josh, *The Taste of Tommorrow* (New York: HarperCollins, 2012)

Servan-Schreiber, David, M.D, Ph.D, *Anti-Cancer* (Toronto: Harper Collins, 2007)

Shankle, Willam Rodman, M.S, M.D and Amen, Daniel G, MD, *Preventing Alzheimer's* (New York: The Berkley Publishing Group, 2004)

Shea, Aimee, "Vitamins and Minerals in Maca Root" (July 2011) at *www.livestrong.com*

Shiva, Vandana, *Privatization, Pollution and Profit* (Cambridge: South End Press, 2002)

Shiva, Vandana, *Manifestos on the Future of Food and Seed* (Cambridge, MA: South End Press, 2010))

Shiva, Vandana, *Staying Alive: Women, Ecology, and Devleopment* (Vancouver BC: South End Press, 2010)

Smith, Jeffrey M., *Seeds of Deception: Exposing Industry and Government Lies About the Safety of the Genetically Engineered Foods You're Eating* (Portland, ME: Yes! Books, 2003)

Smith, Rick and Bruce Lourie, *Slow Death by Rubber Duck: How the Toxic Chemistry of Everyday Life Affects Our Health* (Toronto: Random House of Canada. Ltd., 2009)

Stamets, Paul, "Unusual & Interesting Facts About Mushrooms" (December 15, 2009) at *www.fungi.com* on Articles by Paul Stamets; and and Ken Robbins, *Food for Thought: The Stories Behind the Things We Eat* (New York: Roaring Brook Press (Macmillan), 2009)

Stamets, Paul, *Mycelium Running: How Mushrooms Can Help Save the World* (Berkeley: Ten Speed Press, 2005)

Steiner, Emily, "How Reishi Combats Aging" in *Life Extension Magazine*, February 2013, pp. 82-90

Sullivan, Preston, "Sustainable Soil Management" (2004) at *www.attra.ncat.org*

Suszkiw, Jan, "Phytochemical Profilers Investigate Potato Benefits" from research of Duroy A. Navarre and Charles R. Brownare at the USDA-ARS Vegetable and Forage Crops Research Laboratory in *Agricultural Research* magazine (September 2007)

Suzuki David and Boyd, David, *David Suzuki's Green Guide* (Vancouver: Douglas & McIntyre Publishing Group, 2008)

Tick, Heather, MD, *Holistic Pain Relief* (Novato: New World Library, 2013)

Tortora, G.J., B.R. Funke, and C.L. Case, *Microbiology: An Introduction, 10th ed. (Pearson Education, 2010)*

University of Arkansas, Food Safety Consortium, "To Block the Carcinogens, Add a Touch of Rosemary When Grilling Meats" *(May 24, 2008)* at *www.dailyscience.com*

University of Greenwich,. "Drugs for Diabetes? Scientists Test the Power of Plants" (January 16, 2013) at *www.sciencedaily.com*

University of Illinois College of Agricultural, Consumer and Environmental Sciences, "Lower Nitrogen Losses with Perennial Biofuel Crops" (January 10, 2013) at *www.sciencedaily.com*

University of Maryland Center for Celiac Research and Celiac (July 9, 2010) at *www.umm.edu/celiac*

University of Toronto, Rotman School of Management, "Like Some Happiness with That? Fast Food Cues Hurt Ability to Savor Experience" (June 2, 2014), at *www.dailyscience.com*

US Food and Drug Administration at *www.fda.gov*

Vanta, Brindusa, "Vitamin D Deficiency in Autoimmune Disease" at *www.livestrong.com*

Vasil, Adria, *Ecoholic Body: The Ultimate Earth-Friendly Guide to Living Healthy and Looking Good* (Toronto: Vintage Canada, a division of Random House, 2012)

Webber, Roxanne, "7 Shocking Food Waste Statistics" (June 2, 2011) at *www.chow.com/food-news*

Weil, Andrew, MD, "Tea and Health" at *www.inpursuitoftea.com*

Weil, Dr Andrew, "Intermittent Fasting: A Healthy Choice" at *Huffingtonpost.com*

Weil, Dr., "Balanced Living – Herbal Remedies" at *www.drweil.com*

Wolfe, David, Jeff Beem-Miller, Allison Chatrchyan, and Lauren Chambliss, "Climate Change Facts: Farm Energy, Carbon, and Greenhouse Gases" (November 2011) Cornell Climate Change

Wong, Cathy, "Top 15 Conditions for which People Seek Complementary/Alternative Therapies" (August 11, 2006) at *about.com*

Xaxx, Jagg, "The History of Root Cellars" at *eHow.com*

Yeager, Selene and the editors of *Prevention* magazine, *The Doctors Book of Food Remedies* (Emmaus, PA: Rodale Books, 2008)

Zuckerman, Larry, *Potato* (US: Faber and Faber Inc., 1999)

Websites

Annesremedies.com

en.wikipeida.org

www.all4naturalhealth.com/dandelion-facts.html#ixzz2x1RWzioI

www.anxietycentre.com

www.australianspirulina.com.au

www.buzzle.com

www.care2.com/greenliving/16-health-benefits-of-lemons

www.cdc.gov/pdf/factsaboutobesityin

www.ecotherapyheals.com

*www.healwithfood.org/health-benefits/red-oak-
leaf-lettuce.php#ixzz3GYCM3qFg*

*www.naturalnews.com/028203_nature_deficiency_self_healing.
html#ixzz2J695yuaZ*

*www.naturaltherapypages.com.au/article/drinking_water_to_
manage_inflammation#ixzz35OcZUkEd*

www.painkillerabuse.us

www.steviauniversity.com

Index

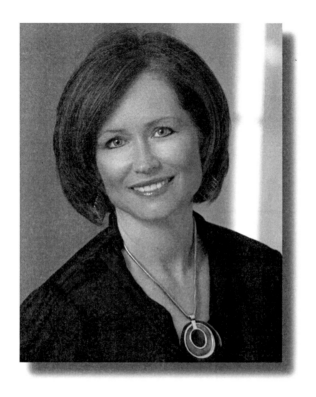

About the author

Patricia Conlin attended the University of Western Ontario with an entrance scholarship in Food Science and graduated with an honors degree (HBA).

Patricia founded Global Consulting Group Inc. in 1991 with the vision of creating a company that provides strategic human resources services. For the past two decades she has delivered quality solutions for recruitment, retention, and transition for a long list of loyal clients ranging from large, national corporations to small, local innovators. Her passion, strategic focus, and professionalism has established her as an outstanding leader, mentor, and enduring business professional.

Patricia also heads up the Workplace Wellness Solutions Division of Global Consulting Group (GCG). Her passion for health and personal development led Patricia to become an energetic and engaging public speaker on Improving Success through Health Strategies. Patricia became a Registered Holistic Nutritionist (RHN) to help others achieve their highest health and career potential. She coaches business professionals all over North America with a comprehensive Health and Success six-session program. In 2015, she was nominated for a Toronto Business Leader Award for Wellness.

Patricia speaks French, German, and some Spanish. After 10 years of dedicated training and competition, she was the first woman in Canada to earn a Black Belt in the Martial Art of Shoot Wrestling. She was selected in 1992 to be a part of the Canadian Olympic Team going to Barcelona as an administrator and to represent Canada as part of an International contingent assisting youth development in Russia through UNESCO.

She plays competitive soccer and is an active member of her community. She has two boys and is a dedicated mother.

To book Patricia for an inspirational public speaking engagement or to learn more about the Health and Success Coaching program for your organization, please contact her at **patricia@globalconsultinggroup.ca** or **905-472-9677 x241**.